KT-480-599

Clinics in Developmental Medicine No. 157
BEHAVIOURAL PHENOTYPES IN
CLINICAL PRACTICE

© 2002 Mac Keith Press

High Holborn House, 52–54 High Holborn, London WC1V 6RL

Senior Editor: Martin CO Bax

Editor: Hilary M Hart

Managing Editor: Michael Pountney

Sub Editor: Pat Chappelle

The views and opinions expressed herein are those of the authors and do not necessarily represent those of the publisher

All rights reserved. No part of this publication may be reproduced, stored in a retrieval system, or transmitted in any form or by any means, electronic, mechanical, photocopying, recording or otherwise, without the prior permission of the publisher

First published in this edition 2002

British Library Cataloguing-in-Publication data:
A catalogue record for this book is available from the British Library

ISSN: 0069 4835
ISBN: 1 89868327 1

Printed by The Lavenham Press Ltd, Water Street, Lavenham, Suffolk
Mac Keith Press is supported by Scope

Clinics in Developmental Medicine No. 157

Behavioural Phenotypes in Clinical Practice

Edited by

GREGORY O'BRIEN

Department of Developmental Psychiatry
University of Northumbria
and Northgate Hospital
Morpeth, Northumberland, England

2002
Mac Keith Press

Distributed by 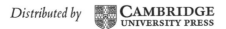 CAMBRIDGE
UNIVERSITY PRESS

CONTENTS

AUTHORS' APPOINTMENTS

Louise Barnard — Research Psychologist, Developmental Psychiatry Research Unit, University of Newcastle, Newcastle upon Tyne, England

Martin Bax — Emeritus Reader in Paediatrics, Imperial College of Medicine, Department of Child Health, Chelsea and Westminster Hospital, London, England

David Clarke — Consultant Psychiatrist, Department of Developmental Psychiatry, Lea Castle Centre, Kidderminster, Worcestershire, England

Robert M Hodapp — Professor, Graduate School of Education and Information Studies, UCLA, Los Angeles, USA

Patricia Howlin — Professor, Department of Psychology, St George's Hospital Medical School, London, England

Kirsty R Lowe — Consultant Clinical Psychologist, Psychology Services, Northgate Hospital, Morpeth, Northumberland, England

Gregory O'Brien — Professor of Developmental Psychiatry, University of Northumbria and Northgate Hospital, Morpeth, Northumberland, England

Joanne Pearson — Research Psychologist, Developmental Psychiatry Research Unit, University of Newcastle, Newcastle upon Tyne, England

Leila A Ricci

Graduate Student, Graduate School of Education and Information Studies, UCLA, Los Angeles, USA

Lisa Rippon

Specialist Registrar, Northgate Hospital, Morpeth, Northumberland, England

Gregory Stores

Professor of Developmental Neuropsychiatry, University of Oxford Department of Psychiatry (Child and Adolescent Section), Oxford, England

Jeremy Turk

Senior Lecturer in Child and Adolescent Psychiatry, Department of Psychiatry, St George's Hospital Medical School, University of London, London, England

Kirk Zimbelman

Chartered Clinical Psychologist, Learning Disability Service, NHS Lothian – Lothian Primary Care, Edinburgh, Scotland

FOREWORD

William Yule

The past 20 years have witnessed major changes in the ways in which biologically based mentally disabling conditions in children are investigated and treated. It is not so long since major textbooks reported that 'the causes' of such conditions were known in only a minority of cases. Now, with more sophisticated techniques for detecting microscopic gene deletions and subtle enzyme deficiencies, that picture is rapidly developing. Paralleling these high-tech advances has been a quieter revolution in the ways that the behaviour of the children has been investigated, contributing to both diagnosis and treatment.

In the early 1980s, I was asked by Tom Oppé to meet with the parents of children with what was then called 'infantile hypercalcaemia' to see what advice I might be able to give them to help with the unusual behaviour their children presented. I still recall that first meeting with a group of 30 individuals, all of whom looked as if they were related, although none of them were. I was used to meeting people with Down syndrome, but had never encountered such a group with another condition who shared so many superficial similarities.

The similarities were not solely in their appearance. The warmth, the friendliness and the superficial chatter made one realize why teachers were reported to say they had never met children like these before and why parents thought the children should be educated in normal as opposed to 'special' schools.

That encounter began a 20 year association. The tiny literature of the time contained a few clinical descriptions of the condition. As a clinical psychologist, I undertook a pilot study of the psychological and behavioural characteristics of a group of children with the disorder, and then followed this with a larger study that identified a number of very characteristic behaviours.

Discussing the findings at scientific meetings brought me in contact with colleagues of different disciplines who were also studying the characteristics of children with particular conditions. Soon, Orlee Udwin and I, who were collaborating on the study of infantile hypercalcaemia (later renamed Williams syndrome), met with Martin Bax and Gillian Colville who were studying the mucopolysaccharide disorders and Jennifer Dennis and Anne Hunt who were studying tuberous sclerosis. As more colleagues joined us, informal meetings became a little more formal and frequent. A few years on, the Society for the Study of Behavioural Phenotypes was born.

The impetus for all these developments was the curiosity of the clinical researchers, each of whom was working very closely with a parent support organization. The parents were wanting to know how best to help their own child, but also wanted to find out more about the causes of each condition so as to develop early detection, prevention and early intervention. Researchers worked closely with parents in what is now seen as an excellent model for user–professional collaboration.

The issues that were raised concerned how to refine observations and reports of children's behaviour and adjustment. Existing rating scales were too crude and often not developed for application to children with these disorders. We wanted to know which behaviours were in common across syndromes and which appeared to be unique. Were there behaviours that would help in making diagnoses?—indeed there were. At the same time, the upsurge of interest in and the technical possibilities heralded by the human genome project gave a new spur to the work. Conditions such as Williams syndrome, which had previously been diagnosed clinically, were now linked to specific tests for microdeletions.

Of course, we were not expecting a one-to-one correspondence between genotype and phenotype. We recognized how complex the interplay is between genes and environment. But we were always mindful of the needs of parents to have better information on the cause of their child's disorder. Better diagnoses should lead to better management. Parents wanted to know what they were facing in the future and also how to deal with it. As William Nyhan said in the previous book on *Behavioural Phenotypes* (O'Brien and Yule 1995), ". . more important are the behaviors that must be lived with day-to-day. It is behavior that can destroy a family or lead to admission to institution, not IQ or cytogenetic or enzymatic status. Appropriate counseling as to what to expect, and introduction to parent support groups and to others with children with the same phenotype lead to the development of realistic ways of coping with an unusual child."

Hence this second volume, one that is complementary to the earlier one and which develops the theme of implications for clinical practice based on a burgeoning literature on behavioural phenotypes. Self-injury, aggression, sleep disorders and odd, autistic-like behaviours are often the problems parents bring to the attention of professionals, and these are highlighted in Chapter 2 after an introductory overview of the clinical relevance of the study of behavioural phenotypes as a whole.

Once the existence of an underlying disorder is suspected from the history or initial observations, then more detailed clinical investigations are required. These are described in detail in Chapter 3, which helpfully includes details of appropriate diagnostic schedules for clinicians working outside specialist centres to use. All of this sophisticated assessment would be of little value without advice on intervention. Parents require information on the nature of their child's disorder and support and counselling if they are to manage their children at home, and this is discussed in Chapter 7, while more specific behavioural management techniques are discussed in Chapter 4. Advice on educational practice is given in Chapter 6, while pharmacological interventions are described in Chapter 5. The book finishes with a lengthy Chapter 8 summarizing the behavioural phenotypes of a myriad of rare conditions, giving not only clear descriptions of each condition and its behavioural characteristics, but also guidance on management and therapy.

The study of behavioural phenotypes has indeed come a long way from the early days when a small group, meeting in each others' offices over instant coffee and curly sandwiches, debated how best to investigate the similarities and differences among groups of children presenting with puzzling and fascinating behaviours. From description to intervention in less than 20 years is no mean feat. This volume is testament to the hard work and dedication of many professionals and many parents. It truly extends and complements the earlier volume. It makes the hard-won findings accessible to clinicians of many disciplines, and that can only be to the benefit of parents and children alike.

William Yule, PhD
London
May 2002

REFERENCE

O'Brien G, Yule W (eds) (1995) *Behavioural Phenotypes. Clinics in Developmental Medicine No. 138.* London: Mac Keith Press.

1
THE CLINICAL RELEVANCE OF BEHAVIOURAL PHENOTYPES

Gregory O'Brien

"Very interesting, but what do I do about it?" So went the response of many colleagues to *Behavioural Phenotypes* (O'Brien and Yule 1995), which was the first textbook on the subject of the behavioural characteristics of genetic syndromes of disability. This earlier edition in the *Clinics in Developmental Medicine* series provided an introduction to the field of behavioural phenotypes, focusing on the behavioural characteristics of a range of syndromes. In describing the developments in which a growing group of researchers had been involved, we concentrated on detailed descriptions of the behaviours encountered in the respective conditions. In this respect, *Behavioural Phenotypes* was a summary of the state of knowledge at that time. It also included a rationale and review of the research approaches employed, and an account of some of the thinking and debate that surrounds this area of inquiry. Pleasingly, the book was warmly welcomed, to the extent that a translation has recently appeared in Italian (*Caratteristiche Compartamentali delle Malattie Genetiche*, O'Brien and Yule 2000).

In the present text, the aim is to build on the success of the previous book by concentrating on the management implications of behavioural phenotypes. As in *Behavioural Phenotypes*, a substantial proportion of the text comprises an account of those syndromes on which substantial behavioural, developmental and related data are available, especially those conditions on which results have been communicated via the *Society for the Study of Behavioural Phenotypes*. Where there is new information on the respective behavioural phenotypes, this is detailed. However, in other respects the descriptions of the syndromes in this edition are quite different from the earlier edition. The accounts of each behavioural phenotype are more brief than before, being summaries of those features that are of particular relevance to the management of affected individuals. The previous edition included detailed descriptions of the general health of people with the conditions in question. In the present text, the emphasis is on the management of health problems, where these are relevant to the management of behaviour and development. Overall, therefore, the syndrome-by-syndrome summaries in the present edition are focused on some of the key principles of managing individuals affected by the behavioural phenotypes of the genetic syndromes of learning disability.

Management of the behavioural problems of children and adults whose disabilities are caused by one specific syndrome should not be considered in isolation. There are well-established approaches to the understanding of the cause, nature and treatment-responsiveness of behaviour disorders presenting among individuals with such disabilities (Gillberg and O'Brien 2000). The most successful and appropriate strategies are multimodal, employing coordinated intervention methods, often over a considerable period of time—especially for some of the more persistent and refractory problems. These include, among other themes: (i) detailed consideration of the topography and determinants of the behaviours presenting in this individual at this time; (ii) discerning whether any diagnosable, treatable, psychiatric disorder is present, and the associated decisions on treatment strategy—including psycho-pharmacology; (iii) delineation of any developmental delays that may underlie the presenting behavioural problems, and design of the appropriate compensatory intervention strategies; (iv) identification of any specific functional deficits, with ensuing plans for interventions to meet needs arising; and (v) consideration of the individual in the wider social context. These issues are explored in context, in the themed chapters that precede the closing syndrome-based section of the text.

From behavioural phenotypes to interventions: the implications of definition
The following definition of 'behavioural phenotype' is proposed (modified from that suggested in O'Brien and Yule 1995):

The behavioural phenotype is a characteristic pattern of motor, cognitive, linguistic and social observations that is consistently associated with a biological disorder. In some cases, the behavioural phenotype may constitute a psychiatric disorder; in others, behaviours which are not usually regarded as symptoms of psychiatric diagnoses may occur.

When we begin to plan interventions for the management of individuals affected by behavioural phenotypes described according to this definition, there are important implications.
1. Behavioural phenotypes are described as a *"characteristic pattern"*. There is a grouping, or a co-occurrence of behaviours, which has a typical, distinct nature that to some extent informs the appropriate interventions. There is rarely, if ever, a single pathognomonic behaviour, although in many syndromes there is a dominant or more prominent clinically important behaviour. In planning intervention strategies for such characteristic patterns of behaviour, the clinician is well-placed to anticipate that certain problems may present, and especially to be aware of the likely co-occurrence of certain sets of behaviours. For example, overeating dominates the picture in Prader–Willi syndrome. The appropriate intervention strategies that are of established use for this difficult behaviour include careful dietary planning and supervised restriction of carbohydrate foods. In addition, it is important to be aware of other common elements of the characteristic pattern of the behavioural phenotype of this syndrome, including skin-picking, for which a cognitive–behavioural-based system using self-monitoring may be applicable, and—in a significant minority of patients—adult-onset paranoid psychosis, which will respond to antipsychotic medication.
2. Behavioural phenotypes are described in terms of their *"motor, cognitive, linguistic and social observations"*. By considering the behaviours in this way, two themes emerge. First, there are pointers toward potential areas of intervention, whether in respect of physio-therapeutic attention to motor functioning; educational programme planning to address or ameliorate cognitive deficits; speech and language therapeutic attention to linguistic functioning; or a behavioural programme designed to address some issue in social or

interpersonal functioning. But the key word here is *observations*: in the approaches to management that follow the adoption of this definition, it is stressed that behavioural phenotypes are empirically based on naturalistic observations of these facets of behaviour. By systematic consideration of motor, cognitive, linguistic and social functioning, the clinician adopts a valid framework, from which is derived the particular set of behaviours that comprise the behavioural phenotype of this person at this time, free of theoretical bias or preconception. Also, the use of the keyword *observations*, as opposed to 'anomalies' or 'abnormalities', carries a message regarding the extent to which the behavioural findings are a natural feature of the condition in question. The term *observations* carries further implications for intervention, in that by accepting that some of these observations are natural features of the conditions in question, one adopts what is technically a normalized approach to management: through recognition that it is in the nature of the disorder in question to present with particular patterns of social and cognitive functioning, it becomes appropriate to plan interventions in keeping with the developmental trajectory of the behavioural phenotype. For example, in an individual with fragile X syndrome, assessment will clarify the nature of cognitive functioning, both in general and specific terms. Obviously, this will carry important implications for education planning, and here the findings in the individual case may be corroborated by published data. In addition, psychological and psychiatric assessment, primed by a familiarity with the common features of the typical pattern of social functioning of people with fragile X syndrome, will focus on the nature and extent of any elements of social anxiety or autistic-type social withdrawal. In planning, say, the elements of an educational programme for a child with fragile X syndrome, it will be important to recognize and accept the social functioning characteristics observed in the child, and to include mechanisms for dealing with these in the child's programme. Such planning will recognize that many activities that characterize normal everyday activities within the school setting may be quite aversive and threatening to the child with fragile X syndrome, because of the traits of social anxiety and autistic-type behaviour which are typical of the condition. Such a normalizing, specialist approach is in contrast to one that assumes that all children will show similar patterns of social functioning to others with the same intellect or ability level. The principles of including such specialist insights into the planning for education, on the basis of an acceptance of the child's own characteristics, are elaborated in Chapter 6.

3. Behavioural phenotypes are *"consistently associated with a biological disorder"*. In planning the management of an individual affected child, once the biological disorder is identified—whether or not by genetic investigation—it is reasonable to anticipate that certain behaviours may ensue, where these have been described as common or typical of the disorder. There is a degree of consistency in this regard. But the clinician responsible for planning in the individual case needs to be mindful of the extent of individual variation. Behavioural phenotypes are here defined as *consistently* associated with a biological disorder, but *not universally*. Take the examples of the two major genetic syndromes cited above. In Prader–Willi syndrome, adult-onset paranoid psychosis is common, more so than in other individuals of matched intelligence. But it is by no means universal—in fact, while this pattern of psychopathology is indeed consistently

associated with Prader–Willi syndrome, the consistent association in question occurs in only around 10% of cases. In fragile X syndrome, autistic symptomatology is common, and indeed relatively stable longitudinally over development, but there are many exceptions, again emphasizing the importance of balancing the knowledge of the common features of the condition with the expression of the phenotype in the individual (see Figs. 1.1–1.4, below).

4. *"In some cases, the behavioural phenotype may constitute a psychiatric disorder; in others, behaviours which are not usually regarded as symptoms of psychiatric diagnoses may occur."* This principle is central to the management of behavioural phenotypes. In all considerations of the management of behavioural phenotypes this issue is emphasized. In the present text it is equally evident in the chapter on the management of behavioural domains (Chapter 2), in the chapters exploring the basic principles of management of all behavioural phenotypes from different, complementary frames of reference (Chapters 3–7), and in the closing section, where the management of the behavioural phenotypes of a range of individual syndromes is reviewed (Chapter 8). Consequently, in a child who presents with autism or attention deficit hyperactivity disorder (ADHD) as part of the behavioural phenotype of a given syndrome, the management strategies to be employed will be informed by the available evidence base on the management of these two diagnoses. However, in the management of behavioural phenotypes, the clinician commonly faces a pattern of behaviour—such as a sleep disorder or a specific pattern of self-injury—that does not amount to a diagnosable psychiatric disorder. The evidence base for the management of such cases typically derives from a wealth of sources, including psycholinguistics, behavioural theory and educational insights into social learning. Moreover, although autism and ADHD figure prominently in the clinical experience of behavioural phenotypes, when these disorders present in children affected by behavioural phenotypes they are commonly only a part of the behavioural picture. In tuberous sclerosis, for example, autism and ADHD are commonly diagnosed, but a case series of 100 children with tuberous sclerosis who present with autism and ADHD will show marked contrasts with another series of 100 children with autism and ADHD drawn from the general population, even where matched for ability level. The management strategies for the children with tuberous sclerosis, while having much in common with those for children from the broader population, will need to be specially adapted towards the needs of the individual child, in her/his context. The clinician dealing with children and adults affected by behavioural phenotypes needs to be mindful of the extent to which these behavioural patterns may be usefully regarded as psychiatric diagnoses—whose management may be facilitated by the available evidence base—and the extent to which, in the field of behavioural phenotypes, we are dealing with specific behaviour disorders, with established aetiologies.

The labelling debate in the management of behavioural phenotypes

The labelling of children as cases of behavioural phenotypes can be controversial. This is for good reason. In *Behavioural Phenotypes* (O'Brien and Yule 1995) we reviewed this theme in the context of the age-old nature/nurture controversy. Issues that figured highly

4

TABLE 1.1
Some pros and cons of labelling in behavioural phenotypes

Cons	Pros
Stigma	Long history of observations
Eugenics revisited	Wide corroboration
Self-fulfilling prophecy	Enhance holistic approach
Encourages therapeutic nihilism	Predictive validity
Unnecessary-genetic influences abound	Academic interest in disability fostered

there included the pitfalls and dangers that arise when one overemphasizes either the genetic or the environmental basis of problems, one at the expense of the other. In either case, an incomplete understanding of the cause of the problem emerges—crucially important where the clinician approaches the management of behaviour problems in which some genetic predisposition operates. Such an approach is useful in any exploration of the basic cause and nature of disorder, which was the aim of that text.

As we proceed to consider the management of individuals affected by behavioural phenotypes, the issue of labelling needs to be addressed. Some of the points that most frequently arise in discussion of these matters are summarized in Table 1.1.

CONS: THE POTENTIAL FOR LABELLING BEHAVIOURAL PHENOTYPES TO ADVERSELY IMPACT ON MANAGEMENT

Of all of the themes that most frequently concern clinicians, educators, carers, support groups, policy advisors, service planners and all who are interested in the maximal development and social adjustment of individuals affected by behavioural phenotypes, the general issue of *stigma* is perhaps the greatest concern. This is understandable. Traditionally, when a condition, *e.g.* Down syndrome, was diagnosed, discussion and clinical management focused on those medical conditions and intellectual disabilities that were known to figure prominently in the phenotype. If any mention was made of behavioural matters, it was most probably centred on assurance that individuals with Down syndrome were held to be passive and pleasant in character. Now, based on recent research on the behavioural and psychiatric features of Down syndrome, such discussions are likely to be different. Not only is it important to be mindful that the rates of psychiatric disorder in children with Down syndrome are similar to those among children of similar ability, it also likely that discussion will turn to considerations of the possibility and problems of premature dementia in middle age. In essence, by highlighting the features of the behavioural phenotype of Down syndrome, we are saying that not only does the condition result in learning disability, a typical pattern of dysmorphology and a high rate of serious medical problems, it also carries a predisposition to adverse behavioural outcomes. It is therefore desirable that we should be acutely aware of the adverse potential for stigma, particularly for the growing child's self esteem, and for ensuing concern on the part of parents and carers. In all such considerations, an acceptance of this possibility is the preferred strategy, along with discussion of how it should be addressed—for example, by emphasizing that one person's stigma is another's opportunity for support and intervention. Efforts to resolve this concern by bland reassurance will meet little success.

One theme that emerges alongside stigma in consideration of behavioural phenotypes is the extent to which there is a danger of *revisiting eugenics*. This criticism has some basis; in the above example, we are stating that the genetic 'anomaly' we call Down syndrome is characterized not only by learning disability, a particular appearance and a set of medical problems, it also carries a high risk of psychopathology, and risk of premature ageing. From the standpoint of eugenics, all of this would be taken to indicate that the genetic predisposition here is one that is inherently 'inferior'. This was the thesis on which Down (1866) based his thinking, when he argued that the individuals he observed were "subnormal", according to a variety of parameters. Taken at face value, all of this has a certain warped logic. However, in acknowledging the real danger of such labelling, we are reassured by maintaining a clear, long-term perspective on the management of affected individuals. Through anticipation of behavioural problems in childhood, and knowledge of the nature and timing of the presentation of dementia in middle age, the clinician maximizes the outcome for people with Down syndrome. Such reactive approaches to the recognition and intervention of emerging problems, coupled with proactive programmes of education and developmental inputs, are the way forward. In this way, the insights from behavioural phenotypes enhance the situation of affected individuals by facilitating management, rather than add to the negative stereotypes that many rightly fear.

The latter argument also serves as one counter to the concern that behavioural phenotypes may carry the danger of creating *self-fulfilling prophecy*. Once again, this is a real concern, and an understandable one. Once a condition is recognized as carrying a predisposition towards a set of behaviours, then parents and carers (and others) who anticipate emerging problems may in a sense promote them. Concerned parents, on identifying some behaviour that is known to be characteristic of a given condition, may well give the behaviour some notice and attention. This attention will substantially influence the child's behaviour, particularly towards maintaining the behaviour. Through such reward cycles, behaviours that may have had less inherent liability to endure may be maintained, and become entrenched. This may be especially likely to occur if there is an approach to the behavioural phenotype that is essentially one of *therapeutic nihilism*. Here, the response to the recognition and description of the behavioural phenotype is one that erroneously accepts the phenotype as inevitable, and not a focus for intervention. In fact, the reverse is true. As emphasized throughout the present text, the diagnosis and delineation of a behavioural phenotype in any one individual does not detract from management endeavours, it adds to them. Where sleep is a problem in one condition, perhaps known to be difficult to manage, then the response is to be more proactive, not less so. Where eating behaviour is an issue, the same applies. Also, in all considerations of behaviour that is to some extent genetically driven, the possibility of biologically based interventions arises. Certainly, many of the behavioural patterns described here pose substantial management challenges. But these are facilitated by the accumulating evidence, which emphasizes behavioural phenotypes as enabling catalysts in the management of affected individuals.

Additionally, one intriguing critique of labelling in behavioural phenotypes proposes that they are *unnecessary* and unhelpful, given that it is now established that *genetic influences abound*. According to this proposal, now that it is recognized that all biological traits have, ultimately, some kind of genetic substrate, why should it add to the understanding of Down syndrome to talk about a behavioural phenotype? Is it not sufficient to describe the behavioural and psychiatric features of the condition, rather than raise them up to some separate status, as a disorder in their own right, to which we then ascribe all features of behaviour we observe (Einfeld and Hall 1994)? Of all the concerns, this one may be the most cogent. It may well be that, in future, there will be no separate discussion of behavioural phenotypes. Descriptions and management plans for genetic disorders in disability may well include behaviour as a major issue, perhaps organized in the four domains described above (cognitive, motor, social, linguistic). If the insights from the initiative that is the study of behavioural phenotypes turn out to be as enduring as this, then far from a criticism of the approach, that will be a powerful indicator of its importance.

PROS: THE POTENTIAL FOR LABELLING BEHAVIOURAL PHENOTYPES TO FACILITATE MANAGEMENT
In the preceding discussion of how labelling may be deleterious for management, and in answering these concerns, many of the benefits of labelling behavioural phenotypes have been highlighted. Management of behavioural phenotypes is based on recognition and systematic diagnosis, and comprises a long-term strategy in which the informed clinician anticipates that certain problems may occur, and acts accordingly. As detailed in the syndrome-by-syndrome descriptions of behaviour and its management that comprise the latter part of this text, these observations have a *long history*, and have been *widely corroborated*. That corroboration has come from a wide variety of scientific and clinical disciplines. Geneticists, paediatricians, physiotherapists, psychologists, psycholinguicists, psychiatrists, speech therapists, specialist surgeons and teachers figure prominently here. It seems that, from whatever frame of reference one approaches the behaviour of these individuals, important insights emerge. It therefore follows that our management response to behavioural phenotypes should be an *holistic* one. In this sense, the label can be seen once again as an enabler, which encourages us to think beyond our own field and to take on the insights from elsewhere.

In addition to one pragmatic spin-off of the study of behavioural phenotypes—that there has been an ensuing general *fostering of academic interest in disability*—one of the most powerful indicators of the positive impact of behavioural phenotypes on management lies in their insights into long-term management: in other words their *predictive validity*. This major theme is next explored with reference to one of the major genetic conditions of learning disability, fragile X syndrome.

The long-term clinical relevance of behavioural phenotypes: fragile X syndrome as an example
To what extent can behavioural phenotypes predict long-term outcomes for affected individuals? Failing that, can they at least give some insight into long-term outcomes? This question raises several issues. In general, which trajectories of behaviour and development

7

can we discern in genetic syndromes of learning disability? To what extent do these trajectories show a distinct nature that is syndrome-specific? Or are behaviours more closely related to the degree, or severity, of the learning disability in individual cases? Can we see continuities between the behavioural phenotype in the child and in the adult? Or is there evidence that some problems are more apparent in childhood—or indeed in adulthood? (On the latter issue, in Down syndrome—see above—advancing age carries major cognitive and behavioural changes in many individuals.) As an illustration of the extent to which consideration of behavioural phenotypes demonstrates that some behavioural characteristics endure, while others are altered over the course of development, a study of fragile X syndrome is described.

Sample
In collaboration with the UK Fragile X Society, two groups of affected individuals (all having had *FraX-A* identification by known centres) were studied, in childhood and adulthood. Both comprised 35 individuals. The child group comprised boys aged 6–9 years, while the adults were men aged 20–40 years.

Questionnaire
The study employed the parent and child versions of the SSBP (Society for the Study of Behavioural Phenotypes) questionnaire (O'Brien 1992). This widely used measure was designed to assess behavioural phenotypes. It is intended for use in postal surveys, for completion by parents or principal carers. The questionnaire explores behaviours over the domains of: feeding; sleep; social behaviour; language; motor functioning; unusual interest; self-injury and aggression; anxiety and mood.

Results
Developmental differences: developmental continuities
In terms of basic self-care and self-organization skills, the adults showed significant improvements over the children (Fig. 1.1). In such abilities as washing and dressing, bowel and bladder control, and capacity to use a pencil appropriately, there is evidence of considerable improvement with age. However, there is far less evidence of improvements in language function. Both in terms of verbal language use to express basic needs ('needs communication', Fig. 1.1), and in respect of communication for reasons other than basic needs ('social communication', Fig. 1.1) there is only marginally improved function in the older group. These findings demonstrate that, as in all children with developmental disability, substantial improvements in basic self-care and organization may be observed with increasing age over the course of development, but that certain specific developmental disabilities—here, language—may endure in certain genetic syndromes.

In designing management strategies to address these patterns of development, the implications are that:
• conventional strategies geared towards the acquisition of basic social, self-care and organizational skills are appropriate, in that maturation over the course of development will facilitate such work

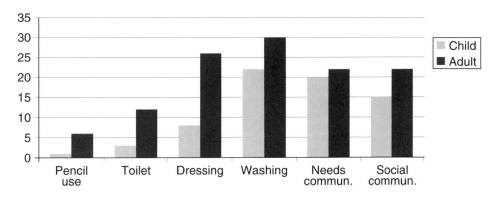

Fig. 1.1. Fragile X syndrome: numbers of children and adults showing age-appropriate development in various skills (both groups, N = 35). (Needs/Social commun. = Needs/Social communication.)

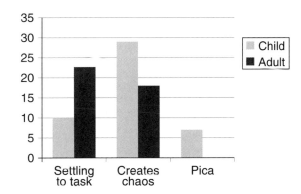

Fig. 1.2. Fragile X syndrome: behavioural differences between children and adults (both groups, N = 35)

- in designing, and especially in implementing, such programmes, it is important to adapt the content of the schedules and interactions with the growing child, towards the affected individual's language skills, which in some conditions (here, in fragile X syndrome) will be persistently delayed over the course of development, more so than will the acquisition of basic self-care and organization skills
- the persistence of the marked language deficit over the course of development highlights the need for speech and language therapeutic involvement in the individual's programme.

Behavioural differences

In some respects, behaviours that were prominent problems in the children were less apparent in the adults. Figure 1.2 summarizes the key changes in behaviour between the children and adults with fragile X syndrome. 'Settling to task'—which is a marker of the individual's

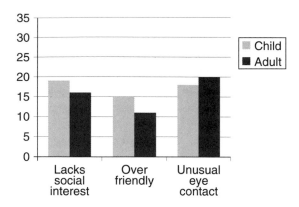

Fig. 1.3. Fragile X syndrome: behavioural continuities across children and adults: social behaviours (both groups, N = 35)

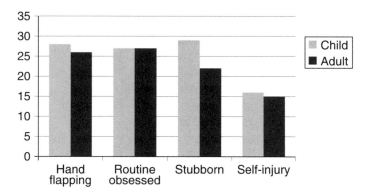

Fig. 1.4. Fragile X syndrome: behavioural continuities across children and adults: 'peripheral autistic' features (both groups, N = 35)

observed capacity to attend and to complete an activity—was markedly deficient in the children, but showed substantial improvement in the adults. In keeping with this maturational change, the adults were far less likely to 'create chaos' in their immediate environment than were the children, by being unsettled, noisy, and interfering with the activities of others. These findings are in keeping with other reports of a high prevalence of ADHD in children with fragile X syndrome (Turk 1992), and evidence that ADHD and related overactive behaviours among children usually diminish with maturation (McArdle *et al.* 1995). Seven of the 35 boys had persistent pica, the eating of non-nutrient material, while none of the 35 adults showed this difficult to manage behaviour. This is also in line with previous research, which emphasizes that where pica presents among people with learning disabilities it is typically developmentally determined, in that it is more common in children than in adults, and in more severely learning disabled individuals (O'Brien and Whitehouse 1990).

Behavioural continuities

The most striking findings were of similarities between the boys and the men with fragile X syndrome in their social behaviour and in certain observations that may be broadly regarded as 'peripheral autistic' behaviours, in that these are behaviours which are more common among autistic individuals, while not being diagnostic of autism. In terms of social behaviour, the boys and men with fragile X syndrome were both characterized by a lack of social interest in others, a proneness to be over-familiar toward strangers, and a pattern of unusual eye contact (Fig. 1.3). This last behavioural trait is gaze avoidance, most marked in affected individuals at the onset of any social encounter or interaction, as previously described in fragile X syndrome (Turk 1992). The 'peripheral autistic' behaviours which were common among both the boys and men with fragile X syndrome and which showed little or no evidence of any reduction in intensity among the older group, were hand-flapping, obsessional behaviour and self-injury (Fig. 1.4).

In designing management strategies to address these behavioural findings, the implications are:

- Behavioural problems that are known to be more common among children in general are also more common among children with genetic syndromes of learning disability. Many common disorders such as ADHD, which reduces in prevalence with increasing age though childhood into adulthood, show the same trajectory among people with genetic learning disability syndromes. It is therefore appropriate to apply the same treatment modalities to such disorders. In this example, orthodox approaches such as prescribing stimulant medication coupled with behavioural management would be indicated.
- Certain behavioural problems are persistent from childhood into adulthood among individuals affected by genetic syndromes of learning disability. Long-term strategies are therefore required to address this central issue. Where this is known to be typical of a given condition, once the behavioural pattern is identified in a given child, one of the first tasks is to advise and prepare parents and carers accordingly (see Chapter 7). Contact with the respective support society is recommended. In some such behavioural phenotypes of individual genetic syndromes, there is already evidence on the effectiveness of particular management and treatment strategies (see Chapter 8 for a review of the management of the behavioural phenotypes of common syndromes of learning disability). In many cases, management is informed more by experience and knowledge derived from wide experience of the management of the behaviour or psychiatric diagnosis in question.

Conclusion

Managing behavioural phenotypes among children and adults with genetic syndromes of learning disability poses challenges. While bearing in mind the issues of stigma, labelling and creation of self-fulfilling prophecies through anticipation of problems as here reviewed, it is recommended that clinicians and other specialists who deal with affected individuals maintain an approach of keen awareness of the occurrence of certain behavioural patterns in particular genetic conditions. Based on such an approach, coordinated multimodal treatment programmes may be appropriately employed. These treatment programmes will often need to be framed on a long-term basis. Here, three themes are apparent over the course of managing behavioural phenotypes in clinical practice. First, the mechanisms of the links between genetic syndromes and behaviour are typically complex. Intervention therefore needs to be informed by comprehensive assessment. Second, it is crucial to recognize where behaviours are related to the severity of learning disability and developmental level of the individual, rather than being based on the genetic condition in question. Finally, all of the known causes of behaviour also apply to the behaviour of those affected by genetic syndromes of learning disability. Toothache, personal environmental changes and personal distress are among the host of issues that figure prominently, and regularly merit our close attention.

REFERENCES

Down JL (1866) 'Observations on an ethnic classification of idiots.' *London Hospital Reports*, **3**, 259–262. [Reprinted in Down JL (1990) *Mental Affectations of Childhood and Youth. Classics in Developmental Medicine No. 5*. London: Mac Keith Press, pp 127–131.]

Einfeld SL, Hall W (1994) 'When is a behavioural phenotype not a phenotype?' *Developmental Medicine and Child Neurology*, **36**, 467–470.

Gillberg C, O'Brien G (eds) (2000) *Development Disability and Behaviour. Clinics in Developmental Medicine No. 149*. London: Mac Keith Press.

McArdle P, O'Brien G, Kolvin I (1995) 'Hyperactivity: prevalence and relationship with conduct disorder.' *Journal of Child Psychology and Psychiatry*, **36**, 279–303.

O'Brien G (1992) 'Behavioural phenotypy in developmental psychiatry.' *European Child and Adolescent Psychiatry*, Suppl. 1, 1–61.

O'Brien G, Whitehouse A (1990) 'A psychiatric study of deviant eating behaviour among mentally handicapped adults.' *British Journal of Psychiatry*, **157**, 281–284.

O'Brien G, Yule W (eds) (1995) *Behavioural Phenotypes. Clinics in Developmental Medicine No. 138*. London: Mac Keith Press.

O'Brien G, Yule W (eds) (2000) *Caratteristiche Compartamentali delle Malattie Genetiche*. Milan: McGraw-Hill.

Turk J (1992) 'The fragile X syndrome. On the way to a behavioural phenotype.' *British Journal of Psychiatry*, **160**, 24–35.

2
COMMON PROBLEMS IN BEHAVIOURAL PHENOTYPES

A. OVERVIEW

Gregory O'Brien

What kinds of problems commonly present as behavioural phenotypes? One answer might be 'any behaviour observed'. This comment, however trite, does emphasize a few key themes. Firstly, we do indeed see a very wide variety of behaviours among the people we study in this field. These include many behaviours that are far less common among other, non-disabled populations, in addition to problems more typical of individuals of normal intelligence. In many of the conditions with which we deal in this area of clinical practice, it is the *combinations*, or profiles, of behaviours encountered that are of particular interest, in that the behaviours that come together in some of these conditions do not constitute patterns of behaviour seen widely in other populations. The low intelligence that characterizes these children goes some considerable way to giving an explanation for the occurrence of these behaviours. However, the wide differences we see between different behavioural phenotypes drawn from different genetic conditions, even allowing for IQ, emphasize that other factors associated with individual genetic conditions are also important.

Always in considering genetic influences on behaviour, we need to bear in mind other influences—and in this respect we note that different individuals with the same genetic conditions often present with quite different behavioural profiles, particularly according to a host of environmental and developmental influences. However, the fundamental message concerns the nature of 'phenotype' as defined in the *Oxford English Dictionary*: "the sum-total of the observable or detectable characteristics of an individual or group, as determined by its genotype and by genetic or environmental factors". In other words, it is not just that the behavioural phenotype is a genetically determined entity, liable to be moulded by environmental influences. By this definition, the behavioural phenotype we observe at any one time in an individual is the product of genetic and environmental influences; and on that basis, any behaviour we see may be construed as part of the behavioural phenotype.

Behavioural domains
Once we accept that any behaviour may be included under the rubric of 'behavioural pheno-types', there is a need to adopt some kind of systematic consideration and classification of the behaviours in question. One approach favoured by many is to take the actual observable behaviours as the starting point. In this way, no assumptions are made about whether a set

of behaviours might constitute a psychiatric disorder—very much in line with our preferred definition of behavioural phenotype (see Chapter 1, p 2), which states that while "In some cases, the behavioural phenotype may constitute a psychiatric disorder; in others, behaviours which are not usually regarded as symptoms of psychiatric diagnoses may occur."

Currently, work in this field recognizes certain important domains or groupings of behaviour, which have utility in classification, clinical practice and research. The domains are: aggression; self-injury; sleep and circadian problems; eating behaviour; mood; language; motor; and sexual function (O'Brien 1992). The advantages of such an approach include: (i) these domains provide for a wide view of behaviour; (ii) the behaviours are observable; (iii) these behavioural domains have clinical relevance; (iv) findings of behaviours on these domains go some way to inform intervention planning; (v) these sets of behaviours are of crucial importance to the lives of the children concerned, and consequently to their families. It is therefore recommended that some consideration of behaviours arranged into these domains should always be given—in this way, the clinician is less likely to 'miss', or underestimate the importance of, any additional or coincidental behaviours that may be present alongside any presenting or already identified behavioural problem.

Classification
Throughout the present text, it is emphasized that conventional psychiatric diagnostic approaches—such as the ICD or DSM—are of limited applicability to the consideration of behavioural phenotypes. For this reason, an empirical approach to the observation and recording of behaviour is here recommended. In addition, in some cases it is quite possible to ascribe clinically useful diagnostic labels, and this in turn can, of course, be invaluable in planning interventions. Some recent initiatives in this connection are of considerable interest, notably the development of the new *Diagnostic Criteria for Psychiatric Disorder for Adults with Learning Disability/Mental Retardation* (Royal College of Psychiatrists DCLD Development Group 2001), which provides guidelines and a framework for the use of ICD-10 psychiatric diagnoses among adults with moderate to severe learning disability (*i.e.* those with IQ <50; the conventional ICD-10 criteria may be used for those with mild learning disability, corresponding to IQ 50–69). This approach does include consideration of behavioural phenotypes, and also of other problem behaviours, for which operational definitions are given. In clinical practice, it is hoped that the adoption of the behavioural and psychiatric measurement schedules reviewed in Chapter 3 will both facilitate the derivation of diagnoses, and aid in monitoring treatment effects and progress.

Three common problems considered
Sections B–D of this chapter concentrate on three of the most important of the problems encountered in clinical practice with children affected by behavioural phenotypes: sleep, self-injury and autism. As can be seen in Chapter 8, where consideration is given to the management of people affected by the different syndromes in question, these problems are particularly common in this area of clinical practice. The selection of these three as foci for attention also says something about the basic mechanisms of derivation of behavioural phenotypes. In some cases, our focus of attention is on disruption or disorder of a normal

or adaptive behaviour pattern—here exemplified by sleep. On the other hand, in some we must concentrate on behaviours that are of themselves essentially deviant or maladaptive, *e.g.* self-injury. In others, we find that psychiatric diagnoses present, such as autism. Recognition of these different orders of behavioural phenotypes is useful, whether through efforts to promote adaptive behaviour, to minimize maladaptive behaviour, or to adopt treatment strategies of proven benefit for specific disorders.

REFERENCES

O'Brien G (1992) 'Behavioural phenotypy in developmental psychiatry.' *European Child and Adolescent Psychiatry*, Suppl. 1, 1–61.
Royal College of Psychiatrists' DCLD Development Group (Bailley N, Cooper SA, Clarke D, Holland A, Gravestock S, Matthews M, O'Brien G, Simpson N) (2001) *Diagnostic Criteria for Learning Disability/Mental Retardation. Occasional Paper No. 46.* London: Gaskell Press.

B. SELF-INJURIOUS AND AGGRESSIVE BEHAVIOURS

David Clarke

The nature and definition of self-injury associated with genetic disorders
The definition of self-injurious behaviour varies markedly between studies, making estimates of the prevalence of the problem among people with genetic disorders associated with behavioural phenotypes difficult. Many definitions centre on actual or potential tissue damage (*e.g.* Oliver *et al.* 1987), but the severity of such damage varies markedly from syndrome to syndrome at the population level, and may vary between individuals with any one syndrome. The compulsive lip- and finger-biting associated with Lesch–Nyhan disease (Christie *et al.* 1982, Anderson and Ernst 1994) is usually severe, and case reports of Smith–Magenis syndrome also suggest severe self-injury is a problem for at least some people (Colley *et al.* 1990; Greenberg *et al.* 1991, 1996; Stratton *et al.* 1986). Prader–Willi syndrome is associated with skin-picking that usually causes relatively mild tissue damage (Clarke *et al.* 1989, 1996) but may also be associated with more severe forms of self-injury, or with complications of self-injury such as cellulitis (Warnock and Kestenbaum 1992, Bhargava *et al.* 1996). The tissue damage resulting from self-injury in Rett syndrome is often mild, and a consequence of midline hand stereotypies, self-biting or hitting (Coleman *et al.* 1988, Sansom *et al.* 1993).

The relationship between self-injury and age is complex: adolescents and young adults are usually shown to have higher rates than children or the elderly in most studies. Self-injury becomes more prevalent with increasing severity of intellectual disability, and also tends to be more severe and resistant to treatment. The prevalence is slightly greater among males than females, and is higher among people living in institutions than those living with their families or in small community facilities (Borthwick-Duffy 1994; Rojahn 1986, 1994).

Influences on the initiation and maintenance of self-injury
There have been many attempts to explain one of the most puzzling paradoxes of human behaviour—why should people repeatedly engage in behaviour that is damaging and painful? The hypotheses and factors suggested as influences on self-injury discussed below are those prominent in the literature concerning self-injury associated with developmental disability. Other forms of self-injury occur, including culturally sanctioned behaviours such as tattooing, the self-cutting behaviours associated with personality abnormalities in young people, and self-mutilation secondary to severe mental disorders such as schizophrenia. The link, if any, between these forms of self-injury/self-mutilation and those associated with developmental disability is obscure.

Psychological influences on self-injury include the (operant) conditioning of behaviour by reinforcement, the behaviour (*e.g.* head banging) being followed by a response (such as the provision of staff attention, or avoidance of an undesired activity) that is rewarding. Such reinforcement may be apparent in clinical settings, but may be difficult to avoid. Not attending to self-injurious behaviour may result in an increase in its frequency and severity, with severe tissue damage as a consequence. Other functions of self-injury may include communication of needs, and improving communication has been suggested as a way of reducing such behaviours (Bird *et al.* 1989). A need for an optimal level of stimulation has been suggested as a factor in self-stimulatory behaviours associated with autistic spectrum disorders and with sensory impairments. Self-stimulation may take the form of rocking, head rolling or seeking firm pressure, and if severe may be associated with tissue damage (Thurrell and Rice 1970). Self-injury may serve the function of communicating distress arising from pain, and possibly of alleviating pain (in a manner similar to the effect of rubbing a painful joint). Upper respiratory tract infections causing otitis or sinusitis and dental pain may provoke head banging. Other physical causes such as epilepsy (Gedye 1989), the adverse effects of anticonvulsant medication (Kalachnik *et al.* 1995) or menstruation (Taylor *et al.* 1993) may be associated with self-injury.

Aggressive behaviours

Sigafoos *et al.* (1994) surveyed aggressive behaviours among a population of people with developmental disability living in Queensland, Australia. They found that 11% of the population studied had aggressive behaviours, most of whom (54%) had profound learning disorder. Aggressive behaviours were more prevalent among people living in institutions (35%) than among those living in group homes (17%) or other community facilities. Harris (1993) studied 1362 people with developmental disability in a single health district. The prevalence of aggressive behaviour was 18%, with differing rates in hospitals (38%) and day facilities (10%). Sigafoos *et al.* (1994) found aggression to be commoner among males, but Harris (1993) found no significant gender difference. Once established, aggressive behaviours are one of the most persistent of challenging behaviours associated with developmental disability (Leudar *et al.* 1984).

The relationship between aggressive and self-injurious behaviours

In the study by Sigafoos *et al.* (1994) referred to above, over a third of the people with aggressive behaviours also had self-injurious behaviours. Griffin *et al.* (1986) also found, in a statewide survey of people with mental retardation resident in institutions, that about 14% of the study population had self-injurious behaviours, and of these 55% also had aggressive behaviours. Read (1998) reviewed the evidence concerning the co-occurrence of self-injurious and aggressive behaviours among people with developmental disability, and found it so persuasive that he postulated the existence of the syndrome of "organic behaviour disorder", which "is understood to be a biological psychiatric condition which produces a characteristic clinical picture of violence associated with self-injury in severely and profoundly learning-disabled people and which is expressed as a final common pathway imposed upon a number of different aetiologies."

Self-injurious and aggressive behaviours associated with genetic syndromes
LESCH–NYHAN SYNDROME
The majority of children with Lesch–Nyhan syndrome "show verbal and physical aggression

towards other people and objects" (Deb 1998), and over 85% of affected children have compulsive self-injurious behaviour, often taking the form of lip, mouth or finger biting. Other behaviours seen in association with the disease include hitting the ears and face, banging the head against objects, skin-picking and attempting to trap fingers in wheelchair spokes (Nyhan 1976, Turk and Hill 1995). The self-injury often starts around the age of 2–3 years and tends to become less severe in adolescence and early adult life. The self-injury may occur in episodes, often lasting a few weeks, with a marked reduction in the behaviour for several weeks followed by worsening again. Although self-injurious and externally directed aggressive behaviours are so prevalent among men with Lesch–Nyhan disease as to suggest a link to the underlying metabolic abnormality (hypoxanthione-guanine phosphoribosyl transferase deficiency), there is also evidence that the self-injury is often precipitated by physical or emotional stressors (Anderson and Ernst 1994).

CORNELIA DE LANGE SYNDROME
Self-injurious behaviour has been widely reported in case series of people with Cornelia de Lange syndrome (Bryson *et al.* 1971, Shear *et al.* 1971). Behaviours reported included picking at eyelids; hitting the face with the knuckles; lip-, tongue-, arm-, finger- and knee-biting; scratching, picking and gouging skin over the hands; and beating hands and feet against hard surfaces. Bryson *et al.* (1971) commented that "In each of the patients we have now observed, the self-mutilative behavior was stereotyped. Each repeated the same self-mutilative act over and over again, often reopening a single wound year in and year out. More than one pattern was seen in some of the patients, but each was a particular expression for that patient and was performed repeatedly."

PRADER–WILLI SYNDROME
Behavioural and psychiatric aspects of Prader–Willi syndrome have now been researched in a systematic fashion, and studies show that the disorder is associated with a relatively high rate of problem behaviours, including outbursts of temper that may include aggressive behaviour, and self-injury through skin picking. However, more recent studies tend to show lower overall rates of behavioural disorder than earlier ones, probably because when syndromes are first described the most severely affected people are more likely to be included in such reports. The self-injury associated with Prader–Willi syndrome is mostly a result of skin picking or scratching (Clarke *et al.* 1989), although more severe self-injury, including the use of objects to inflict injury, has also been described (Bhargava *et al.* 1996). There are reports of effective psychopharmacological treatment with fluoxetine and naltrexone (Warnock and Kestenbaum 1992, Benjamin and Buot-Smith 1993), but in clinical practice the author has found that caution is necessary when using psychoactive compounds for people with Prader–Willi syndrome, and advises the use of small doses and gradual dose increases if the situation allows this. The combination of appetite, sleep, sexual and thermoregulatory problems, together with an excess of compulsive and probably mood and psychotic disorders suggests that serotonergic dysfunction may be associated with the syndrome (Clarke *et al.* 1989, 1996, 1998; Dykens *et al.* 1996; Clarke and Boer 1998).

SMITH–MAGENIS SYNDROME

Smith–Magenis syndrome is associated with a constellation of unusual and problematic behaviours. These include a self-hugging stereotypy that tends to occur more when affected people are excited, and may have a very high frequency (up to 100 times an hour) (Finucane *et al.* 1994). The syndrome is also associated with a variety of sleep disorders including reduced REM sleep, problems with sleep initiation, repeated nocturnal wakening and daytime sleepiness, and severe self-injury (Dykens *et al.* 1997; Smith *et al.* 1998a,b). The latter may include head banging, skin picking and scratching, the removal of finger- and toenails and the insertion of objects into body orifices, and are not infrequently associated with externally directed aggressive behaviours (Stratton *et al.* 1986; Colley *et al.* 1990; Greenberg *et al.* 1991; 1996). Clarke and Boer (1998) and Clarke and Marston (2000) surveyed problem behaviours in four chromosome deletion disorders (Smith–Magenis, Prader–Willi, 5p–/cri du chat and Angelman syndromes) using the same carer-rated instrument and found the highest mean ratings of maladaptive behaviour to be associated with Smith–Magenis syndrome. Hodapp *et al.* (1998) reported high levels of stress among the families of children with Smith–Magenis syndrome, and observed that these were comparable to findings for families of children with Prader–Willi and 5p– (cri du chat) syndromes, but far exceeded those reported by the families of children whose developmental disability was of nonspecific origin. Maladaptive behaviours, including self-injury and aggressive behaviours, were the variable most predictive of parental pessimism, reinforcing the view that the effective management of such behaviours must be an urgent goal of behavioural phenotype research.

OTHER SYNDROMES

Self-injurious and aggressive behaviours have been described in association with many other syndromes, including Joubert syndrome (Holroyd *et al.* 1991), FG syndrome (Opitz *et al.* 1988); Aicardi syndrome (O'Brien 1994) and Lowe syndrome (Kenworthy *et al.* 1993). Fragile X syndrome is associated with self-biting, often over the anatomical snuff box near the wrist, and aggressive behaviours that often seem to be manifestations of anxiety or over-arousal (Udwin and Dennis 1995). One report has described self-injury and aggressive behaviours in association with Smith–Lemli–Opitz syndrome (Tint *et al.* 1994).

Managing severe self-injury and aggressive behaviours

Given the multitude of influences on the vulnerability to, precipitation of, and maintenance of self-injury, it is no surprise that many different techniques of management, rationally related to these influences, have been used to manage the behaviour. All are successful in some circumstances and for some people, but none is universally effective. If an obvious precipitant (such as a source of pain) can be identified, it makes sense to remove it if possible. It is sometimes easy to identify possible vulnerability factors (such as a genetic disorder associated with self-injury) and precipitants (such as loss or bereavement) but impossible to reverse them. Basic measures, such as the provision of an optimal level of stimulation of a kind the person finds enjoyable, can be of benefit for many people. In the case of people whose self-injury is associated with an autistic spectrum disorder, a careful assessment of sensory needs and an approach based on sensory integration may be helpful (Reisman 1993).

A systematic approach to evaluating the various factors thought to play a role in the vulnerability to, and initiation and maintenance of self-injurious behaviours is to be commended. Bridgen and Todd (1990) describe one such system for evaluating relevant factors and deciding on interventions, based around a flow chart. It is often the case that some factors can only be guessed at, and an estimate made of their likely importance and amenability to intervention. Having decided what intervention might be possible, it is then important to decide on a measure of outcome. This may be individually tailored to the person's problems (such as a four-point rating scale) or a standardized checklist of problem behaviours that is sensitive to change, such as the Aberrant Behavior Checklist (Aman *et al.* 1985). One intervention should then be made and its effect evaluated before trying the next. However, in clinical practice such a counsel of perfection often has to be tempered by the reality of trying to prevent further physical and mental deterioration. This may be a pressing need; in someone with severe head banging and a history of retinal detachment, for example, the risk of a further retinal detachment or the development of a subdural haematoma must be significant. In such circumstances many changes may have to be made simultaneously, and elements then removed in sequence to try to determine what was effective.

It is important to manage self-injurious and aggressive behaviours optimally; in addition to the risks to physical health created by self-injury, such behaviours, when associated with developmental disability, increase family and carer stress (Quine and Pahl 1985) and the risk of carers inflicting physical abuse (Maurice and Trudel 1982). They are also associated with an increased likelihood of moving from family to other residential care settings (Lakin *et al.* 1983, Tausig 1985, Bromley and Blacher 1991), an increased risk of exclusion from community-based services (Shlalock *et al.* 1985) and a higher rate of prescribing of psychotropic medication (Oliver *et al.* 1987, Chadsey-Rusch and Sprague 1989).

Psychological approaches to the treatment of self-injurious and aggressive behaviours

SELF-INJURY

If analysis of the factors involved in self-injury shows a clear relationship between the behaviour and particular antecedent events, an approach based on altering the influence of antecedent conditions may be appropriate. Interventions may involve enriching the stimulatory nature of the environment (if behaviours seem to result from understimulation) through the use of tactile, visual, olfactory or proprioceptive stimuli. Favell *et al.* (1982) used such an approach to modify self-injury by providing toys, and found that they were used to serve similar functions to the self-injury—people who had previously eye-poked used the toys for visual stimulation, those who had problems with hand-biting and pica chewed the toys. Others have used approaches based on encouraging alternative motor activity, which has the advantage of being more age-appropriate for adults (Baumeister and MacLean 1984). Other approaches include functional equivalence training, the aim of which is to encourage socially appropriate and functionally equivalent replacement behaviours. The behaviours encouraged usually involve motor skills or communicatory responses. Durand

and Kishi (1987) taught young adults with severe intellectual disabilities to sign or present a token to indicate requests for objects or for staff attention. A reduction in self-injury was observed when staff members responded consistently to the newly taught communications. A strategy of encouraging behaviours that are incompatible with self-injury may be helpful, such as using a stress-ball to alleviate skin picking. Noncontingent reinforcement, in which the reinforcer (such as attention) is provided to a timetable that is not influenced by self-injury, has been shown to be effective for some people with intellectual disability (Vollmer *et al.* 1993). Rincover and Devany (1982) showed a reduction in self-injury when the sensory stimulation associated with such behaviour was removed (*e.g.* by wearing gloves to reduce the tactile stimulation from skin-scratching).

If the function of self-injury appears to be task avoidance or a method of avoiding a stimulus or situation that is perceived as aversive, strategies can be devised accordingly. In people with autism, changes in routine, transitions (*e.g.* between rooms or activities) or social interaction may be associated with over-arousal and an increase in self-injury. It is sometimes possible to restructure the environment to minimize stressful situations. Other approaches aim to encourage functionally equivalent behaviours, and include regimes based on functional communication training (FCT) (Carr and Durrand 1985). More controversially, Gardner *et al.* (2001) suggest that "in those patients who do not respond to FCT with a clinically acceptable reduction of their self-injurious and related destructive behaviors, it may be useful to add a mild punishment contingency to increase their motivation to select the alternative communicative response as an alternative to the [self-injurious behaviours]." Gardner *et al.* also discuss the use of differential reinforcement, and relaxation training, in the management of self-injury. An overview of psychological interventions to reduce self-injury associated with developmental disability is given by Halliday and Mackrell (1998).

AGGRESSIVE BEHAVIOURS
The management of aggressive behaviours using psychological treatments employs many of the same concepts as the management of self-injury, but many practitioners draw a distinction between the theoretical 'best' way to treat behaviours with the aim of eliminating them, and the most effective way of managing behaviours in clinical and normal life settings with the aim of containing them. The use of low-arousal approaches may minimize the need for more intrusive strategies such as physical restraint, and interventions such as relaxation training and anger management training may be of benefit, especially for those people with less severe intellectual disabilities (Harvey 1979, Benson *et al.* 1986). Griffiths (2001) has summarized the issues pertaining to the assessment and management of aggressive behaviours, and draws a useful distinction between aggressive behaviours that are reactive, those that are responsive and those that are functional.

Pharmacological approaches to the treatment of aggressive and self-injurious behaviours
Neurochemical hypotheses concerning the initiation and maintenance of self-injury centre largely on the roles of dopamine, serotonin and endogenous opioids (Clarke 1998, Verhoeven and Tuinier 2001). These hypotheses have led to psychopharmacological approaches to self-

injury, some based on an attempt to redress postulated neurotransmitter or neurochemical imbalances, others based on the high level of comorbidity with psychiatric disorders such as depression (e.g. Sovner *et al.* 1993). Most of the interventions are based on relatively little evidence (the same is true for many of the psychologically based strategies referred to above). Evidence is usually gained from case studies, rarely from double-blind placebo-controlled trials. Even where such evidence is available there are often methodological issues that create a need for replication. Tyrer and Hill (2001) have provided a flow-chart to guide prescribing to people with developmental disability and self-injury or aggressive behaviours.

ANTIPSYCHOTICS

The compounds that have historically been used most widely in the management of both aggressive and self-injurious behaviours are the antipsychotics, especially haloperidol and thioridazine (Clarke 1998, Verhoeven and Tuinier 2001). Thioridazine has now been withdrawn from the market in the UK for all indications other than the treatment of schizophrenia. Antipsychotic medications (especially older compounds) are associated with problems such as tardive and withdrawal dyskinesias, sedation and sometimes a worsening of seizure control (Verhoeven and Tuinier 2001). There is some published evidence that zuclopenthixol may have some effect on aggressive behaviour associated with developmental disability (Izmeth *et al.* 1988, Singh and Owino 1992), and Malt *et al.* (1995) suggested that zuclopenthixol was superior to haloperidol for the treatment of aggressive and other problem behaviours associated with learning disability. Evidence from animal studies suggests that the dopamine D_1 receptor system is implicated in the maintenance of some self-injurious behaviours, especially those associated with Lesch–Nyhan syndrome (Breese *et al.* 1984). Most antipsychotic drugs have relatively little D_1 blocking action, and act predominantly on D_2 receptors. This observation has led to the suggestion that fluphenazine or clozapine would be of benefit for people with severe self-injury (Schroeder *et al.* 1995). Unfortunately, the use of fluphenazine is often limited by unpleasant extrapyramidal adverse effects, and the use of clozapine requires very close haematological monitoring. In his review of the concept of 'organic behaviour disorder' comprising the co-occurrence of severe learning disability, self-injury and aggressive behaviours, Read (1998) suggested that the most effective treatment was with antipsychotic D_2 blocking medications, preferably given by depot injection. Others have come to different conclusions: Verhoeven and Tuinier (1999) stated that "reviewing the literature, no specific effects of antipsychotics on challenging behaviour can be inferred. Most probably, their presumed efficacy is restricted to suppressing behaviour in general." Vanden Borre *et al.* (1993) report beneficial effects from treatment with risperidone, an atypical antipsychotic, on problems including aggressive and self-injurious behaviours associated with developmental disability. Lott *et al.* (1996) found a significant reduction in target behaviours including aggression, self-injury and property destruction among adults with learning disability treated with risperidone in an institutional setting. Positive outcomes have also been reported in studies by McDougle *et al.* (1998) and Williams *et al.* (2000). Risperidone has the advantage that extrapyramidal adverse effects are relatively rare compared to those of older antipsychotic compounds. Many clinicians use it in low doses to treat aggressive or self-injurious behaviours that seem to be precipitated by over-arousal and anxiety in people with autistic spectrum disorders, but this use is unlicensed. Brylewski and Duggan (1999) carried out a systematic review of randomized controlled trials of the use of antipsychotic medication to treat challenging behaviours associated with developmental disability. They could find only three papers of a sufficient standard to include in the analysis, and concluded that there was no evidence as to whether antipsychotic medication does or does not help adults with developmental disability and challenging behaviour.

TRICYCLIC AND SSRI ANTIDEPRESSANTS
There is a hypothetical link between some forms of self-injury and compulsive and stereo-typed behaviours (King 1993), for which the tricyclic antidepressant clomipramine has been shown to be effective for people with developmental disability (Lewis *et al.* 1995). Clomipramine has also been found to benefit self-injury (Garber *et al.* 1992, Lewis *et al.* 1996), and other antidepressants acting on the serotonergic system, such as trazodone, have been reported to be of benefit in reducing aggressive behaviour (O'Neal *et al.* 1986). Interest in serotonergic dysfunction and its amelioration through the use of antidepressant compounds such as clomipramine has led to the use of selective serotonin reuptake inhibitors (SSRIs), which have similar effects to clomipramine but with fewer adverse effects. The compound most widely studied is fluoxetine, which has been found to have beneficial effects on self-injurious and aggressive behaviours, whether or not associated with comorbid depressive disorder (Cook *et al.* 1992, Markowitz 1992, Bodfish and Madison 1993, Ricketts *et al.* 1993, Sovner *et al.* 1993). Sertraline has also been employed (Garber *et al.* 1992), and Warnock and Kestenbuam (1992) reported a beneficial effect from fluoxetine on the skin-picking associated with Prader–Willi syndrome.

BUSPIRONE
The 5-HT$_1$ agonist buspirone has been used to treat aggressive and self-injurious behaviours, and many studies have reported positive effects. One study (King and Davanzo 1996) found that people with autism may have increased problems with aggressive behaviour after buspirone treatment. The evidence has been tabulated and reviewed by Verhoeven and Tuinier (1999).

BETA-BLOCKERS
Propranolol, a beta-adrenegic antagonist (beta-blocker) has been found to be of benefit in the treatment of aggressive and self-injurious behaviours, including in people with developmental disability (Ruedrich *et al.* 1990, Ratey and Lindem 1991, Thibaut and Colonna 1993). Beta-blockers are thought to act by reducing anxiety or over-arousal, but they also have effects on serotonergic systems.

OPIATE ANTAGONISTS
The use of opiate antagonist compounds in the management of severe self-injury is based on the opioid hypothesis, which suggests that self-injury leads to the release of endogenous,

opiate-like compounds that reinforce self-injury by providing a rewarding mood state, elevating the pain threshold by reducing the unpleasant emotional aspects of pain, or both. Naturally occurring opioids such as beta-endorphin are derived from the large precursor peptide pro-opiomelanocortin (POMC), which can be split enzymatically into many biologically active peptide fragments including endorphins, melanocyte stimulating hormone (MSH) and adrenocorticotrophic hormone (ACTH). Some evidence to support the opioid hypothesis comes from the accounts of some people with self-injury who can give accurate descriptions of their mood state, and from the finding that beta-endorphin concentrations in venous blood samples rise 2–3 minutes after episodes of self-injury in some people (Sandman and Hetrick 1995). Sandman and Hetrick also noted that ACTH and cortisol concentrations fell after self-injury, contrary to expectation. Such decoupling of the usual co-release of beta-endorphin and ACTH has also been found in long-term users of opiates. The findings suggest that some people with severe self-injury may have an abnormality in the hypothalamic–pituitary axis, or an imbalance in the two enzymes (PC1 and PC2) that 'cut' ACTH and beta-endorphin from POMC. Sandman and Hetrick also noted that those people with the greatest elevation of beta-endorphin after self-injury showed the greatest reduction in the behaviour after treatment with naltrexone, an opiate antagonist. Because the effects of opiates differ in the brain at different stages of development, treatment with opiate antagonists such as naltrexone may be more effective for adults with severe self-injury, and less effective for children. There are now many positive (and a significant number of negative) reports of treatment of self-injury with naltrexone (which can be given by mouth) or the older compound naloxone (which had to be given parenterally); see Verhoeven and Tuinier (2001) for a summary of these studies. Some authors have noted that preferred topographies for self-injury include those traditionally used in acupuncture, "stimulation-produced analgesia body sites" (Symonds and Thompson 1997). This could be interpreted as lending some support to the opioid hypothesis concerning the maintenance of self-injury, although it is equally true that the locations most frequently implicated in self-injury are those that are most accessible to hitting, scratching, etc.

LITHIUM
Lithium has been used treat both self-injurious and aggressive behaviours associated with developmental disability. The largest study is that of Craft *et al.* (1987) but there have also been several other reports of successful treatment, often where the person concerned was thought to have a mood disorder, or where there was a cyclical pattern to the self-injury (*e.g.* Cooper and Fowlie 1973, Micev and Lynch 1974, Dale 1980, Spreat *et al.* 1989, Langee 1990). A disadvantage of lithium treatment is the need for careful monitoring of blood levels, and the low therapeutic index with the risk of lithium toxicity in situations where body fluids are lost rapidly. Verhoeven and Tuinier (2001) concluded that "only equivocal data exist suggesting a place for lithium as a potentially useful agent in the management of mentally retarded patients with aggressive behavior."

ANTICONVULSANTS AND OTHER COMPOUNDS
Carbamazepine has been used to treat aggressive behaviours, especially when EEG abnor-

malities are present, or there is evidence of a syndrome of episodic dyscontrol (Reid *et al.* 1981, Langee 1989, Laminack 1990). Sodium valproate has also been reported to be of benefit for adults with developmental disability and associated aggressive or self-injurious behaviour (Mattes 1992, Ruedrich *et al.* 1999).

Baclofen, a gamma-aminobutyric acid analogue, was found to benefit the majority of 22 people with developmental disability and severe self-injury, in a double-blind trial (Primrose 1979). Benzodiazepines are useful only in situations such as the need to sedate a patient with severely self-injurious or aggressive behaviour prior to a medical or dental procedure; their use is associated with the development of tolerance and dependence, and may be associated with paradoxical excitement and aggression (Barron and Sandman 1985).

Conclusions

Aggressive and self-injurious behaviours are relatively commonly associated with genetic causes of developmental disability. The genetic abnormality presumably creates a vulnerability to such behaviours, sometimes relatively directly through an identifiable metabolic abnormality (as in Lesch–Nyhan disease), sometimes through the influence of intervening variables such as social anxiety (as in fragile X syndrome). Secondary psychological, social and biological factors such as alterations in pain threshold, neurotransmitter or neuropeptide abnormalities, comorbid psychiatric disorder and the effects of development and learning then determine whether the behaviour is expressed at a particular time or not. A structured assessment, with a measure of outcome, is helpful when planning clinical interventions to manage such behaviours. An understanding of factors predisposing to, precipitating and maintaining such behaviours is helpful clinically. Interventions may have to be targeted at factors amenable to change, rather than those most obviously implicated in precipitating the behaviour.

Self-injurious and aggressive behaviours are some of the most problematic aspects of a genetic disorder for a substantial proportion of people and their carers. Research into the causes of, influences on, and management of such behaviours is one of the most pressing issues in the field of behavioural phenotypes.

REFERENCES

Aman MG, Singh NN, Stewart AW, Field CJ (1985) 'The Aberrant Behavior Checklist: A behavior rating scale for the assessment of treatment effects.' *American Journal of Mental Deficiency*, **89**, 485–491.
Anderson LT, Ernst M (1994) 'Self-injury in Lesch–Nyhan disease.' *Journal of Autism and Developmental Disorders*, **24**, 67–81.
Barron J, Sandman CA (1985) 'Paradoxical excitement to sedative–hypnotics in mentally retarded clients.' *American Journal of Mental Deficiency*, **90**, 124–129.
Baumeister A, MacLean WE (1984) 'Deceleration of self-injurious and stereotypic responding by exercise.' *Applied Research in Mental Retardation*, **5**, 385–393.
Benjamin E, Buot-Smith T (1993) 'Naltrexone and fluoxetine in Prader–Willi syndrome.' *Journal of the American Academy of Child and Adolescent Psychiatry*, **32**, 870–873.
Benson BA, Rice CJ, Miranti SV (1986) 'Effects of anger management training with mentally retarded adults in group treatment.' *Journal of Consulting and Clinical Psychology*, **54**, 728–729.
Bhargava SA, Putnam PE, Kocoshis SA, Rowe M, Hanchett J (1996) 'Rectal bleeding in Prader–Willi syndrome.' *Pediatrics*, **97**, 265–267.
Bird F, Dores P, Moniz D, Robinson J (1989) 'Reducing severe aggressive and self-injurious behaviors with

functional communication training.' *American Journal on Mental Retardation*, **94**, 37–48.

Bodfish JW, Madison JT (1993) 'Diagnosis and fluoxetine treatment of compulsive behavior disorder of adults with mental retardation.' *American Journal on Mental Retardation*, **98**, 360–367.

Borthwick-Duffy SA (1994) 'Prevalence of destructive behaviors.' *In:* Thompson, T., Gray DB. (eds) *Destructive Behavior in Developmental Disabilities: Diagnosis and Treatment.* Thousand Oaks, CA: Sage, pp 3–23.

Breese GR, Baumeister AA, McCown TJ, Emerick JG, Frye GD, Mueller RA (1984) 'Neonatal 6-hydroxy-dopamine treatment: Model of susceptibility for self-mutilation in the Lesch–Nyhan syndrome.' *Pharmacology and Biochemistry of Behavior*, **21**, 459–461.

Bridgen P, Todd M (1990) 'Challenging behaviour: introducing a preadmission checklist, problem analysis flow chart, and intervention flow chart to guide decision making in a multidisciplinary team.' *Mental Handicap*, **18**, 99–104.

Bromley BE, Blacher J (1991) 'Parental reasons for out of home placement of children with severe handicaps.' *Mental Retardation*, **29**, 275–280.

Brylewski J, Duggan L (1999) 'Antipsychotic medication for challenging behaviour in people with intellectual disability: a systematic review of randomised controlled trials.' *Journal of Intellectual Disability Research*, **43**, 360–371.

Bryson Y, Sakati N, Nyhan WL, Fisch CH (1971) 'Self mutilative behavior in the Cornelia de Lange syndrome.' *American Journal of Mental Deficiency*, **76**, 319–324.

Carr EG, Durrand VM (1985) 'Reducing behavior problems through functional communication training.' *Journal of Applied Behavior Analysis*, **18**, 111–126.

Chadsey-Rusch J, Sprague RL (1989) 'Maladaptive behaviors associated with neuroleptic drug maintenance.' *American Journal on Mental Retardation*, **93**, 607–617.

Christie R, Bay C, Kaufman IA, Bakay B, Borden M, Nyhan WL (1982) 'Lesch–Nyhan disease: clinical experience with nineteen patients.' *Developmental Medicine and Child Neurology*, **24**, 293–306.

Clarke DJ (1998) 'Psychopharmacology of severe self-injury associated with learning disabilities.' *British Journal of Psychiatry*, **172**, 389–394.

Clarke DJ, Boer H (1998) 'Problem behaviors associated with deletion Prader–Willi, Smith–Magenis and cri du chat syndromes.' *American Journal on Mental Retardation*, **103**, 264–271.

Clarke DJ, Marston G (2000) 'Problem behaviors associated with 15q– Angelman syndrome.' *American Journal on Mental Retardation*, **105**, 25–31.

Clarke DJ, Boer H, Chung MC, Sturmey P, Webb T (1996) 'Maladaptive behaviour in Prader–Willi syndrome in adult life.' *Journal of Intellectual Disability Research*, **40**, 159–165.

Clarke DJ, Boer H, Webb T, Scott P, Frazer S, Vogels A, Borghgraef M, Curfs LMG (1998) 'Prader–Willi syndrome and psychotic symptoms: 1. Case descriptions and genetic studies.' *Journal of Intellectual Disability Research*, **42**, 440–450.

Clarke DJ, Waters J, Corbett JA (1989) 'Adults with Prader–Willi syndrome: abnormalities of sleep and behaviour.' *Journal of the Royal Society of Medicine*, **82**, 21–24.

Coleman M, Brubaker J, Hunter K, Smith G (1988) 'Rett syndrome: A survey of North American patients.' *Journal of Mental Deficiency Research*, **32**, 117–124.

Colley AF, Leversha MA, Voullaire LE, Rogers JG (1990) 'Five cases demonstrating the distinctive behavioural features of chromosome deletion 17 (p11.2) (Smith–Magenis syndrome).' *Journal of Pediatrics and Child Health*, **26**, 17–21.

Cook EH, Rowlett R, Jaselskis C, Leventhal BL (1992) 'Fluoxetine treatment of children and adults with autistic disorder and mental retardation.' *Journal of the American Academy of Child and Adolescent Psychiatry*, **31**, 739–745.

Cooper AF, Fowlie HC (1973) 'Control of gross self-mutilation with lithium carbonate.' *British Journal of Psychiatry*, **122**, 370–371.

Craft M, Ismail IA, Krishnamurti D, Mathews J, Regan A, Seth RV, North PM (1987) 'Lithium in the treatment of aggression in mentally handicapped patients: a double-blind trial.' *British Journal of Psychiatry*, **150**, 685–689.

Dale PG (1980) 'Lithium therapy in aggressive mentally subnormal patients.' *British Journal of Psychiatry*, **137**, 469–474.

Deb S (1998) 'Self-injury and genetic syndromes.' *British Journal of Psychiatry*, **172**, 385–388.

Durand VM, Kishi G (1987) 'Reducing severe behaviour problems among persons with dual sensory impairments: an evaluation of a technical assistance model.' *Journal of the Association for Severely Handicapped*, **12**, 2–10.

26

Dykens EM, Leckman JF, Cassidy SB (1996) 'Obsessions and compulsions in Prader–Willi syndrome.' *Journal of Child Psychology and Psychiatry*, **37**, 995–1002.

Dykens EM, Finucane BM, Gayley C (1997) 'Cognitive and behavioural profiles in persons with Smith–Magenis syndrome.' *Journal of Autism and Developmental Disorders*, **27**, 203–211.

Favell JE, McGimsey JF, Schnell RM (1982) 'Treatment of self-injury by providing alternate sensory activities.' *Analysis and Intervention in Developmental Disabilities*, **2**, 83–104.

Finucane BM, Konar D, Haas-Givner B, Kurtz MD, Scott LI (1994) 'The spasmodic upper-body squeeze: a characteristic behaviour in Smith–Magenis syndrome.' *Developmental Medicine and Child Neurology*, **36**, 78–83.

Garber HJ, McGonigle JJ, Sloma GT, Monteverde E (1992) 'Clomipramine treatment of stereotypic behaviors and self-injury in patients with developmental disabilities.' *Journal of the American Academy of Child and Adolescent Psychiatry*, **31**, 1157–1160.

Gardner WI, Graeber-Whalen JL, Ford DR (2001) 'Self-injurious behaviors: Multimodal contextual approach to treatment.' *In:* Dosen A, Day K (eds) *Treating Mental Illness and Behavior Disorders in Children and Adolescents with Mental Retardation.* Washington, DC: American Psychiatric Association, pp 323–342.

Gedye A (1989) 'Extreme self-injury related to frontal lobe seizures.' *American Journal on Mental Retardation*, **94**, 201–214.

Greenberg F, Guzzetta V, de Oca-Luna RM, Magenis RE, Smith AM, Richter SF, Kondo I, Dobyns WB, Patel PI, Lupski JR (1991) 'Molecular analysis of the Smith–Magenis syndrome: A possible contiguous gene syndrome associated with del (17) (p11.2).' *American Journal of Human Genetics*, **49**, 1207–1218.

Greenberg F, Lewis RA, Potocki L, Glaze D, Parke J, Killian J, Murphy MA, Williamson D, Brown F, Dutton R, McCluggage C, Friedman E, Sulek M, Lupski, J. (1996) 'Multi-disciplinary clinical study of Smith–Magenis syndrome (deletion 17p11.2).' *American Journal of Medical Genetics*, **62**, 247–254.

Griffin JC, Williams DE, Stark MT, Altmeyer BK, Mason M (1986) 'Self-injurious behavior: A state-wide prevalence survey of the extent and circumstances.' *Applied Research in Mental Retardation*, **7**, 105–116.

Griffiths D (2001) 'Strategic behavioural interventions in aggression.' *In:* Dosen A, Day K (eds) *Treating Mental Illness and Behavior Disorders in Children and Adolescents with Mental Retardation.* Washington, DC: APA, pp 305–321.

Halliday S, Mackrell K (1998) 'Psychological interventions in self-injurious behaviour. Working with people with a learning disability.' *British Journal of Psychiatry*, **172**, 395–400.

Harris P (1993) 'The nature and extent of aggressive behaviour among people with learning difficulties (mental handicap) in a single health district.' *Journal of Intellectual Disability Research*, **37**, 221–242.

Harvey JR (1979) 'The potential of relaxation training for the mentally retarded.' *Mental Retardation*, **17**, 71–76.

Hodapp RM, Fidler DJ, Smith ACM (1998) 'Stress and coping in families of children with Smith–Magenis syndrome.' *Journal of Intellectual Disability Research*, **42**, 331–340.

Holroyd S, Reiss AL, Bryan N (1991) 'Autistic features in Joubert syndrome: a genetic disorder with agenesis of the cerebellar vermis.' *Biological Psychiatry*, **29**, 287–294.

Izmeth MG, Khan SY, Kumarajeewa DI, Shivanathan S, Veall RM, Wiley YV (1988) 'Zuclopenthixol decanoate in the management of behavioural disorders in mentally handicapped patients.' *Pharmatherapeutica*, **5**, 217–227.

Kalachnik E, Hanzel TE, Harder SR, Bauernfeind JD, Engstrom EA (1995) 'Anti-epileptic drug behavioural side effects in individuals with mental retardation and the use of behavioural measurement techniques.' *Mental Retardation*, **33**, 374–382.

Kenworthy L, Park T, Charnas LR (1993) 'Cognitive and behavioural profile of the oculocerebrorenal syndrome of Lowe.' *American Journal of Medical Genetics*, **46**, 297–303.

King BH (1993) 'Self-injury by people with mental retardation: A compulsive behavior hypothesis.' *American Journal on Mental Retardation*, **98**, 93–112.

King BH, Davanzo P (1996) 'Buspirone treatment of aggression and self-injury in autistic and nonautistic persons with severe mental retardation.' *Developmental Brain Dysfunction*, **9**, 22–31.

Lakin KC, Hill BK, Hauber FA, Bruininks RH, Heal IW (1983) 'New admissions and readmissions to a national sample of public residential facilities.' *American Journal of Mental Deficiency*, **88**, 13–20.

Laminack L (1990) 'Carbamazepine for behavioral disorders.' *American Journal on Mental Retardation*, **94**, 563–564.

Langee HR (1989) 'A retrospective study of mentally retarded patients with behavioral disorders who were treated with carbamazepine.' *American Journal on Mental Retardation*, **93**, 640–643.

Langee HR (1990) 'Retrospective study of lithium use for institutionalized mentally retarded individuals with behavior disorders.' *American Journal on Mental Retardation*, **94**, 448–452.

Leudar I, Fraser WI, Jeeves MA (1984) 'Behaviour disturbance in mental handicap: typology and longitudinal trends.' *Psychological Medicine*, **14**, 923–935.

Lewis MH, Bodfish JW, Powell SB, Golden RN (1995) 'Clomipramine treatment for stereotypy and related repetitive movement disorders associated with mental retardation.' *American Journal on Mental Retardation*, **100**, 299–312.

Lewis MH, Bodfish JW, Powell SB, Parker DE, Golden RN (1996) 'Clomipramine treatment for self-injurious behavior of individuals with mental retardation: A double-blind comparison with placebo.' *American Journal on Mental Retardation*, **100**, 654–665.

Lott RS, Kerrick JM, Cohen SA (1996) 'Clinical and economic aspects of risperidone treatment in adults with mental retardation and behavioural disturbance.' *Psychopharmacology Bulletin*, **32**, 721–729.

Malt UF, Nystad R, Bache T, Noren O, Sjaastad M, Solberg KO, Tonseth S, Zachariassen P, Maehlum E (1995) 'Effectiveness of zuclopenthixol compared with haloperidol in the treatment of behavioural disturbances in learning disabled patients.' *British Journal of Psychiatry*, **166**, 374–377.

Markowitz PI (1992) 'Effect of fluoxetine on self-injurious behaviour among institutionalised retarded persons.' *Journal of Mental Deficiency Research*, **22**, 27–36.

Mattes JA (1992) 'Valproic acid for nonaffective aggression in the mentally retarded.' *Journal of Nervous and Mental Disease*, **180**, 601–602.

Maurice P, Trudel G (1982) 'Self injurious behavior; prevalence and relationships to environmental events.' *In:* Hollis J, Meyers C (eds) *Life-threatening Behavior*. Washington, DC: American Association for Mental Deficiency, pp 81–103.

McDougle CJ, Holmes JP, Carlson DC, Pelton GH, Cohen DJ, Price LH (1998) 'A double blind study placebo controlled of risperidone in adults with autistic disorder and other pervasive developmental disorders.' *Archives of General Psychiatry*, **55**, 633–641.

Micev V, Lynch DM (1974) 'Effect of lithium on disturbed severely mentally retarded patients.' *British Journal of Psychiatry*, **125**, 110 (letter).

Nyhan WL (1976) 'Behavior in the Lesch–Nyhan syndrome.' *Journal of Autism and Childhood Schizophrenia*, **6**, 235–252.

O'Brien G (1994) 'The behavioural and developmental consequences of corpus callosal agenesis and Aicardi syndrome.' *In:* Lassonde M, Jeeves MA (eds) *Callosal Agenesis*. New York: Plenum Press, pp 235–246.

Oliver C, Murphy GH, Corbett JA (1987) 'Self-injurious behaviour in people with mental handicap: a total population study.' *Journal of Mental Deficiency Research*, **31**, 146–162.

O'Neal M, Page N, Atkins WN, Eichelmann B (1986) 'Tryptophan–trazodone treatment of aggressive behaviour.' *Lancet*, **ii**, 859–860.

Opitz JM, Richieri-da Costa A, Aase JM, Benke PJ (1988) 'FG syndrome update 1988: Note of 5 new patients and bibliography.' *American Journal of Medical Genetics*, **30**, 309–328.

Primrose DA (1979) 'Treatment of self-injurious behaviour with a GABA (gamma-aminobutyric acid) analogue.' *Journal of Mental Deficiency Research*, **23**, 163–173.

Quine L, Pahl J (1985) 'Examining the causes of stress in families with mentally handicapped children.' *British Journal of Social Work*, **15**, 501–517.

Ratey JJ, Lindem KJ (1991) 'β-blockers as primary treatment for aggression and self-injury in the developmentally disabled.' *In:* Ratey J (ed) *Mental Retardation: Developing Pharmacotherapies*. Washington, DC: American Psychiatric Press, pp. 5–81.

Read S (1998) 'Self-injury and violence in people with severe learning disabilities.' *British Journal of Psychiatry*, **172**, 381–384.

Reid AH, Naylor GJ, Kay DS (1981) 'A double-blind, placebo-controlled, cross-over trial of carbamazepine in overactive, severely mentally handicapped patients.' *Psychological Medicine*, **11**, 109–113.

Reisman J (1993) 'Using a sensory integrative approach to treat self-injurious behavior in an adult with profound mental retardation.' *American Journal of Occupational Therapy*, **47**, 403–411.

Ricketts R., Goza AB, Ellis CR, Singh YN, Singh NN, Cooke JC (1993) 'Fluoxetine treatment of severe self-injury in young adults with mental retardation.' *Journal of the American Academy for Child and Adolescent Psychiatry*, **32**, 865–869.

Rincover A, Devany J. (1982) 'The application of sensory extinction procedures to self-injury.' *Analysis and Intervention in Developmental Disabilities*, **2**, 67–81.

Rojahn J (1986) 'Self-injurious and stereotypic behavior of non-institutionalized mentally retarded people. Prevalence and classification.' *American Journal of Mental Deficiency*, **91**, 268–276.

Rojahn J (1994) "Epidemiology and topographic taxonomy of self-injurious behavior.' *In:* Thompson, T, Gray DB. (eds) *Destructive Behavior in Developmental Disabilities: Diagnosis and Treatment.* Thousand Oaks, CA: Sage, pp. 49–67.

Ruedrich SL, Grush L, Wilson J (1990) 'Beta adrenergic blocking medications for aggressive or self-injurious mentally retarded persons.' *American Journal on Mental Retardation*, **95**, 110–119.

Ruedrich S, Swales TP, Fossaceca C, Toliver J, Rutkowski A (1999) 'Effect of divalproex sodium on aggression and self-injurious behaviour in adults with intellectual disability: a retrospective review.' *Journal of Intellectual Disability Research*, **43**, 105–111.

Sandman CA, Hetrick WP (1995) 'Opiate mechanisms in self-injury.' *Mental Retardation and Developmental Disabilities Research Reviews*, **1**, 130–136.

Sansom D, Krishnan VHR, Corbett J, Kerr A (1993) 'Emotional and behavioural aspects of Rett syndrome.' *Developmental Medicine and Child Neurology*, **35**, 340–345.

Schroeder SR, Hammock RG, Mulick JA, Rojahn J, Walson P, Fernald W, Meinhold P, Saphare G (1995) 'Clinical trials of D1 and D2 dopamine modulating drugs and self-injury in mental retardation and developmental disability.' *Mental Retardation and Developmental Disabilities Research Reviews*, **1**, 120–129.

Shear CS, Nyhan WL, Kirman BH, Stern J (1971) 'Self-mutilative behavior as a feature of the de Lange syndrome.' *Journal of Pediatrics*, **78**, 506–509.

Shlalock R, Harper R, Genung T (1985) 'Community integration of mentally retarded adults: Community placement and program success.' *American Journal of Mental Deficiency*, **89**, 352–361.

Sigafoos J, Elkins J, Kerr M, Attwood T (1994) 'A survey of aggressive behaviour among a population of persons with intellectual disability in Queensland.' *Journal of Intellectual Disability Research*, **38**, 369–381.

Singh I, Owino WJE (1992) 'A double-blind comparison of zuclopenthixol tablets with placebo in the treatment of mentally handicapped in-patients with associated behavioural disorders.' *Journal of Intellectual Disability Research*, **36**, 541–549.

Smith ACM, Dykens EM, Greenberg F (1998a) 'Behavioral phenotype of Smith Magenis syndrome (del 17 p11.2).' *American Journal of Medical Genetics*, **81**, 179–185.

Smith ACM, Dykens EM, Greenberg F (1998b) 'Sleep disturbance in Smith–Magenis syndrome (del 17 p11.2).' *American Journal of Medical Genetics*, **81**, 186–191.

Sovner R, Fox CJ, Lowry MJ, Lowry MA (1993) 'Fluoxetine treatment of depression and associated self-injury in two adults with mental retardation.' *Journal of Intellectual Disability Research*, **37**, 301–311.

Spreat S, Behar D, Reneski B, Miazzo P (1989) 'Lithium carbonate for aggression in mentally retarded persons.' *Comprehensive Psychiatry*, **30**, 505–511.

Stratton RF, Dobyns WB, Greenberg F, DeSana JB, Moore C, Fidone G, Runge GH, Feldman P, Sekhon GS, Pauli RM, Ledbetter DH (1986) 'Interstitial deletion of (17) (p11.2). Report of six additional patients with a new chromosome deletion syndrome.' *American Journal of Medical Genetics*, **24**, 421–432.

Symonds FJ, Thompson T (1997) 'Self-injurious behaviour and body site preference.' *Journal of Intellectual Disability Research*, **41**, 456–468.

Tausig M (1985) 'Factors in family decision making about placement for developmentally disabled individuals.' *American Journal on Mental Retardation*, **89**, 352–361.

Taylor DV, Rush D, Hetrick WP, Sandman CA (1993) 'Self-injurious behavior within the menstrual cycle of women with mental retardation.' *American Journal on Mental Retardation*, **97**, 659–664.

Thibaut F, Colonna L (1993) 'Efficacité antiaggressive des beta-bloquants.' *Encephale*, **19**, 263–267.

Thurrell RJ, Rice DG (1970) 'Eye rubbing in blind children: application of a sensory deprivation model.' *Exceptional Children*, **10**, 325–330.

Tint GS, Irons M, Elias ER, Batta AK, Frieden R, Chen TS, Salen G (1994) 'Defective cholesterol biosynthesis associated with the Smith–Lemli–Opitz syndrome.' *New England Journal of Medicine*, **330**, 107–113.

Turk J, Hill P (1995) 'Behavioural phenotypes in dysmorphic syndromes.' *Clinical Dysmorphology*, **4**, 105–115.

Tyrer S, Hill S (2001) 'Psychopharmacological approaches.' *In:* Dosen A, Day K (eds) *Treating Mental Illness and Behavior Disorders in Children and Adolescents with Mental Retardation.* Washington, DC: American Psychiatric Association, pp 45–67.

Udwin O, Dennis J (1995) 'Psychological and behavioural phenotypes in genetically determined syndromes: a review of research findings.' *In:* O'Brien G, Yule W (eds) *Behavioural Phenotypes. Clinics in Developmental Medicine No. 138.* London: Mac Keith Press, pp 90–208.

Vanden Borre R, Vermote R, Buttiens M, Thiry P, Dietrick G, Geutjens J, Sieben G, Heylen S (1993) 'Risperidone as add-on therapy in behavioural disturbances in mental retardation: a double-blind placebo-controlled cross-over study.' *Acta Psychiatrica Scandinavica*, **87**, 167–171.

29

Verhoeven WMA, Tuinier S (1999) 'The psychopharmacology of challenging behaviours in developmental disabilities.' *In:* Bouras N (ed) *Psychiatric and Behavioural Disorders in Developmental Disabilities and Mental Retardation.* Cambridge: Cambridge University Press, pp 295–316.

Verhoeven WMA, Tuinier S (2001) 'Pharmacotherapy in aggressive and auto-aggressive behavior.' *In:* Dosen A, Day K (eds) *Treating Mental Illness and Behavior Disorders in Children and Adolescents with Mental Retardation.* Washington, DC: American Psychiatric Association, pp 283–303.

Vollmer TR, Iwata BA, Zarcone JR, Smith RG, Mazaleski JL (1993) 'The role of attention in the treatment of attention-maintained self-injurious behavior: Noncontingent reinforcement and differential reinforcement of other behavior.' *Journal of Applied Behavior Analysis*, **26**, 9–21.

Warnock JKB, Kestenbaum T (1992) 'Pharmacological treatment of severe skin picking behavior in Prader–Willi syndrome.' *Archives of Dermatology*, **128**, 1623–1625.

Williams H, Clarke R, Bouras N, Martin J, Holt G (2000) 'Use of the atypical antipsychotics olanzapine and risperidone in adults with intellectual disability.' *Journal of Intellectual Disability Research*, **44**, 164–169

C. AUTISM-RELATED DISORDERS

Patricia Howlin

Autism, as defined by DSM-IV (APA 1994) and ICD-10 (WHO 1992) is a pervasive developmental disorder characterized by problems in three main areas: communication, social understanding, and rigid and repetitive patterns of behaviour. It is this *combination* of difficulties that is required for a diagnosis of typical autism, but difficulties associated with some or all of these domains may be found in many other disorders.

Although early research in autism suggested prevalence rates of around 3–4 individuals per 10,000 (Lotter 1966) these studies focused on individuals meeting clear diagnostic criteria for autistic disorder. If cases of atypical autism (in which some but not all of the core criteria for autism are met), those with Asperger syndrome and those with pervasive developmental disorders (not otherwise specified) are included, the figures are far higher. Fombonne (1999), in an overview of epidemiological research from 1966 to 1998, concludes that the prevalence rate for pervasive developmental disorders, *not including Asperger syndrome*, is around 18.7 per 10,000. Data from Gillberg and Gillberg (1989) and Wing (1993) suggest that classic autism may in fact be a much rarer condition than either Asperger syndrome or other autism spectrum disorders more generally. Figures published by the National Autistic Society (1997) indicate that if these other groups are included the rate rises to around 91 per 10,000 (*i.e.* almost 1% of the population!). While these data are based on small samples, which are more prone to error and yield higher estimates (Fombonne 1999), it is clear that autism related disorders are far more common than once thought. Indeed, the dramatic increase in the numbers of cases being diagnosed in some areas has led to claims of an 'epidemic' of autism (California Department of Developmental Services 1999).

Moreover, the frequency of autism spectrum disorders is influenced by a number of different variables. As with almost any condition affecting language related skills, autism is far more common in males than females. The overall ratio is around 4:1 (Fombonne 1999), but amongst those who are more able the excess of males is even more marked (around 9:1; Howlin and Asgharian 1999). There is also a significant relationship between autism and learning disorders. Although the syndrome can occur at all levels of cognitive ability, the majority of cases (about 80%, Fombonne 1999) have some associated intellectual impairment and around 50% have an IQ below 50. The prevalence of autistic features is also significantly increased amongst individuals with an IQ in the severe to profoundly retarded range. Wing and Gould (1979) reported that in the 35–49 IQ range around 40% of children assessed showed severe social impairments. This figure rose to 53% amongst those in the 20–34 IQ range, and in children with an IQ below 20 almost all (95.5%) had impairments of social interaction.

Links with other disorders
Autism spectrum disorders have been noted in association with a range of other syndromes

including Biedl–Bardet syndrome, cerebral palsy, Coffin–Siris syndrome, Cohen syndrome, Duchenne muscular dystrophy, Lawrence–Moon–Biedl syndrome, myotonic dystrophy, oculocutaneous albinism, Noonan syndrome, Sanfillippo syndrome and many more (Gillberg and Coleman 1992, 2000; O'Brien and Yule 1995). Gillberg (1992) has suggested that as many as 37% of cases of autism are associated with other medical or genetic disorders. In contrast, Rutter *et al.* (1994) conclude that comorbidity rates are much lower (probably around 10%).

Over the years the conditions with which autism has been most consistently associated are phenylketonuria, maternal rubella, neurofibromatosis, fragile X syndrome, Rett syndrome and tuberous sclerosis. However, Lord and Rutter (1994) suggest that the association with the first three of these conditions is weak and that the pattern of autistic features found is generally atypical.

Estimates of the association between autism and fragile X syndrome have reduced over recent years, from a high of 60%, to 16% when DSM-III criteria for autism were used (Hagerman 1990, Bailey *et al.* 1993), to current estimates (using advanced genetic testing and stringent diagnostic criteria) of around 2.5% (Bailey *et al.* 1996). Even a 2.5% rate of fragile X in autism, however, is significantly higher than that found in the general population, although the nature of the relationship remains unclear. Since both autism and fragile X are associated with learning disorder, the underlying association may be between fragile X and learning disorder, and hence the link with autism may be secondary (Bailey *et al.* 1996).

Autistic patterns of disorder are also found in Rett syndrome (Kerr 2002). Although this condition is included within the Pervasive Developmental Disorders category of the DSM-IV and ICD-10, it has a known genetic cause, is typically found in females, and has a very different developmental sequence to the other disorders within that category. Communication problems are common, but social interactions and awareness tend to improve with age, and the typical stereotypic and ritualistic patterns of behaviour are rather different to those found in classic autism.

A number of other chromosomal/genetic abnormalities have been associated with autism. Probably around 5% of individuals with autism (in addition to those with fragile X) have some chromosomal anomaly, although the meaning of this association is unclear. Most of the abnormalities reported are of uncertain clinical significance, or are also known to arise in individuals with no apparent disabilities. There *may* be a stronger association with the presence of an extra marker chromosome on chromosome 15 (Gillberg *et al.* 1991, Hotopf and Bolton 1995), but since autism has been associated with anomalies involving almost all chromosomes (Lauritsen *et al.* 1999) these reports provide few clues regarding possible genetic mechanisms.

The one genetic condition that is clearly associated with autism is tuberous sclerosis. Epidemiological studies have shown that 40–80% of individuals with tuberous sclerosis develop autism spectrum disorders (Smalley 1998, Fombonne *et al.* 1997, Harrison and Bolton 1997, Park and Bolton 2001). These rates are several hundred times greater than expected. The association is strongest in individuals with a history of infantile spasms and the presence of tubers in the temporal lobes (Bolton and Griffiths 1997). Comorbidity is reported in individuals of normal intelligence as well as those with learning disorder (Harrison and Bolton 1997).

There are other disorders that, in the past, have been considered to have a very low association with autism but, as diagnostic criteria have been refined, these estimates, too, have been revised. For example, although it was once thought that the co-occurrence of autism and Down syndrome was extremely rare, this is no longer the case. It is true that autism does not seem to occur in children with Down syndrome as often as in other children with nonspecific learning disabilities but there are now a number of reports suggesting that the frequency is probably around 10% (Ghazziuddin *et al.* 1992; Howlin *et al.* 1995, 1995; Kent *et al.* 1999). Individuals with specific developmental language disorders may also show some of the social, communication and ritualistic behaviours associated with autism, with these features sometimes becoming *more* rather than less evident with age (Howlin *et al.* 2000, Mawhood *et al.* 2000). Children with semantic pragmatic syndrome exhibit social and communication difficulties, as well as obsessional interests (Bishop 2000). Those diagnosed as having 'nonverbal learning disabilities' frequently show similar social and cognitive problems to those found in Asperger syndrome (Rourke and Tsatsanis 2000), and there are several characteristics that are common to Asperger syndrome/autism and attention deficit hyperactivity disorder (ADHD) (Ehlers *et al.* 1997, Klin and Volkmar 1997). Gillberg (1992) suggests that there may be links between autism spectrum disorders and a variety of psychological disorders including anorexia, language and reading difficulties, obsessive–compulsive personality disorder and Tourette syndrome. Several other reports of comorbidity of autism and Tourette syndrome have also appeared (*e.g.* Kerbeshian and Burd 1986, Littlejohns *et al.* 1990, Berthier *et al.* 1993, Marriage *et al.* 1993, Baron-Cohen *et al.* 1999). Although Klin *et al.* (2000) suggest that the association is much lower than implied by these publications, the rate of Tourette syndrome in autism still appears to be significantly higher than in the general population.

Problems associated with autism spectrum disorders

COMMUNICATION DIFFICULTIES

Around half of all children with autism fail to develop functional speech (Lord and Rutter 1994) but severe language impairments are also characteristic of almost all children with learning disorder. The discrepancy between verbal and nonverbal skills tends to increase as IQ falls, and amongst children with an IQ below 50 language skills are frequently very limited. In those with severe cognitive impairment (IQ below 20) useful language is almost invariably absent. Many such children will have little or no understanding of spoken language, or any compensatory use of gesture. Severe impairments of language are also commonly associated with many of the other medical and genetic conditions noted above, particularly tuberous sclerosis and Rett syndrome.

Amongst children with autism related disorders who do develop language, the acquisition of first words or phrases is frequently delayed. There may also be many unusual linguistic features, including repetitive and stereotyped language; semantic errors, such as neologisms and pronoun reversal; abnormalities in voice tone and modulation; and often, especially amongst those who are more able, a formal and pedantic style of speaking. Particularly characteristic is the lack of reciprocal conversation and the failure to use communication for purely *social* purposes. Receptive skills are often of an even lower level than spoken language, and in the case of children who are echolalic, expressive language may give a very misleading impression of how much they are actually able to understand. Interpretation of speech may be very literal, and abstract concepts present particular difficulties. Imaginative play, too, is frequently extremely limited.

SOCIAL ABNORMALITIES

Although the nature and extent of autistic-type social difficulties varies between individuals, and may also change with age (Wing and Gould 1979, Szatmari 2000), certain core features tend to prevail, whatever the child's developmental level. These include impairments in nonverbal communication, such as gesture, eye-gaze and greeting behaviours. However, in certain conditions, notably fragile X syndrome, the severity of such problems is related to environmental factors and the demands of the social situation (Turk and Graham 1997). Other typical problems are lack of reciprocity, difficulties in initiating social interactions, impaired empathy, failure to share enjoyment or activities with others, and, in particular, an inability to understand other people's feelings, beliefs or emotions or to respond to these in an appropriate way. Whilst once considered to be specific to autism, problems related to 'theory of mind' (Baron-Cohen 1995) tend to be mediated by intellectual and verbal ability, and have been identified in many other groups of children including those with learning disorder, fragile X syndrome, ADHD and developmental language disorders (Buitelaar *et al.* 1999). Difficulties in executive functioning, which affect social interactions as well as many other aspects of behaviour, have also been reported in a variety of different conditions, as well as ICD/DSM defined autism (Ozonoff 1977). Because of their lack of understanding of social rules, the behaviour of individuals with autism spectrum disorders is frequently inappropriate or unacceptable, and can give rise to many difficulties for families. The deficit also means that very few are able to develop close reciprocal relationships, especially with their peers.

RITUALISTIC AND STEREOTYPED INTERESTS OR BEHAVIOURS

Problems in this area can span a very wide range. The nature and severity are likely to vary both with cognitive levels, and, to some extent, with the underlying disorder. Stereotyped motor behaviours, such as rocking, hand flapping, spinning, flicking, or lining up objects are characteristic of children who are more severely cognitively impaired. In addition, there is a greater risk of this group developing self-injurious behaviours, such as head banging, eye poking, skin picking and biting (Hall 1997). Certain stereotyped motor movements are also associated with particular disorders, such as the hand wringing of girls with Rett syndrome and the hand flapping and hand biting of children with fragile X syndrome (Hagerman and Hagerman 2002, Kerr 2002).

Some children insist on acquiring extensive collections of particular objects (*e.g.* leaves of a particular shape, miniature car models, Star Trek videos, stick insects, sunglasses, etc.). Although the type of object collected is not *necessarily* unusual, it is the number of items collected, or the child's overwhelming interest in these that gives rise to problems.

Many young children with autism spectrum disorders also develop intense attachments to certain objects, again often of an unusual nature. If these are lost, broken or otherwise unobtainable, severe distress may result. Insistence on routines and marked resistance to change can also lead to severe disruption to normal family life. Other children become distraught by even minor changes to their environment (such as an ornament being moved, or door left open at a different angle). Occasionally, too, compulsive behaviours involving handwashing or constant checking can emerge in later childhood, as may obsessional and intrusive thoughts.

More able children may try to involve other people in their routines. Verbal routines and questioning, in particular, can be very difficult to deal with. These children are also more likely to develop intense preoccupations with certain topics, and although such interests may be age appropriate, as for example in football or computer games, it is their intensity that gives rise to difficulties.

Intervention strategies
TREATMENT CLAIMS

Over the past 50 years various treatments have been claimed to bring about 'recovery' from autism and related disorders, or at least significantly to improve outcome (for a review, see Howlin 1998). Among the most recent of these are the reduction of mercury levels in the child's body, the use of a 36-ingredient vitamin/mineral/antioxidant supplement (Rimland 2000), and secretin infusions (Horvath 1998, Rimland 1998). Sensational accounts of the effects of other therapies, from swimming with dolphins to swinging around in nets also appear frequently in the press, leading to much confusion and doubt amongst parents (Muller 1993). However, few such claims have been subject to any form of experimental investigation. Of those that have, Facilitated Communication is now generally discredited (APA 1994, Bebko *et al.* 1996); Auditory Integration Therapy has been found to have no positive effects (Dawson and Watling 2000, Mudford *et al.* 2000); fenfluramine, previously widely used in the USA, has been virtually withdrawn because of adverse side-effects; while initial control trials of secretin (Sandler *et al.* 1999, Chez *et al.* 2000) indicate no advantages over placebo.*

While certain therapies that have been found to have positive effects—notably the early developmental programmes reviewed by Rogers (1998) or the intensive home-based behavioural programmes of McEachin *et al.* (1993) and Smith *et al.* (2000)—the number of cases involved in these evaluative studies remains very small, and blind, randomized control trials are virtually nonexistent (see Lord 2000). In a recent review of therapies specifically for autism Prizant and Rubin (1999) conclude that, given the current state of research in the field, no one approach has been demonstrated to be superior to all others or to be equally effective for all children.

Over recent years it has become increasingly evident that the number of individuals with autism-related disorders is far greater than the number who meet diagnostic criteria

---

*For a more detailed review of pharmacological treatments for autism and pervasive developmental disorder, see the special issue of *Journal of Autism and Developmental Disorders*, Vol. 30, October 2000.

for typical autism (Gillberg and Gillberg 1989, Wing 1993). There is an equally clear need for therapeutic approaches that are effective in ameliorating the associated, fundamental deficits (communication and social impairments and ritualistic/stereotypic behaviours), in preventing the development of secondary problems, and in reducing the burden on families. Autism itself is a highly complex condition, and autism-related disorders associated with other behavioural phenotypes may be even more complicated. Given the heterogeneity of autism-related disorders it would be particularly foolish to accept the 'one size fits all' view of therapy. Interventions need to be matched to the nature of the disorder, and to its determinants, as well as being adapted to suit differing family needs. Complex disorders demand a flexible approach to treatment and the use of a *combination* of different strategies. As far as possible these should be hypothesis-led, and subject to careful monitoring, so that ineffective or harmful interventions are avoided, or abandoned without delay. Unfortunately there are no well-controlled treatment trials on which to base decisions about which approach may work best with which child or with which set of problems. However, it is possible to extrapolate, both from well designed single case reports and small group studies, certain principles that are likely to be effective for a wide range of problems, with children of differing levels of ability, and across very different behavioural profiles (Dawson and Osterling 1997, Prizant and Rubin 1999).

THERAPEUTIC GUIDELINES

Individualized approaches to treatment

There is evidence from a number of review studies of the effectiveness of individually designed intervention programmes. These should take account of the child's cognitive level, the severity of autistic symptomatology, and overall developmental level (Anderson and Romanczyk 1999, Prizant and Rubin 1999). Social and communication problems, although characteristic of all autism spectrum disorders, vary widely from child to child as do the extent and pervasiveness of ritualistic and obsessional behaviours. Cognitive abilities, too, can range from profound impairment to superior intelligence, and problems may also change with age. An intervention programme that is appropriate for a nonverbal 3-year-old with severe learning disabilities will need to be very different from one that is suitable for a verbally fluent 13-year-old with Asperger syndrome and an IQ of 130.

It is also important to recognize that problem behaviours may arise for many different reasons. For example, the child may lack the ability to communicate her/his needs, or distress and confusion, in any other way; problem behaviours may be maintained because of the response they receive from others, or arise because they are the child's most effective way of controlling her/his environment. Before any attempt to intervene takes place, it is essential to try to determine: why the behaviour occurs; what it achieves for the child; how others respond to it, and what might be done to replace it? In other words, the focus of intervention should be on the underlying cause, not on the surface behaviour.

Addressing core 'autism' deficits

Although certain autism-related disorders may require syndrome-specific interventions [for example, the physical therapy needed by women with Rett syndrome (Kerr 2002), or the specific teaching strategies that appear to benefit children with fragile X syndrome (Saunders 2000)], effective treatments must also address the core 'autistic' deficits of communication and social impairments, and ritualistic and stereotypic behaviours.

- Communication difficulties, which can be found at all levels of intellectual ability, will never be totally eliminated, but much can be done by ensuring that the communication used by parents and other carers is appropriate for the individual's *comprehension* level and that verbal messages are augmented as far as possible by visual or other means (Howlin 1998). It is also important to recognize that much anxiety, confusion or distress may occur because of the child's failure to understand what is happening, or why. Many apparently inappropriate behaviours may be the child's only effective means of communication. It is crucial, therefore, to try to establish the purpose of problem behaviour (to avoid/escape situations; gain objects/food/attention) and to teach the child equally effective ways to communicate her/his needs, *e.g.* by pictures, objects, symbols or simple gestures/actions (Koegel 2000).

- Lack of understanding of social rules, and deficits in empathy and 'theory of mind' mean that individuals with autism-related disorders will be frequently unaware of how to initiate interactions or how to respond to others in an acceptable way. Again, while the core social deficits may remain throughout life, many unacceptable behaviours can be minimized if attention is paid to ensuring that even the very young child is taught simple invariable rules (*e.g.* never to take off clothes in public, except in the swimming pool or at the doctor's; not to approach strangers; not to touch things in shops; not to talk about certain topics). More able children can be helped by teaching basic social behaviour such as how to approach others, how to respond to greetings/simple requests and how to join in (structured) activities with peers, as well as by ensuring that the basic rules of hygiene and self-care are established from an early age.

- Obsessional and ritualistic tendencies may often be the underlying cause of many behaviour problems, and frequently become progressively more unacceptable with age (Howlin and Rutter 1987, Schopler 1995, Howlin 1998). From early childhood, it is important to set clear limits on when, where, with whom, and how often these behaviours are allowed, so that disruption to other activities is minimized. If obsessional or ritualistic behaviours begin to interfere with other activities (or other people), the most successful solution is to try gradually to reduce the amount of time the child spends in a particular ritualistic activity or to limit the number of places/people where it is allowed. Resistance to change is often best dealt with by helping the child to predict change and by gradually introducing planned change into daily routine. Similarly the problems caused by attachments to specific objects can be reduced by gradually reducing the amount of time spent with the object, the number of places where the object is allowed, or the actual size of the object. However, it is important when dealing with ritualistic behaviours that the aim of intervention should be to modify not eliminate them. This is because routines, special interests, etc. can be used as very effective rewards, are an important source of comfort for the child, and can help reduce anxiety and distress. Moreover, in certain cases they may form the basis for social contacts as the child gets older.

The combination of behavioural, developmental and educational approaches
Behaviourally based strategies have been shown to be effective in very many studies (see Howlin 1998) but these seem to be more generally effective if combined with appropriate educational approaches, so that gains acquired in one setting can generalize across multiple situations and hence be more readily maintained (Koegel and Koegel 1995, Schopler 1995, Howlin 1998, Schreibman 2000). The application of findings from research with typically developing young children, particularly in the areas of social engagement and communication (Wetherby *et al.* 1997) has also been shown to be important.

Numerous single case reports, and a few small group studies, also indicate the benefits of structured educational or daily living programmes, that place particular emphasis on visually based instruction and cues. These provide the individual with autism with a predictable and readily understandable environment, which helps to minimize confusion and distress and hence to accelerate the acquisition of new skills (Jordan and Powell 1995, Quill 1995, Schopler and Mesibov 1995, Bondy and Frost 1996, Prizant and Wetherby 1998).

Specialist interventions focusing on the development of social–communication and play activities, especially with peers, have been found to be effective in a number of studies (Wolfberg and Schuler 1993, Quill 1995, Lord 1996, Rogers 2000). The implementation of highly specialized training programmes, for example to improve 'mind-reading' skills (Ozonoff and Miller 1995, Swettenham 1995, Howlin *et al.* 1998) or social understanding (Mesibov 1984, Williams 1989, Gray 1995) may also prove of value.

Teaching functional equivalence
It is well established that many so-called undesirable or challenging behaviours are frequently a reflection of limited behavioural repertoires or poor communication skills. A focus on skill enhancement, and the establishment of more effective communication strategies is, therefore, often the most successful means of reducing difficult or disruptive behaviours (Durand and Carr 1991, Prizant *et al.* 1997). A principal goal of therapy should be to develop functionally equivalent, but socially acceptable responses, rather than simply the elimination of so-called 'maladaptive' or 'challenging' behaviours.

Environmental factors
Much can often be achieved by focusing intervention efforts on changing the environment rather than the child. Many problems can be minimized if care is taken simply to avoid situations that trigger problems. For example, at school, playtimes or games lessons, which frequently require considerable social, communication and motor expertise, can be replaced by time in the library or computer room, or just tidying the classroom. It is also crucial to try to improve knowledge and awareness amongst those working with individuals with autism spectrum disorders. The *consistent* application of intervention strategies is particularly important. Many problems can be reduced or even eliminated by ensuring that the child's environment and daily routine are as predictable and as controllable as possible. This does not mean that the same regime must be followed every day, but to avoid disruption or distress the child must be forewarned of changes in advance (by visual means if appropriate).

The implementation of treatment approaches that are family centred, rather than exclusively child oriented, will also help to ensure generalization and maintenance of skills (Marcus *et al.* 1997, Schreibman 2000). The development of management strategies, which can be implemented consistently but in ways that do not demand extensive sacrifice in terms of time, money or other aspects of family life, seems most likely to offer benefits for all involved.

The need for early identification
Whatever the benefits of different treatments it is clear that diagnostic provision needs to improve considerably if individuals with autism or related difficulties are to receive the help they need. The average age at which children with typical autism are diagnosed is still far too high, at around 5 years. Diagnosis of those who are more able, or in whom the diagnosis is less certain, may not be obtained until much later (Howlin and Moore 1997, Howlin and Asgharian 1999). Late diagnosis can result in inadequate support for parents and teachers, an escalation of behavioural problems, increasing exclusion and isolation, and perhaps severe emotional and psychiatric problems in later life. Wider implementation of appropriate screening techniques, such as the CHAT (Baron Cohen *et al.* 1996), which can be used by health visitors and GPs with minimal training, *could* benefit very many young children with developmental problems. However, such tools are only worthwhile if backed by sufficient funding to ensure that possible cases receive a prompt and detailed diagnostic assessment, and that this, in turn, is backed up by practical advice and assistance for families.

REFERENCES

Anderson SR, Romanczyk RG (1999) 'Continuum-based behavioral models.' *Journal of the Association for Persons with Severe Handicaps*, **24**, 162–173.
APA (1994) *Diagnostic and Statistical Manual of Mental Disorders, 4th Edn. (DSM-IV)*. Washington, DC: American Psychiatric Association.
Bailey A, Bolton P, Butler L, Le Couteur A, Murphy M, Scott S, Webb T, Rutter M (1993) 'Prevalence of the fragile X anomaly amongst autistic twins and singletons.' *Journal of Child Psychology and Psychiatry*, **34**, 673–688.
Bailey A, Phillips W, Rutter M (1996) 'Autism: towards an integration of clinical, genetic and neurobiological perspectives.' *Journal of Child Psychiatry and Psychology*, **37**, 89–126.
Baron-Cohen S (1995) *Mindblindness: An Essay on Autism and Theory of Mind*. Cambridge, MA: MIT Press.
Baron-Cohen S, Cox A, Baird G, Swettenham J, Nightingale N, Morgan K, Drew A, Charman T (1996) 'Psychological markers in the detection of autism in a large population.' *British Journal of Psychiatry*, **168**, 158–163.
Baron-Cohen S, Mortimore C, Moriarty J, Izaguirre J, Robertson M (1999) 'The prevalence of Gilles de la Tourette's syndrome in children and adolescents with autism.' *Journal of Child Psychology and Psychiatry*, **40**, 213–218.
Bebko JM, Perry A, Bryson S (1996) 'Multiple method validation study of facilitated communication: II. Individual differences and subgroup results.' *Journal of Autism and Developmental Disorders*, **26**, 19–42.
Berthier ML, Bayes A, Tolosa ES (1993) 'Magnetic resonance imaging in patients with concurrent Tourette's disorder and Asperger's syndrome'. *Journal of American Academy of Child and Adolescent Psychiatry*, **32**, 633–639.
Bishop DVM (2000) 'What's so special about Asperger syndrome? The need for further exploration of the borderlands of autism.' *In:* Klin A, Volkmar FR, Sparrow SS (eds) *Asperger Syndrome*. New York: Guildford Press, pp 254–278.
Bolton PF, Griffiths PD (1997) 'Association of tuberous sclerosis of temporal lobes with autism and atypical autism.' *Lancet*, **349**, 392–395.

Bondy A, Frost L (1996) 'Educational approaches in pre-school: Behavior techniques in a public school setting.' *In:* Schopler E, Mesibov GB (eds) *Learning and Cognition in Autism.* New York: Plenum Press, pp 311–334.

Buitelaar JK, van der Wees M, Swaab-Barneveld H, van der Gaag RJ (1999) 'Verbal memory and Performance IQ predict theory of mind and emotion recognition ability in children with autistic spectrum disorders and in psychiatric control children.' *Journal of Child Psychology and Psychiatry,* **40,** 869–881.

California Department of Developmental Services (1999) *Changes in the Population of Persons with Autism and Pervasive Developmental Disorders in California's Developmental Services System: 1987–1998. A Report to the Legislator.* Sacramento: California Department of Developmental Services.

Chez MG, Buchanan CP, Bagan BT, Hammer MS, McCarthy KS, Ovrutskaya I, Nowinski CV, Cohen ZS (2000) 'Secretin and autism: a two-part clinical investigation.' *Journal of Autism and Developmental Disorders,* **30,** 87–94.

Dawson G, Osterling J (1997) 'Early intervention in autism.' *In:* Guralnick M (ed) *The Effectiveness of Early Intervention.* Baltimore: Brookes, pp 307–326.

Dawson G, Watling R (2000) 'Interventions to facilitate auditory, visual and motor integration in autism: a review of the evidence.' *Journal of Autism and Developmental Disorders,* **30,** 415–422.

Durand BM, Carr EG (1991) 'Functional communication training to reduce challenging behaviour: Maintenance and application in new settings.' *Journal of Applied Behavior Analysis,* **24,** 251–254.

Ehlers S, Nyden AM, Gillberg C, Sandberg AD, Dahlgren SO, Hjelmquist E, Oden A (1997) 'Asperger syndrome, autism and attention disorders.' *Journal of Child Psychology and Psychiatry,* **308,** 207–217.

Fombonne E (1999) 'The epidemiology of autism: a review.' *Psychological Medicine,* **29,** 769–786.

Fombonne E, du Mazaubrun C, Cans C, Grandjean H (1997) 'Autism and associated medical disorders in a large French epidemiological sample.' *Journal of the American Academy of Child and Adolescent Psychiatry,* **36,** 1561–1569.

Ghazziuddin M, Tsai LY, Ghaziuddin N (1992) 'Autism in Down's syndrome: presentation and diagnosis.' *Journal of Intellectual Disability Research,* **36,** 449–456.

Gillberg C (1992) 'The Emanuel Miller Memorial Lecture 1991. Autism and autistic-like conditions: Subclasses among disorders of empathy.' *Journal of Child Psychology and Psychiatry,* **33,** 813–842.

Gillberg C, Coleman M (1992) *The Biology of the Autistic Syndromes, 2nd Edn. Clinics in Developmental Medicine No. 126.* London: Mac Keith Press.

Gillberg C, Coleman M (2000) *The Biology of the Autistic Syndromes, 3rd Edn. Clinics in Developmental Medicine No. 153/154.* London: Mac Keith Press.

Gillberg C, Steffenburg S, Wahlström J, Gillberg IC, Sjostedt A, Matrtinsson Y, Liedgren S, Eeg Olofsson O (1991) 'Autism associated with marker chromosome.' *Journal of the American Academy of Child and Adolescent Psychiatry,* **30,** 489–494.

Gillberg IC, Gillberg C (1989) 'Asperger syndrome-some epidemiological considerations: a research note.' *Journal of Child Psychology and Psychiatry,* **30,** 631–638.

Gray CA (1995) 'Teaching children with autism to "read" social situations.' *In:* Quill A (ed) *Teaching Children with Autism: Strategies to Enhance Communication and Socialization.* New York: Delmar, pp 219–242.

Hagerman R.J (1990) 'The association between autism and fragile X syndrome.' *Brain Dysfunction,* **3,** 219–227.

Hagerman RJ, Hagerman PJ. (2002) 'Fragile X syndrome.' *In: Outcomes in Neurodevelopmental and Genetic Disorders.* Cambridge: Cambridge University Press (in press).

Hall S (1997) 'The early development of self-injurious behaviour in children with developmental disabilities.' PhD thesis, University of London.

Harrison JE, Bolton PF (1997) 'Tuberous sclerosis.' *Journal of Child Psychology and Psychiatry,* **38,** 603–614.

Horvath K (1998) 'Improved social and language skills after secretin administration in patients with autistic spectrum disorders.' *Journal of the Association of the Academy of Minority Physicians,* **9,** 1–15.

Hotopf M, Bolton P (1995) 'A case of autism associated with partial tetrasomy 15.' *Journal of Autism and Developmental Disorders,* **25,** 41–49.

Howlin P (1998) *Treating Children with Autism and Asperger Syndrome: A Guide for Parents and Professionals.* Chichester: Wiley.

Howlin P, Asgharian A (1999) 'The diagnosis of autism and Asperger syndrome: findings from a survey of 770 families.' *Developmental Medicine and Child Neurology,* **41,** 834–839.

Howlin P, Moore A (1997) 'Diagnosis in autism: a survey of over 1200 parents in the UK.' *Autism: International Journal of Research and Practice,* **1,** 135–162.

Howlin P, Rutter M (1987) *Treatment of Autistic Children.* Chichester: Wiley.

Howlin P, Wing L, Gould J (1995) 'The recognition of autism in children with Down syndrome—implications for intervention and speculations about pathology.' *Developmental Medicine and Child Neurology*, **37**, 406–414.

Howlin P, Baron-Cohen S, Hadwin J, Swettenham J (1998) *Teaching Children with Autism to Mindread. A Practical Manual for Parents and Teachers.* Chichester: Wiley.

Howlin P, Mawhood LM, Rutter M (2000) 'Autism and developmental receptive language disorder. A follow-up comparison in early adult life. II. Social, behavioural and psychiatric outcomes.' *Journal Of Child Psychology and Psychiatry*, **41**, 561–578.

Jordan R, Powell S (1995) *Understanding and Teaching Children with Autism.* Chichester. Wiley.

Kent L, Evans J, Paul M, Sharp M (1999) 'Comorbidity of autistic spectrum disorders in children with Down syndrome.' *Developmental Medicine and Child Neurology*, **41**, 153–158.

Kerbeshian J, Burd L (1986) 'Asperger's syndrome and Tourette syndrome: the case of the pinball wizard.' *British Journal of Psychiatry*, **148**, 731–736.

Kerr A (2002) 'Rett's syndrome.' *In: Outcomes in Neurodevelopmental and Genetic Disorders.* Cambridge: Cambridge University Press (in press).

Klin A, Volkmar FR (1997) 'Asperger's syndrome.' *In:* Cohen D, Volkmar F (eds) *Handbook of Autism and Pervasive Developmental Disorders, 2nd Edn.* New York: Wiley, pp 94–122.

Klin A, Sparrow SS, Marans WD, Carter A, Volkmar FR (2000) 'Assessment issues in children and adolescents with Asperger syndrome.' *In:* Klin A, Volkmar FR, Sparrow SS (eds) *Asperger Syndrome.* New York: Guildford Press, pp 309–339.

Koegel LK (2000) 'Interventions to facilitate communication in autism.' *Journal of Autism and Developmental Disorders*, **30**, 383–392.

Koegel RL, Koegel LK (1995) *Teaching Children with Autism: Strategies for Initiating Positive Interactions and Improving Learning Opportunities.* Baltimore: Brookes.

Lauritsen M, Mors O, Mortensen PB, Ewald H (1999) 'Infantile autism and associated autosomal chromosome abnormalities: a register-based study and a literature survey.' *Journal of Child Psychology and Psychiatry*, **40**, 335–346.

Littlejohns CS, Clarke DJ, Corbett JA (1990) 'Tourette-like disorder in Asperger's syndrome.' *British Journal of Psychiatry*, **156**, 430–443.

Lord C (1996) 'Facilitating social inclusion: Examples from peer intervention programs.' *In:* Schopler E, Mesibov G (eds) *Learning and Cognition in Autism.* New York: Plenum Press, pp 221–242.

Lord C (2000) 'Achievements and future directions for intervention research in communication and autism spectrum disorders.' *Journal of Autism and Developmental Disorders*, **30**, 393–398.

Lord C, Rutter M (1994) 'Autism and pervasive developmental disorders.' *In:* Rutter M, Taylor E, Hersov B (eds) *Child and Adolescent Psychiatry: Modern Approaches, 3rd Edn.* Oxford: Blackwell, pp 569–591.

Lotter V (1966) 'Epidemiology of autistic conditions in young children. I: Prevalence.' *Social Psychiatry*, **1**, 163–173.

Marcus LM, Kunce LJ, Schopler E (1997) 'Working with families.' *In:* Cohen D, Volkmar F (eds) *Handbook of Autism and Pervasive Developmental Disorders, 2nd Edn.* New York: Wiley, pp 631–649.

Marriage K, Miles T, Stokes D, Davey M (1993) 'Clinical and research implications of the co-currence of Asperger's and Tourette syndrome.' *Australian and New Zealander Journal of Psychiatry*, **30**, 666–672.

Mawhood LM, Howlin P, Rutter M (2000) 'Autism and developmental receptive language disorder – a follow-up comparison in early adult life. I: Cognitive and language outcomes.' *Journal of Child Psychology and Psychiatry*, **41**, 547–559.

McEachin JJ, Smith T, Lovaas OI (1993) 'Long-term outcome for children with autism who received early intensive behavioral treatment.' *American Journal on Mental Retardation*, **97**, 359–372.

Mesibov GB (1984) 'Social skills training with verbal autistic adolescents and adults: a treatment model.' *Journal of Autism and Developmental Disorders*, **14**, 395–404.

Mudford OC, Cross BA, Breen S, Cullen C, Reeves D, Gould J, Douglas J (2000) 'Auditory integration training for children with autism: no behavioral benefits detected.' *American Journal on Mental Retardation*, **105**, 118–129.

Muller J (1993) 'Swimming against the tide.' *Communication*, **27**, 6.

National Autistic Society (1997) *Statistics Sheet 1. How Many People Have Autistic Spectrum Disorders?* London: National Autistic Society.

O'Brien G, Yule W (1995) *Behavioural Phenotypes. Clinics in Developmental Medicine No. 138.* London: Mac Keith Press.

41

Ozonoff S (1977) 'Components of executive function in autism and other disorders.' *In:* Russell J (ed) *Autism as an Executive Disorder.* New York: Oxford University Press, pp 179–211.

Ozonoff S, Miller JN (1995) 'Teaching theory of mind: A new approach to social skills training for individuals with autism.' *Journal of Autism and Developmental Disorders*, **25**, 415–433.

Park RJ, Bolton PF (2001) 'Pervasive developmental disorder and obstetric complications in children and adults with tuberous sclerosis.' *Autism*, **5**, 237–248.

Prizant BM, Rubin E (1999) 'Contemporary issues in interventions for autism spectrum disorders: a commentary.' *Journal of the Association for Persons with Severe Handicaps*, **24**, 199–208.

Prizant B, Wetherby A (1998) 'Understanding the continuum of discrete-trial traditional behavioral to social–pragmatic developmental approaches in communication enhancement for young children with autism/PDD.' *Seminars in Speech and Language*, **19**, 329–337.

Prizant B, Schuler A, Wetherby A, Rydell P (1997) 'Enhancing language and communication development: Language approaches.' *In:* Cohen D, Volkmar F (eds) *Handbook of Autism and Pervasive Developmental Disorders, 2nd Edn.* New York: Wiley, pp 572–605.

Quill KA (1995) *Teaching Children with Autism: Strategies to Enhance Communication and Socialization.* New York: Delmar.

Rimland B (1998) 'First secretin efficacy study produces positive results!' *Autism Research Review International*, 15 (2), insert page 1 (editorial).

Rimland B (2000) 'Promising therapies revealed at DAN conference.' *Autism Research Review*, **1**, 6.

Rogers .J (2000) 'Interventions that facilitate socialization in children with autism.' *Journal of Autism and Developmental Disorders*, **30**, 399–410.

Rourke BP, Tsatsanis KD (2000) 'Non-verbal learning disabilities and Asperger syndrome.' *In:* Klin A, Volkmar FR, Sparrow SS (eds) *Asperger Syndrome.* New York: Guildford Press, pp 254–278.

Rutter M (1999) 'Autism: two-way interplay between research and clinical work.' *Journal of Child Psychology and Psychiatry*, **40**, 169–188.

Rutter M, Bailey A, Bolton P, Le Couteur A (1994) 'Autism and known medical conditions: Myths and substance.' *Journal of Child Psychology and Psychiatry*, **35**, 311–322.

Sandler, A.D., Sutton, K., De Weese, J., Girardi, M.A. Sheppard, V., Bodfish, J.W. (1999) 'A double blind placebo controlled trial of synthetic human secretin in the treatment of autism and pervasive developmental disorder.' *Journal of Developmental and Behavioral Paediatrics*, **20**, 400.

Saunders S (2000) *Fragile X Syndrome. A Guide for Teachers.* London: David Fulton.

Schopler E (ed) (1995) *Parent Survival Manual: A Guide to Crisis Resolution in Autism and Related Developmental Disorders.* New York: Plenum.

Schopler E, Mesibov GB (eds) (1995) *Learning and Cognition in Autism.* New York: Plenum Press.

Schreibman L (2000) 'Intensive behavioral/psychoeducational treatments for autism: research needs and future directions.' *Journal of Autism and Developmental Disorders*, **30**, 373–378.

Smalley S (1998) 'Autism and tuberous sclerosis.' *Journal of Developmental Disorders*, **28**, 407–414.

Smith T, Groen AD, Wynn JW (2000) 'Randomized trial of early intensive intervention for children with pervasive developmental disorder.' *American Journal on Mental Retardation*, **105**, 269–285.

Swettenham J (1995) 'Can children with autism be taught to understand false beliefs using computers?' *Journal of Child Psychology and Psychiatry*, **37**, 157–166.

Szatmari P (2000) 'Perspectives on the classification of Asperger syndrome.' *In:* Klin A, Volkmar FR, Sparrow SS (eds) *Asperger Syndrome.* New York: Guildford Press, pp 403–417.

Turk J, Graham P (1997) 'Fragile X syndrome, autism and autistic features.' *Autism: The International Journal of Research and Practice*, **1**, 175–198..

Wetherby A, Prizant B (1999) 'Profiles of communicative and cognitive–social abilities in autistic children.' *Journal of Speech and Hearing Research*, **27**, 364–377.

Wetherby A, Schuler A, Prizant B (1997) 'Enhancing language and communication development: Theoretical foundations.' *In:* Cohen D, Volkmar F (eds) *Handbook of Autism and Pervasive Developmental Disorders. 2nd Edn.* New York: Wiley, pp 513–538.

Williams T.I (1989) 'A social skills group for autistic children.' *Journal of Autism and Developmental Disorders*, **19**, 143–156.

Wing L (1993) 'The definition and prevalence of autism: A review.' *European Child and Adolescent Psychiatry*, **2**, 61–74.

Wing L, Gould J (1979) 'Severe impairments of social interaction and associated abnormalities in children: epidemiology and classification.' *Journal of Autism and Developmental Disorders*, **9**, 11–29.

Wolfberg PJ, Schuler AL (1993) 'Integrated play groups: A model for promoting the social and cognitive dimensions of play.' *Journal of Autism and Developmental Disorders*, **23**, 1–23.

WHO (1992) *International Classification of Diseases, 10th Edn (ICD-10). Diagnostic Criteria for Research.* Geneva: World Health Organization.

D. SLEEP AND ITS DISORDERS

Gregory Stores

Why bother about sleep?

It is paradoxical that, although much of life is spent asleep (especially in childhood), so little informed attention is paid to it.

The majority of people, without any serious sleep problem, take sleep for granted without regard to its importance for ensuring effective daytime functioning. There have been various theories proposed for why sleep is necessary (including energy conservation, memory consolidation, discharge of emotions, brain growth, and maintenance of immune systems) no one of which is entirely adequate in itself, but what is incontrovertible is that sleep is essential for physical and psychological restoration because without it daytime activities and well-being are seriously affected in many ways.

Despite these possible consequences, many opportunities to improve matters are missed because the importance of satisfactory sleep and the prospects of achieving it are not appreciated. Even when sleep is persistently disturbed, as happens in perhaps a fifth or more of the general public (Partinen and Hublin 2000), and despite the distress and disability that such disturbance can cause, sufferers often do not seek help.

Two examples illustrate this point. First, obstructive sleep apnoea (which often carries risks of severe impairment of daytime functioning and also cardiovascular complications) is said to occur in the general population in perhaps 4% of adult men, 2% of adult women and at least 1% of children, but only a very small minority of cases come to medical attention. As explained later, the condition is much more prevalent than this in various neurodevelopmental disorders but the signs are that this serious complication is frequently not considered and treated. A second example also concerns children with neurodevelopmental disorders, whose parents often seem not to seek help even when their child's sleep is extremely disturbed (Wiggs and Stores 1996). The various reasons for this include a mistaken belief (shared by many professionals) that sleep disturbance is an inevitable and largely untreatable part of the child's basic condition. In fact, correctly chosen and properly implemented, treatment (mainly of a behavioural type) can be quite quickly effective even in severe and long-standing cases (Wiggs and Stores 1998).

Many further instances could be cited to illustrate the unfortunate fact that the subject of sleep and its disorders is widely neglected. There is considerable room for improvement on the part of the general public and healthcare professionals in understanding the fundamental ways in which satisfactory sleep is important and that disturbed sleep must not (and need not) be tolerated. The educational changes by which these improvements can be achieved will be discussed later.

Before the types of sleep disturbance reported in various neurodevelopmental disorders are reviewed, the basic issues of ways in which sleep can be disturbed and the consequences

TABLE 2.1
Average sleep duration at different ages

Term birth	16–18 hours
1 year	15 hours
2 years	13–14 hours
4 years	12 hours
10 years	8–10 hours
Mid-adolescence	8.5 hours
Later adolescence	7–8 hours

of such disturbance will be considered, followed by an outline of normal sleep and its disorders.

More detailed information (including references in addition to those provided in this chapter) on these and other issues raised in this chapter is available in the clinical account of sleep disorders in children and adolescents in general by Stores (2001) and the detailed review of sleep disturbance in various forms of developmental disorder by Stores and Wiggs (2001).

Sleep disturbance and its consequences
TYPES OF SLEEP DISTURBANCE

The restorative properties of sleep depend not only on the length of time for which a person sleeps but also on the quality of sleep obtained. The timing of the period of sleep is also important.

The *length of time* children of different ages usually sleep is shown in Table 2.1. Sometimes parents have a mistaken idea of how long their child should sleep, and it can be therapeutic to simply acquaint them with these normal values. Although there are individual differences in sleep requirements (*i.e.* in order to function at maximum efficiency), if a child persistently sleeps at least one hour less than the average for the child's age, s/he may be sleep deprived and capable of benefiting from a longer period of sleep.

The most important aspect of *sleep quality* seems to be the extent to which overnight sleep is consolidated, *i.e.* free from frequent interruptions. So called 'fragmented' sleep is caused by repeated awakenings and/or by very brief subclinical 'microarousals' in which (as shown by physiological recording) the depth of sleep is interrupted without actual awakening. Sleep fragmentation is a feature of sleep-related breathing problems.

Inappropriate timing of the overnight sleep period is best exemplified by night-shift work. Because activities are undertaken at night when the brain is biologically set to be asleep, impaired performance at this time is often accompanied by discomfort and distress. Daytime sleep is often inadequate in both duration and quality. A comparable situation to occupational night-shift work can exist for parents who frequently attend to their child at night.

Combinations of short duration sleep, poor quality sleep and inappropriate timing of sleep are particularly damaging to child and parent alike. All three possible impairments of sleep should be considered when assessing their sleep patterns.

CONSEQUENCES OF SLEEP DISTURBANCE

The effects of persistent severe sleep disturbance can be very wide-ranging, involving various aspects of a child's psychological state, sometimes physical development, and also functioning of the family as a whole.

Mood and behaviour

Review of adult studies of the effects of sleep deprivation suggest that mood is affected more than other aspects of psychological function, although significant changes are reported in many domains. The main general effects are irritability, aggression and depressed mood. In children a number of observations suggest that various behaviour and cognitive problems occur, including symptoms of attention deficit hyperactivity disorder (ADHD). Perhaps especially in younger children, it is important to explore the possibility (suggested by some reports) that ADHD-type symptoms are the result of a primary sleep disorder, if only in a minority of cases. Children may become emotionally upset because of distress about their sleep problem, confrontation with their parents, or from fear or embarrassment depending on the nature of the sleep disorder.

Cognitive function and educational performance

Again from adult studies, it appears that sleep deprivation can adversely affect attention (especially sustained attention), memory and other aspects of cognitive function. Comparable effects have been reported in children, and there are consistent accounts of sleep loss in children and adolescents being associated with daytime sleepiness and impaired performance at school. Also, in keeping with adult studies, sleep-related breathing difficulties (caused by sleep apnoea or asthma) and consequent impairment of sleep quality have been linked with impaired cognitive and academic performance as well as behavioural problems.

Family functioning

A child's sleep disturbance can affect other members of the family. Siblings may develop sleep problems and their consequences but the main effect is likely to be on parents who can become chronically sleep deprived. Mothers of children with a learning disability and severe sleep problems have been described as more irritable, concerned about their own health and less affectionate towards their children (with greater use of physical punishment) than mothers of such children without sleep problems (Quine 1992). Marital discord and separation (and even physical abuse of children) has sometimes been attributed to children's sleep problems. There is evidence that successful treatment of a child's sleep disorder can improve parental functioning and well-being.

Physical development

Impaired growth and failure to thrive are associated with obstructive sleep apnoea starting early in life. Growth hormone deficiency, linked to abnormal sleep physiology, has been implicated in the origin of 'psychosocial dwarfism'. There is increasing interest in the possible physical and psychological effects of immune system dysfunction associated with sleep disturbance.

Much more research is needed to fill the gaps in current knowledge about the adverse effects of persistent sleep disturbance. However, even the above outline account provides compelling reason to believe that the possible developmental consequences for children of persistently unsatisfactory sleep are very important. That being so, it is regrettable that so little attention is paid in professional training to sleep including its developmental importance. A survey undertaken in recent times indicated that in UK medical schools, out of a typical 5-year course a median of only 5 minutes was being devoted to formal teaching about sleep and its disorders (Stores and Crawford 1998). There is no particular reason to believe that this situation is rectified in postgraduate medical training including that required for general paediatrics or paediatric neurology, or in the training of nurses, psychologists and others involved in the provision of child healthcare services.

Efforts have been made in some countries to correct these omissions but much more consistent attempts are required. Various relevant books have been written in recent years. The present chapter is intended to be a further contribution specifically in relation to neurodevelopmental disorders.

Normal sleep in childhood and adolescence
THE PHYSIOLOGY AND STRUCTURE OF SLEEP

There are two physiologically distinct forms of sleep: non-rapid eye movement (NREM) sleep and rapid eye movement (REM) sleep. Conventionally, NREM sleep is divided according to standard criteria into four levels or stages. The first two are light sleep; levels 3 and 4 are called deep sleep because awakening from these levels is most difficult. Stages 3 and 4 NREM are also called slow wave sleep (SWS) or delta sleep because their main EEG characteristic is prominent slow (delta) activity in the EEG. SWS is largely confined to the first third of the night. REM sleep is also called 'dreaming sleep' because most dreaming occurs during it; it occurs increasingly as overnight sleep progresses. Brain metabolism is at a high level in REM sleep, other main features of which are the characteristic eye movements and the absence of skeletal muscle tone.

As can be seen from Figure 2.1, NREM and REM sleep alternate with each other (NREM/REM cycles) several times during overnight sleep. Table 2.1 demonstrates that duration of sleep is greatest in infancy (averaging 16–18 hours at term birth) and gradually reduces by adolescence to the usual adult level of 7–8 hours.

The reason for these two forms of sleep is unclear. The prominence of REM sleep in early life suggest it is important in early brain development. SWS has been considered the most restorative form of sleep but this is not particularly supported by experimental studies and it is thought that the combination of NREM and REM sleep in the first few NREM/REM cycles of overnight sleep is particularly important for satisfactory daytime functioning. Continuity of sleep is important because, as mentioned earlier, fragmentation of sleep by repeated awakenings or subclinical arousals significantly impairs the restorative quality of sleep.

The timing of sleep is regulated by the circadian clock in the suprachiasmatic nuclei, which is influenced by melatonin mainly produced in the pineal gland during darkness. This clock also controls other biological rhythms including body temperature and cortisol

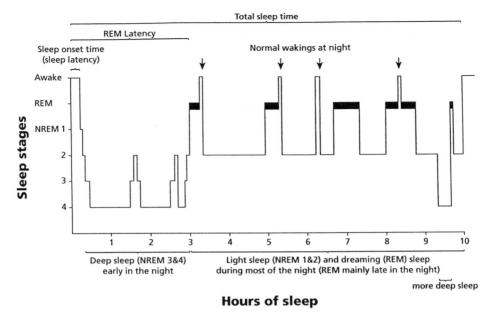

Fig. 2.1. Hypnogram showing characteristic progression of sleep stages overnight in healthy school-age child. (Reproduced by permission from Stores and Wiggs 2001.)

production with which the sleep–wake rhythm is normally synchronized. From an early age, the sleep–wake rhythm has to be entrained to the day–night cycle. The main cue (or *'zeitgeber'*) for this process is light perception, but social cues (*e.g.* mealtimes and social activities) are also important.

Within each 24 hour period the level of alertness and tendency to sleep varies, sleep tendency being greatest in the early hours of the morning and (to a less extent) in the early afternoon (the 'post-lunch dip'). Alertness level is generally highest in the evening before the onset of sleepiness (the 'forbidden zone'). However, individual differences are seen (even in children). Some people are very alert early in the day ('larks') and others in the evening perhaps until late ('owls').

Most children sleep soundly at night and are very alert during the day. This contrasts with postpubertal adolescents who are sleepy during the day partly because of lifestyle (including staying up late) but also because of biological changes in sleep at that age.

Sleep problems and disorders
There are three basic sleep problems or complaints: not sleeping enough (sleeplessness), sleeping too much (excessive daytime sleepiness) and episodes of disturbed behaviour during or related to sleep (parasomnias). Although often not attempted, it is essential to try to identify the exact sleep *disorder* (of which over 80 are recognized) underlying these sleep problems. Treatments based on symptoms alone are likely to be ineffective, if not harmful.

TABLE 2.2
Main structure of the International Classification of Sleep Disorders—Revised*

Dyssomnias
Difficulty getting off to sleep/staying asleep, or excessive daytime sleepiness caused by:
  • intrinsic conditions such as sleep apnoea or narcolepsy
  • extrinsic factors such as sleep environment or parenting practices
  • circadian sleep–wake cycle disorders (mistiming of the sleep period)

Parasomnias
Episodic behaviour intruding into sleep. Grouped according to stage of sleep with which they are usually associated:
  • arousal disorders (deep NREM sleep)
  • sleep–wake transition parasomnias
  • REM-related parasomnias
  • other parasomnias

Sleep disorders associated with physical or psychiatric disorders
e.g. depression
      dementia
      nocturnal epilepsy
      asthma

Proposed sleep disorders
Sleep-related conditions needing further research before being accepted as definitive sleep disorders

*American Sleep Disorders Association (1997).

This basic point is illustrated by the common problem of sleeplessness in young children, for which hypnotic medication is commonly prescribed. Failure to go to sleep at a satisfactory time may be the result of parents' failure to establish good sleep habits from an early age, including overpermissiveness or inconsistency. Alternatively, children may be put to bed too early (in the forbidden zone) so that they are physiologically unable to sleep, or their sleep phase may have become delayed (see later) so that, again, their brain does not allow them to fall asleep until later. Otherwise, bedtime fears may prevent him going to sleep. It is clear that these and other reasons require different forms of treatment (and rarely hypnotic medication).

CLASSIFICATION OF SLEEP DISORDERS
There is merit in using the International Classification of Sleep Disorders (American Sleep Disorders Association 1997), although it needs to be modified to some extent for use with children and its account of sleep disturbance in the learning disabled is understated. Table 2.2 provides an outline of its main structure.

Sleeplessness
In one form or another this is the most common form of sleep problem, affecting 20–30% of children in the general population and many more children with a developmental disorder. It is essential to establish the details of the problem and to distinguish between bedtime difficulties, troublesome waking during the night and early morning waking, as the causes

TABLE 2.3
**Examples of factors to consider in sleepless children of
different ages***

Infancy
'Colic'
Cow's milk intolerance
Frequent night-time feeds

Early childhood (1–3 years)
Inappropriate napping
Poor bedtime routine
Stressful or otherwise undesirable sleep onset associations
Poor limit-setting by parents
Too early bedtime
Middle ear disease

Middle childhood (4–12 years)
Difficulty getting to sleep
• Persistence of earlier problems
• Night-time fears
• Overarousal
• Worry and anxiety
Night waking
• Parasomnias
Early morning waking
• Environmental disturbance

Adolescence
Erratic sleep–wake schedule
Delayed sleep phase syndrome
Sleep-disrupting substances (recreational, illicit)
Worry and anxiety
Psychiatric disorder

---

*Modified by permission from Stores (2001).

tend to be different, although these forms of sleeplessness can occur in combination with each other.

General factors that contribute to sleeplessness include aspects of parenting (such as inconsistent or otherwise unsatisfactory parenting factors), inappropriate sleeping environment, and medical disorders affecting sleep. However, more specific influences can be identified in many cases, their nature varying somewhat with the age of the child (Table 2.3). In general, behavioural forms of treatment are the most appropriate and can be rapidly effective in contrast to medication which is usually ineffective and possibly harmful.

Excessive sleepiness
This is by no means a rare sleep problem but is frequently overlooked or misconstrued as laziness, boredom or some other psychological state not amenable to treatment. Again there are many possible explanations to consider in the individual case. Table 2.4 gives some examples. As mentioned earlier, disrupted sleep from upper airway obstruction, including obstructive sleep apnoea, is important in children in general (affecting possibly 1% or

TABLE 2.4

Differential diagnosis of excessive sleepiness in older children and adolescents*

Insufficient sleep (including circadian sleep–wake cycle disorders)
Causes of sleeplessness
Disturbed circadian sleep–wake patterns

Disturbed sleep
Upper airway obstruction
Recreational drugs (caffeine, alcohol, nicotine)
Illicit drugs, including withdrawal
Medical and psychiatric disorders
Medication effects
Other sleep disorders (frequent parasomnias, periodic limb movements)

Increased need for sleep
Narcolepsy
Idiopathic CNS hypersomnia
Neurological disease or other physical illness
Kleine–Levin syndrome (intermittent sleepiness)

*Adapted by permission from Stores (2001).

more) but should be very carefully considered in children with neurodevelopmental disorders, in some forms of which it is particularly common. The main features and factors to consider are listed in Tables 2.5 and 2.6. Disorders of the circadian sleep–wake cycle are also common in such children and a cause of both sleeping difficulties and abnormal sleepiness during the day.

Episodic disturbances of sleep (parasomnias)
Parasomnias (of which there are many different types) are also of special significance in children with neurodevelopmental disorders because of the special risk within this group of misdiagnosis and inappropriate treatment. In particular, there is a risk that nocturnal epileptic attacks will be confused with other forms of parasomnia especially those of a dramatic nature (Stores 1991). In addition to primary parasomnias (*i.e.* primary disorders of sleep), there are many parasomnias that are secondary in the sense of being nocturnal manifestations of medical or psychiatric disorders. Examples of both groups of parasomnias are given in Table 2.7).

ASSESSMENT OF SLEEP DISORDERS
The essential requirement for identifying and characterizing sleep disorders is an adequate clinical enquiry about sleep, which is not usually included in conventional history-taking protocols. Routinely, the following basic questions should be asked about any child:
• Does s/he have difficulty getting off to sleep or staying asleep?
• Is s/he very sleepy during the day?
• Does s/he have any disturbed episodes at night?

A positive answer to any of these questions calls for a detailed sleep history, including a review of the child's 24 sleep–wake pattern, and overall developmental review. Physical

TABLE 2.5

Night-time and daytime features of upper airway obstruction*

During sleep
Chronic loud snoring
Other sounds of breathing difficulty (gasping, snorting)
Other evidence of increased respiratory effort (retractions of chest wall muscles, paradoxical inward movement of the chest during inspiration with outward movement of the abdomen)
Rapid breathing
Apnoeic episodes
Nasal flaring
Mouth breathing
Cyanosis
Unusual sleeping positions including kneeling or neck extension
Very restless sleep
Profuse sweating
Enuresis
Awakenings and associated parasomnias (sleep terrors, nightmares)

On waking
Difficulty waking up, disorientation, grogginess
Bad mood
Headache
Dry mouth

Daytime
Sleepiness
Concentration and memory problems, poor school progress
Irritability and other emotional or behavioural problems

*Reproduced by permission from Stores (2001).

TABLE 2.6

Main factors to consider on physical examination of a child with upper airway obstruction*

Nasal obstruction
Congenital stenosis
Deviated septum
Nasal polyps
Foreign body
Rhinitis (seasonal or perennial)

Nasal and oropharynx
Enlarged tonsils and adenoids
Large tongue
Abnormal hard palate including cleft palate repair
Abnormal soft palate including abnormal uvula

Craniofacial structures
Micrognathia
Midface hypoplasia

General
Obesity
Adenoidal facies
Growth
Muscle tone
Evidence of neurodevelopmental syndrome (*e.g.* Down syndrome)
Chest, cardiac or neurological abnormalities

*Reproduced by permission from Stores (2001).

and mental state examination is also essential. Sleep diaries kept over a period of two weeks or so can give important insights into a child's typical sleep pattern and associated circumstances. Objective sleep studies are required in only a minority of cases and can often be performed in the home environment. Audiovisual recordings may be very instructive about night-time events; actigraphy (body movement monitoring) can provide useful information about basic sleep–wake patterns. Polysomnography is indicated when the details of sleep physiology and architecture are required. Other special investigations may be appropriate depending on diagnostic possibilities.

TREATMENT
Sometimes explanation and reassurance (if appropriate) are therapeutic in themselves. General principles for promoting satisfactory sleep ('sleep hygiene') are important. These

TABLE 2.7
Examples of primary and secondary parasomnias*

PRIMARY PARASOMNIAS	SECONDARY PARASOMNIAS
Sleep onset	**Nocturnal epilepsies**
Sleep starts	**Other physical disorders**
Hypnagogic hallucinations	Headaches
Sleep paralysis	Respiratory disorders
Rhythmic movement disorder (*e.g.* head banging)	Gastrointestinal conditions
Nocturnal muscle cramps	Cardiac arrhythmias
Light NREM sleep	Some cases of restless legs syndrome or periodic limb movements in sleep
Bruxism	
Periodic limb movements in sleep	**Psychiatric disorders**
Deep NREM sleep	Post-traumatic stress disorder episodes
Arousal disorders (confusional arousals, sleepwalking, sleep terrors)	Nocturnal panic attacks
Other (including psychogenic dissociative states and 'pseudoparasomnias')	Dissociative states
	Other 'pseudoparasomnias'
REM sleep	
Nightmares	
REM sleep behaviour disorder	
Waking	
Hypnopompic hallucinations	
Sleep paralysis	
Inconsistently related to stage of sleep	
Sleep talking	
Nocturnal enuresis	
Other primary parasomnias	
Overlap parasomnia disorder	

*Adapted by permission from Stores (2001).

include ensuring a satisfactory sleeping environment, encouraging consistent sleep–wake patterns, avoiding the child's overdependence on the parents' presence in order to sleep, and avoiding activities and sleeping circumstances unconducive to sleep.

Table 2.8 sets out some of the specific measures known to be effective in different types of sleep disorder, assuming they have been diagnosed accurately. A detailed account of the various behavioural treatments (often relevant in children with neurodevelopmental disorders) is beyond the scope of this chapter. Further information is available in Stores (2001), and in specialized reviews of such treatments—*e.g.* Owens *et al.* (1999), which is concerned with children in general, and Lancioni *et al.* (1999) and Wiggs and France (2000) which concentrate on patients with disability of one type or another. The behavioural treatment chosen for sleeplessness, for example, must be one with which parents feel comfortable and within their ability to implement consistently. In general, letting the child cry itself to sleep is not acceptable and, indeed, inadvisable especially if s/he has a medical condition that might worsen at night. Instead, methods which gradually reduce parental contact with the child, or which avoid reinforcing unwanted behaviour, are much more appropriate. Rewarding satisfactory behaviour might also be effective.

TABLE 2.8
Examples of treatment approaches for sleep disorders

Psychological
Bedtime routine
Appropriate associations with bedtime
Promotion of self-soothing (ability to fall asleep without
    parents being present)
Setting limits to resistant behaviour
Reinforcement of good behaviour

Chronobiological (circadian sleep–wake cycle disorders)
Sleep phase retiming
Light therapy

Medication
Hypnotics (selectively and short-term)
Stimulants (excessive sleepiness)
Melatonin (some circadian cycle disorders)

Physical measures
Continuous positive airway pressure (OSA)

Surgery
Adenotonsillectomy (OSA)

*Adapted by permission from Stores (2001).

General comorbid factors affecting sleep in children with neurodevelopmental disorders

Before describing the types of sleep disturbance reported in particular neurodevelopmental disorders, it is appropriate to mention certain conditions commonly associated with such disorders, and which themselves often predispose to sleep problems.

LEARNING DISABILITY

A number of surveys have consistently shown that sleep problems are very common in children with a learning disability (mental retardation) (Stores 1992), irrespective of the precise aetiology of the learning disability. However, some learning disability syndromes commonly involve particular types of sleep disturbance.

Extreme degrees of brain malformation causing severe degrees of learning disability also produce grossly disturbed sleep physiology and sleep–wake patterns. Lesser degrees of learning disability are mainly associated with serious and often persistent sleeplessness problems of the various types just described, *i.e.* settling and night-waking difficulties and/or early morning wakening. The reasons for this may include some degree of brain dysfunction but, perhaps more often, there may be difficulties in teaching an intellectually impaired child good sleep habits (because of communication problems, for example). Other factors include lack of discipline (perhaps out of parental compassion for the child) or the child's behavioural disturbance which itself is often accompanied by sleep problems. It is worth emphasizing that even severe and long-standing sleep disorders in children with a learning disability can usually be treated effectively.

Polysomnographic studies of learning disabled children in general suggest that, also regardless of the cause of the basic condition, abnormalities of REM sleep and of sleep spindles (a feature of stage 2 NREM sleep) are prominent and may be interpreted as a possible indication of intellectual impairment at a given age.

EPILEPSY

Epilepsy of various types and degrees of severity is often associated with sleep disturbance. The problems include difficulty getting off to sleep, disturbed overnight sleep and daytime sleepiness. Impaired quality of overnight sleep seems to be particularly prominent, even in relatively mild cases of childhood epilepsy (Stores *et al.* 1998).

Sometimes the sleep disturbance is the result of underlying brain dysfunction or the occurrence of seizures during sleep, but other factors can again include psychological problems or parenting practices. Modern antiepilepsy medication does not generally seem to be important as a cause. Indeed, improved seizure control appears to lessen sleep disturbance.

OTHER PHYSICAL FACTORS

Visual impairment accompanying a neurodevelopmental disorder might well affect sleep because high rates of sleepiness are described in severely visually impaired children. Because light perception is the main cue to day or night, it is the main factor in entraining sleep–wake rhythms. Therefore severely visually impaired children may have irregular or non-24-hour sleep–wake cycles. However, parenting factors or associated psychiatric disturbance might also play a part. Accordingly, treatment may need to be either chrono-biological, behavioural or both.

Hearing impairment has also been linked to sleep disturbance, including that apparently caused by the disturbing effect of tinnitus at night.

Physical deformity or immobility causing discomfort at night may contribute to sleep difficulties in some children.

It has been mentioned already that sleep-related breathing problems, especially *upper airway obstruction*, occurs widely in children with neurodevelopmental disorders.

COMORBID PSYCHIATRIC DISORDERS

Developmental disorders of neurological origin are often complicated by psychological disturbance such as anxiety and depression, difficult behaviour and overactivity. As sleep disturbance is a common feature of psychiatric disorder, the nature and extent of abnormal sleep in children with neurodevelopmental disorders may well be partly determined by this further complication to their lives.

Sleep disorders in specific neurodevelopmental disorders

In this section, the sleep problems and disorders described in various neurodevelopmental syndromes are outlined. Further details can be found in Stores and Wiggs (2001), including extensive referencing. The scope of the review and the relative length of the outline for each condition are limited by the available information, which is patchy. Some syndromes are not mentioned simply because no findings seem to have been reported. Emphasis has been placed on clinically apparent sleep abnormalities rather than polysomnographic findings of uncertain clinical significance. It is assumed that the earlier sections will have been read before this part of the chapter.

DOWN SYNDROME

Surveys have consistently shown that parents report sleep problems in a significantly higher proportion of children with Down syndrome compared with children in the general population. The emphasis in these reports is on sleeplessness, mainly in the form of difficulty going to sleep and troublesome night-waking, but many parents have also reported symptoms suggestive of upper airway obstruction (UAO) during sleep such as noisy breathing or apnoeic episodes. These UAO-type symptoms differentiate children with Down syndrome from those with a variety of other forms of learning disability when their sleep abnormality profiles are compared. Other studies have suggested that the sleep of at least some children with Down syndrome is fragmented (and therefore less likely to be restorative, as discussed earlier) in a way that is only partly attributable to sleep-related breathing problems. Additional potentially disruptive influences on sleep include psychological disturbance and, in a proportion of cases, cardiovascular problems, epilepsy or hypothyroidism.

The UAO to which children with Down syndrome seem particularly prone (because of a combination of anatomical abnormalities of the upper airway or related structures and also hypotonia of the pharyngeal musculature) has been the subject of a number of physiological studies. These have reported obstructive sleep apnoea (OSA) or hypoventilation during sleep as a contributory factor in between 50% and 80% of children. Central sleep apnoea has also been reported in a proportion, possibly caused by brainstem dysfunction. In some cases atlantoaxial subluxation could be responsible. Pulmonary hypoplasia has also been described. These various ways in which respiration can be affected are obviously of particular significance in children with congenital heart disease.

In Down syndrome and other neurodevelopmental disorders, the early detection and (whenever possible) correction of the sleep disturbance, whether behavioural or physical in origin, at an early stage is extremely important because of its harmful psychological or physical effects on the child and the family. The means by which this is achieved depends essentially on the exact nature of the sleep disorder. As outlined earlier, one or other behavioural method is capable of being effective for sleeplessness of behavioural origin. Sleep-related breathing problems in Down syndrome can be difficult to treat but good results have been reported with adenotonsillectomy or other physical methods in some cases.

FRAGILE X SYNDROME

Sleep problems are also consistently reported in this disorder, but the underlying cause is not clear for lack of sufficiently detailed assessment. By the same token the contribution of comorbid conditions such as ADHD, autistic behaviour or epilepsy is unclear. Behavioural sleep problems again feature prominently but OSA has also been described in some cases, sometimes responding to nasal continuous positive airway pressure.

PRADER–WILLI SYNDROME

Excessive daytime sleepiness (EDS) has been reported in a number of studies as a common and often disabling symptom in patients with this syndrome. Although OSA has been demonstrated as the cause in certain cases, in probably the majority of such patients the cause of their EDS is uncertain and much debated. Suggestions have included intrinsic hypothalamic dysfunction and also obesity as at least a compounding factor. A narcolepsy-like condition has been postulated by some authors but the evidence for this is not conclusive. This aetiological uncertainty makes choice of treatment difficult other than appropriate measures for OSA where it is convincingly diagnosed, or weight reduction as a general measure. The value of stimulant drugs or other medication has not been established.

CRANIOFACIAL SYNDROMES

UAO has been described in many syndromes characterized by craniofacial deformity, of which there are many (Betancourt and Beckerman 1992). Cor pulmonale and sudden death caused by UAO are acknowledged risks in infants with Pierre–Robin syndrome, although such complications are often preventable, and some of the anatomical abnormalities affecting respiratory function may improve with age. Because of the complexity of the anatomical abnormalities, treatment may be difficult, especially in the presence of additional lower airway problems as in some children with Apert or Pfeiffer syndromes. Behavioural sleep disorders can be expected in many children with craniofacial deformities but they do not seem to have been reported in any systematic way.

MUCOPOLYSACCHARIDOSIS

Yet again, UAO features prominently in the reported sleep abnormalities in this group of disorders but there appear to be differences in both the type and severity of sleep problems from one form of mucopolysaccharidosis to another. High prevalence rates (40% or more) have been reported in all four main syndromes (i.e. Hurler, Hunter, Morquio and Sanfilippo), with particularly high rates in the last of these (up to 86%).

As in other children with disturbed sleep, settling and night-waking problems and short duration sleep are often reported. UAO is common and sometimes accounts for severe morbidity or even death according to some reports. In general, the predisposition to UAO is caused by a number of anatomical abnormalities compromising the upper airway, made worse by widespread glycosaminoglycan deposits in the upper and sometimes lower airway, together with varying degrees of skeletal deformity (including scoliosis and thoracic hyper-kyphosis) affecting respiratory function. Other factors include chronic pulmonary disease.

Obstructive problems seem to be less common in Sanfilippo syndrome, where the commonly disorganized sleep patterns may result from abnormalities of metabolism within the central nervous system. The high rate of epilepsy may itself contribute to the problem.

Colville et al. (1996) describe a number of desperate measures used by parents in an attempt to cope with the sleep problems of children with Sanfilippo syndrome. Hypnotics had been used for many children in their series but often ineffectively. Various surgical measures to relieve upper airway obstruction have been described, but, because of the complicated elements involved, such treatment can be very difficult. Behavioural methods are indicated for non-physical sleep problems but do not seem to have been used with any regularity.

TUBEROUS SCLEROSIS

Parents of children with the tuberous sclerosis complex (TSC) report high rates of sleep disturbance, mainly taking the form of the ubiquitous problem of settling and night-waking problems. Polysomnographic findings have been in keeping with these reports but have also suggested disrupted sleep architecture, especially in those children with seizures.

The origins of these sleep disturbances can be complex because of the various comorbid conditions in TSC. Behavioural factors are likely to be relevant in many cases because of the impact of the condition on the family, but other possibly contributing factors are co-existing epilepsy (which is common in TSC), autistic-like behaviour and other psychiatric disturbance associated with the condition, and learning disability which in various degrees is also a usual accompaniment.

Clearly, careful analysis of the nature of the sleep disturbance and its likely causes is essential for appropriate choice of treatment.

RETT SYNDROME

It has been reported that over 80% of children with this condition develop sleep problems, which are often of a multiple nature. The problems described consist of difficulty getting off to sleep, recurrent awakenings, early morning waking and excessive daytime sleepiness. A peculiar feature is the occurrence of laughing, crying or screaming during the night. The sleep disturbance (perhaps especially daytime sleepiness) may worsen as the condition progresses.

The cause of these various sleep problems is not clear. Some believe that CNS dysfunction is responsible, affecting basic circadian sleep–wake rhythms or causing a more generalized disturbance as demonstrated by the widespread EEG abnormalities seen (in both the waking state and during sleep) as the disorder worsens. Abnormal breathing patterns (which are common in Rett syndrome) do not seem to be closely related to the sleep disturbance. Behavioural sleep problems are highly likely in view of the effects of the condition on both the child and parents.

There have been reports of some success with behavioural methods and with melatonin, but treatment of the sleep disturbance in Rett syndrome has not been studied systematically.

SMITH–MAGENIS SYNDROME

The various types of sleeplessness described in Rett syndrome have also been reported in Smith–Magenis syndrome with the exception of the night-time laughing, crying or screaming. However, an apparently distinctive feature of children with this condition is that from an early age they tend to sleep in short bursts of about 2 hours with prolonged awakenings terminating in very early waking with very active and possibly destructive or hazardous behaviour. The reported daytime sleepiness is presumably the result of disrupted sleep. There has been some suggestion that patients with the Smith–Magenis syndrome have an abnormality of the biological clock (of possibly genetic origin) associated with abnormal melatonin production. This is thought to produce an advanced sleep phase with early onset of overnight sleep in some children and early morning wakening.

Choice of treatment will obviously depend on the type of sleep disorder in the individual child.

ANGELMAN SYNDROME

Repeatedly, surveys have described sleep disturbance as a prominent feature of this syndrome but its exact nature remains to be clarified. At present, it seems that nonspecific types of sleeplessness predominate. It is uncertain whether reports of destructive behaviour during the night indicate a peculiarly characteristic feature of the condition.

Various form of treatment have been described (behavioural, and medication in the form of sedative antihistamines or low dose melatonin) but none has been comprehensively evaluated in children with this disorder.

WILLIAMS SYNDROME

The nature and aetiology of the sleep problem often associated with this syndrome have been difficult to judge from the reports, but the indications are again that the problems are of a similar type to those in other neurodevelopmental disorders and that behavioural factors are often responsible. However, there is some evidence that at least part of the sleep disturbance may be biological in origin. Features suggesting disordered breathing during sleep have been reported by parents of some children. More often, abnormal movements during sleep, especially periodic limb movements in sleep (PLMS), have been described and verified by polysomnography. Such movements, if frequent, are thought to disrupt sleep and affect daytime behaviour. Treatment of the PLMS by means of clonazepam is said to have been effective.

OTHER NEURODEVELOPMENTAL DISORDERS

Piecemeal information is available from published reports on a number of other neurodevelopmental disorders.

The characteristic self-mutilation by children with *Lesch–Nyham syndrome* is said to occur in all stages of sleep, and the various nonspecific abnormalities demonstrated during sleep have included abnormal limb movements. The uncertain relationship between disturbed sleep and self-mutilation is illustrated by the claim that 5-hydroxytryptophan can improve sleep without affecting the abnormal behaviour.

Sleep studies in children with *phenylketonuria* seem to have been confined to polysomnographic investigations which have demonstrated abnormalities (for example, sleep spindles) seen in various other conditions characterized by learning disability.

Sleep-related breathing disorders have been reported to a limited extent in some cases of *neurofibromatosis* (in which sleep problems are said to be very common), *Joubert syndrome* and *Rubenstein–Taybi syndrome*.

Conclusions

Clearly, there are very many gaps that need to be filled in what is known about sleep disturbance in the neurodevelopmental disorders, but certain basic clinically important points can already be made with confidence.

- Sleep disturbance is very common indeed in such disorders but relatively little attention has been paid to it in either clinical practice or research.
- This is a serious neglect because such disturbance is highly likely to be a significant additional complication to affected children and their families, not only at the time of the sleep disturbance itself but also because of its harmful long-term psychological (and sometimes physical) effects.
- Enough is known about sleep and its disorders to permit accurate diagnosis and often effective treatment in the individual case. However, this will only happen if those involved in the care of affected children become better acquainted with modern practice in the field of sleep disorders. Achieving this requires considerable improvement in professional training.

The need for a greater awareness of the sleep disturbances associated with neurodevelopmental disorders, and a more detailed evaluation of such disturbances, is also relevant to the question of whether certain behavioural phenotypes include characteristic and specific types of sleep disturbance attributable to basic biological influences. At present, there is very limited evidence of this but that might well be the result of inadequate documentation. As described earlier, tantalizing possibilities are raised that some aspects of sleep disturbance in Smith–Magenis syndrome, Sanfilippo syndrome and Rett syndrome (including the curious emotional manifestations at night) might be ascribable to neurophysiological dysfunction. It is interesting that somewhat similar unaccountable emotional displays also seem to occur in some children with autistic spectrum disorders (Wiggs and Stores 2000).

These are just some of the many interesting possibilities of clinical and theoretical importance that need to be explored in children with neurodevelopmental disorders.

REFERENCES

American Sleep Disorders Association (1997) *International Classification of Sleep Disorders, Revised: Diagnostic and Coding Manual.* Rochester, MN: American Sleep Disorders Association.
Betancourt D, Beckerman RC (1992) 'Craniofacial syndromes.' *In:* Beckerman RC, Brouillette RT, Flunt CE (eds) *Respiratory Control Disorders in Infants and Children.* Baltimore: Williams & Wilkins, pp 294–305.
Colville GA, Watters JP, Yule W, Bax MCO (1996) 'Sleep problems in children with Sanfilippo syndrome.' *Developmental Medicine and Child Neurology*, **38**, 538–544.
Lancioni GE, O'Reilly MF, Basili G (1999) 'Review of strategies for treating sleep problems in persons with severe or profound mental retardation or multiple handicaps.' *American Journal on Mental Retardation*, **104**, 170–186.
Owens JL, France KG, Wiggs L (1999) 'Behavioural and cognitive–behavioural interventions for sleep disorders in infants and children: a review.' *Sleep Medicine Reviews*, **3**, 281–302.
Partinen M, Hublin C (2000) 'Epidemiology of sleep disorders.' *In:* Kryger MH, Roth T, Dement WC (eds) *Principles and Practice of Sleep Medicine, 3rd Edn.* Philadelphia: WB Saunders, pp 558–579.
Quine L (1992) 'Severity of sleep problems in children with severe learning difficulties: description and correlates.' *Journal of Community and Applied Social Psychology*, **2**, 247–268.
Stores G (1991) 'Confusions concerning sleep disorders and the epilepsies in children and adolescents.' *British Journal of Psychiatry*, **158**, 1–7.
Stores, G (1992) 'Sleep studies in children with a mental handicap.' *Journal of Child Psychology and Psychiatry*, **33**, 1303–1317.
Stores, G (2001) *A Clinical Guide to Sleep Disorders in Children and Adolescents.* Cambridge: Cambridge University Press.

Stores G, Crawford C (1998) 'Medical student education in sleep and its disorders.' *Journal of the Royal College of Physicians of London*, **32**, 149–153.

Stores G, Wiggs L (2001) *Sleep Disturbance in Children with Disorders of Development: its Significance and Management. Clinics in Developmental Medicine No. 155.* London: Mac Keith Press.

Stores G, Wiggs L, Campling G (1998) 'Sleep disorders and their relation to psychological disturbance in children with epilepsy.' *Child: Care, Health and Development*, **24**, 5–19.

Wiggs L, France K (2000) 'Behavioural treatments for sleep problems in children and adolescents with physical illness, psychological problems or intellectual disabilities.' *Sleep Medicine Reviews*, **4**, 299–314.

Wiggs L, Stores G (1996) 'Sleep problems in children with severe intellectual disabilities: what help is being provided?' *Journal of Applied Research in Intellectual Disabilities*, **9**, 160–165.

Wiggs L, Stores G (1998) 'Behavioural treatment for sleep problems in children with severe learning disabilities and daytime challenging behaviour: effect on sleep patterns of mother and child.' *Journal of Sleep Research*, **7**, 119–126.

Wiggs L, Stores G (2000) 'Sleep disorders in children and adolescents with autistic spectrum disorders.' *Journal of Sleep Research*, **9**, Suppl. 1, S209 (abstract).

3
CLINICAL INVESTIGATION OF BEHAVIOURAL PHENOTYPES

Gregory O'Brien and Martin Bax

In this chapter, we outline some of the principle routine investigations that should be undergone once the diagnosis of a behavioural phenotype is established. Our review is not exhaustive, nor even comprehensive. In any one individual syndrome, an extensive array of investigations is possible, and indeed likely. These are the province of specialist clinics, and no attempt is made here to go into such detail. The intention of the present review is to indicate the areas of assessment and investigation that are important in most conditions encountered in clinical practice of behavioural phenotypes, with reference to the role of the personal physician or clinician with ongoing responsibility for the affected child.

The chapter includes a review of the most frequently used checklists and measurement schedules for the assessment of behaviour. With very few exceptions, these schedules are not diagnostic, in that they cannot be relied upon to yield a comprehensive behavioural assessment or clinical diagnosis. Advice on their strengths, limitations and applicability is therefore included. For a more detailed review of these behavioural measurement schedules, see O'Brien *et al.* (2001).

One of the problems encountered when working in the field of genetic disease or behavioural phenotypes is that many of the conditions are relatively rare, and it is therefore difficult for an individual clinician to acquire experience in all of them. In addition, the specialized nature of academic interest means that often there will be a particular centre where the diagnostic process is well developed, and to which parents will gravitate. Reaching such centres can often prove difficult for parents, and may entail travelling long distances and involve some considerable expense. Although telephone consultation is useful, it is not in fact practical for many of the behavioural issues to be managed readily at a distance. It is very important therefore to be clear to the parents from the outset of the extent of one's personal familiarity with the particular condition, and also to make it clear that if the family are seeing a distant, tertiary 'expert' clinic, then a shared care arrangement is acceptable. Increasingly, many families derive much of their knowledge of their child's condition from a variety of internet sites. It is well-recognized that these sites are of variable quality (O'Brien 2000). Many of the most reputable sites incorporate information on the special resources and assessment services available in specialist centres. It is only to be anticipated, therefore, that families of children who have rare genetic disorders will endeavour to access specialist services for the assessment and investigation of their child's condition. It can similarly be expected that 'shared care' arrangements are likely to become an increasingly prominent feature of clinical practice in behavioural phenotypes.

General clinical assessment

As always, assessment begins with a full history and a physical examination. These are vital both for diagnostic purposes and to establish which medical features of a particular genetic syndrome are present. Problems identified in specific organ systems in the history will naturally inform the full clinical examination of the child—as will the established known features of the individual genetic condition. Appendix 3.4 (pp 94–103) summarizes the common clinical findings on examination and assessment of the conditions whose management is reviewed in Chapter 8, and details these according to whether the features fall under the headings of the musculoskeletal, neurological and neuromuscular, cardiovascular, genito-urinary/sexual, respiratory, gastrointestinal or sensory systems, and also gives descriptions of the typical facies and other important miscellaneous features of each syndrome.

Consultation with Appendix 3.4 may serve as an *aide-mémoire* for systematic examination and assessment in clinical practice with children affected by behavioural phenotypes. In addition, there are certain issues in this area of work that are worthy of special mention, based on accumulated clinical experience with children affected by the genetic syndromes of disability. In considering the health problems of such children, it is important to constantly revisit and reassess any such problems, always bearing in mind the situation of parents and carers. It is widely recognized that parents and carers are often so familiar with their child's persistent physical health problems that they may not mention them in a routine consultation. It is therefore incumbent on the clinician to be proactive in exploration and examination of these children, and to be keenly aware that new health problems come and go, in addition to maintaining a major focus on the emergence and progression of the major features of the condition in question. Also, while the thrust of this present volume is behavioural issues in children with genetic diseases, the actual physical findings may play a significant role in relationship to behaviour and function. For example, untreated and unrecognized glue ear can account for delays in speech and language development that may be ascribed to the phenotype when in fact they have a more direct cause. Clearly, physical health changes will always exert a major influence on behaviour. On the other hand, many of the common findings on physical examination in these children are in fact a reflection of the behavioural phenotypes of the conditions in question. Whether as a direct result of self-injury in Lesch–Nyhan, Cornelia de Lange or fragile X syndrome, or of overeating in Prader–Willi syndrome, findings on physical examination are routinely important markers of behaviours, and may be especially informative on severity of such behaviour.

In general, close attention should be paid to any history of neurological, cardiovascular and respiratory difficulties—these are all common in many of the conditions under consideration, and have major implications for the general health and situation of the developing child. For similar reasons, it is important to maintain a keen awareness of any feeding problems and difficulties the child may have in the development of bowel and bladder control. Of particular interest in the neurological history would be any account of epilepsy. In some phenotypes such as tuberous sclerosis there is an association between the type of epilepsy and outcome. In tuberous sclerosis where infantile spasms have occurred, cognitive outcome is very much worse and there is often an increased incidence of autistic features and hyperactivity, compared to those in whom this seizure type is not present.

It is helpful to give close consideration to the interaction between the child's development and disabilities and parental concerns and management. For example, bowel and bladder functions are often emotive issues for parents. These important facets of development often raise understandable anxieties. In turn, such parental anxieties will affect management of all kinds of everyday challenges, such as feeding problems, in addition to impacting on the management of the bowel or bladder problem. These issues are indicative of the importance of informed parental involvement at all stages of examination and investigation, and a cautionary indication of the time that may routinely be required for the clinical consultation.

It is important to reevaluate the physical condition on a regular basis. Physical growth and development may be changing. For example, in Sanfilippo and Rett syndromes, tightening of the achilles tendon seems to occur at a certain stage of development, and orthopaedic referral may be appropriate. In Rett syndrome tightening of the achilles tendon and equinus may reach such severity as to prevent the girl walking, and surgery may be required to maintain mobility. Careful measurements throughout childhood are important, particularly in those conditions where there is concern about growth. Height, weight and head circumference should be measured. Many child development centres now include dieticians as a key element in the team, and in conditions where there are concerns regarding weight, such as Prader–Willi syndrome, monitoring the nutritional impact is mandatory.

Genetic investigations

Genetic investigation should not be considered in isolation. A full systematic clinical history should be taken even if a genetic diagnosis has been established. This should include the family history, the clinical course of the pregnancy and the delivery and birth of the index child, and an account of the early infant behaviour.

It is recommended that the clinician should clarify and ensure that the genetic diagnosis is the correct one, and is made as precisely as possible. This entails having sight of the diagnostic investigation results directly, and not trusting mention of diagnosis in, for example, a letter of referral. In those conditions in which different diagnostic laboratories are producing different rates of investigation of gene deletions it is important to document from which centre the diagnosis was made. These points are of practical importance. Often, parents of children affected by behavioural phenotypes choose to contact more than one clinic in order to obtain second opinions or a more precise diagnosis. In all such cases, in addition to carrying out the appropriate genetic analysis, it is important to gain sight of the original investigations.

In this field, we are constantly seeing new techniques becoming available, and with completion of the human genome project, this will proceed apace. Consequently, even in cases where diagnosis seems to be clear-cut, the clinician should always be open to instigating repeat investigations.

Physical appearance

It is important to record and document the affected child's physical appearance. This is probably most reliably done by photography, which many clinicians carry out at regular periods, over years of follow-up. In those conditions that are known to have involvement of certain body areas (hands, feet, etc.), photography is clearly indicated, as appropriate. In addition, it is probably more valuable to gain copies of photos of children in natural settings, perhaps interacting with friends and siblings, as well as stand-alone photos in the clinic. Most authorities now agree that, except in very special cases, there is no need for full-length photographs of affected individuals undressed, as was the norm in previous years.

Anterior and profile photos of the face are standard. In many genetic diseases the dysmorphology of the face is a characteristic feature; however, there is often variation in the dysmorphology which can make identification of a particular syndrome difficult (see Appendix 3.4). In some conditions, this may be recorded systematically. The shape and structure of the mouth and jaw should always be noted. Disorders of dentition are common across many syndromes, and merit early identification and careful assessment with potential view to specialist referral. Abnormal genitalia are seen very commonly throughout this area of clinical practice—not only in the sex chromosome aneuploidies, but also in other common conditions such as fragile X and Prader–Willi syndromes. It is important to raise the significance of any such findings and to discuss them with the family.

Assessment of intelligence and ability

Intellectual assessment by standard intelligence tests is an essential part of assessment. As with genetic investigations, particularly where there are any discrepancies over the period of testing, the source and also the social and personal context of the tests need to be recorded carefully. These matters particularly concern the clinical psychologist, who will choose, administer and interpret the appropriate tests. With more severely intellectually disabled children, it is often not possible to derive IQ levels as such—in these cases, the psychologist will select and administer the appropriate tests of ability level.

Motor ability

Assessment of motor function is a recommended element of the initial diagnostic assessment in behavioural phenotypes practice. Indeed, as with the other issues covered in this brief review, it is an element of routine developmental paediatric practice. However, in order to understand many of the behavioural anomalies, and in particular some of the motor features of conditions on the autistic spectrum, close attention to motor function is recommended. Motor assessment is also a requisite in order to fully appreciate complex developmental facets of behaviour, such as present in delayed acquisition of self-care functions, *e.g.* dressing. In some conditions and contexts—for example the assessment of feeding and eating—attention to motor functioning is a major enterprise in itself, involving specialist referral and sophisticated procedures, which are not within the province of routine practice of most clinicians.

Sensory functioning

Initial diagnostic and developmental assessment of any child with a behavioural phenotype should include careful attention to sensory functioning. Hearing and visual impairments are common across a wide variety of conditions. Also, auditory and visual processing problems are prominent. Consequently, it is important to clarify as early as possible the nature of any deficits, so that specialist referral may be arranged.

Language assessment

Assessment of speech and language function is an important element of diagnostic investigation in behavioural phenotypes. The common occurrence of autistic problems in this area of practice, the range of other language anomalies, and indeed the high rates of feeding and other orofacial problems indicates the need for such assessment. It is recommended that a speech and language therapist should be involved early on in the assessment of any child affected by a behavioural phenotype.

Neuropsychological assessment

In addition to basic intelligence testing, other neuropsychological assessments are commonly required in clinical practice of behavioural phenotypes. As with the choice of intelligence testing, the precise measurements to be employed are the province of the specialist psychologist. Issues that figure prominently include attention and concentration, information processing and memory problems. Insights from neuropsychological testing are often crucial to understanding the significance of a range of behavioural problems encountered in this area of clinical practice. Indeed, precise identification of certain neuropsychological deficits is often the key to understanding some of the more puzzling social and interpersonal behaviours one encounters in practice.

Assessment of social skills and self-care

Systematic assessment of social and self-care functioning is recommended as part of baseline investigation in behavioural phenotypes practice, and is of particular value in monitoring treatment effects over the medium to long term. Schedules such as the Vineland Adaptive Behavior Scales (reviewed in this chapter) are among the more widely used in this respect. Such assessment is complimentary to the other assessments already cited (intelligence/ ability level, motor functioning, sensory functioning, language assessment and neuropsychological testing). An independent, systematic test of self-care skills and social functioning offers a different level of assessment, being somewhat more holistic in its synopsis of the individual.

Recording of social behaviour in its natural settings

It is recommended that the clinician should obtain a record of the child's natural social behaviour. Many clinicians obtain video recordings of the child (*e.g.* at play) for this purpose. This is actively encouraged by many of the parent support societies, and is often welcomed by parents and carers because it offers an opportunity to have a direct account of child behaviours that will often not be seen in more formalized settings such as the clinic or school.

Electrophysiological assessment

The most commonly employed electrophysiological assessment in behavioural phenotypes clinical practice is electroencephalography. The type of recordings to be used will vary, according to the type and nature of the epilepsy, particularly in certain conditions in which pronounced or refractory epilepsies present. In addition, in many cases an EEG is one possible investigation to be carried out in the face of behavioural change, possibly where behaviours of an intermittent stereotypical pattern are accompanied by any altered consciousness. Some authorities would maintain that an EEG investigation should now be a routine element of assessment in autistic spectrum disorder, and in a range of patterns of paroxysmal behavioural change.

Radiological investigations on brain imaging
In some conditions, X-ray and brain imaging investigations are a crucial feature of diagnosis. While this is by no means true for all conditions encountered in clinical practice in behavioural phenotypes, increasingly there is an expectation that some investigations of this type, particularly brain imaging, will be carried out. Parents and carers often anticipate that particular procedures, such as functional imaging, should be carried out—perhaps prompted by mention of findings on some website. While it is not recommended that these investigations should be carried out unselectively, it is fair to say that, increasingly, the norm is to arrange brain imaging in all cases where there is conceivably some benefit to be derived for the affected individual. As our technical sophistication develops and neuroimaging techniques emerge, undoubtedly more benefits will be reported. Recently, for example, a careful examination of individuals with Williams syndrome has revealed abnormalities in brain development in both parietal and temporal lobes (Reiss *et al.* 2000). While at the moment these findings are of more academic than clinical significance, families who hear about them will want to discuss their possible significance with their physicians.

Developmental behavioural assessment
It is useful to obtain an account of early infant behaviour. Clinicians should consider the principle behavioural domains in which behaviours commonly present in this field, namely: feeding; sleep; social behaviour; language; motor functioning; unusual interest; self-injury and aggression; anxiety and mood disturbance. All of these domains represent patterns of behaviour that commonly present in behavioural phenotypes clinical practice, and in which there is evidence of a developmental trajectory over the years. In most cases there is some degree of maturation, and some improvement occurs. In consideration of these behaviours, it is recommended that—according to the problems presenting—the clinician select the appropriate measurement schedule from the lists that follow (Tables 3.1–3.3, Appendices 3.1–3.3).

SELECTING BEHAVIOURAL MEASURES
Tables 3.1–3.3 list the most commonly used schedules, on which published information is available, for the measurement of behaviour in behavioural phenotypes. These schedules were derived from a systematic review, the methodology of which is detailed in O'Brien *et al.* (2001), which also incorporates a more detailed description of each measuring instrument.

All of the schedules described have their strengths and their limitations. Clinicians should be aware that the majority of the schedules listed are not diagnostic, in that a psychiatric diagnosis, or even a comprehensive behavioural profile, cannot be yielded by their application. However, all schedules have applicability to some aspect of behavioural measurement, as detailed in the tables and descriptions of each schedule. Many of the schedules rely on special training, or are limited to use by trained clinicians, while others are not so limited. These matters are detailed in the descriptions given of each schedule.

It is therefore suggested that particular care should be taken in the selection of assessment schedules. Where the clinician is interested in the assessment of autism, careful study of Table 3.1 and of the descriptions of the schedules outlined in Appendix 3.1—considered in the context of the patient in question—will suggest which schedule(s) might be appropriate. It will then need to be clarified whether/which specialist training or other input may be required. Similar considerations apply to schedules for other psychiatric measurement (Table 3.2, Appendix 3.2), that is, for psychiatric diagnoses other than autism—notably attention deficit hyperactivity disorder, depression and anxiety problems. Where the focus is on behavioural measurement, either in terms of global assessment of disturbed behaviour or measurement of specific behaviours—*e.g.* sleep problems, self-injury—consultation with Table 3.3 and the schedule summaries in Appendix 3.3 is recommended.

REFERENCES

O'Brien G (2000) 'Is the future of medical publishing on (the) line?' *Developmental Medicine and Child Neurology*, **42**, 651 (editorial).
O'Brien G, Yule W (eds) (1995) *Behavioural Phenotypes. Clinics in Developmental Medicine No. 138.* London: Mac Keith Press.
O'Brien G, Pearson J, Berney T, Barnard L (2001) 'Measuring behaviour in developmental disability: a review of existing schedules.' *Developmental Medicine and Child Neurology*, **43**, Suppl. 87, 1–72.
Reiss AL, Eliez S, Schmitt JE, Straus E, Lai Z, Jones B, Bellugi U (2000) 'Neuroanatomy of Williams syndrome: a high-resolution MRI study.' *Journal of Cognitive Neuroscience*, **12**, Suppl. 1, 65–73.

TABLE 3.1
Schedules for the detection, diagnosis and assessment of autistic spectrum disorder

Asperger Syndrome Screening Questionnaire
Australian Scale for Asperger Syndrome
Autism Behavior Checklist
Autism Diagnostic Interview—Revised
Autism Diagnostic Observation Schedule—Generic
Autism Screening Questionnaire
Behavioral Summarized Evaluation Scale—Revised
Checklist for Autism in Toddlers
Childhood Autism Rating Scale
Diagnostic Interview for Social and Communication Disorders
Handicaps, Behaviour and Skills
Parent Interview for Autism
Pre-Linguistic Autism Diagnostic Observation Schedule
Scale for Pervasive Developmental Disorder in Mentally Retarded Persons

TABLE 3.2

Schedules designed for the purpose of detection, diagnosis and assessment of psychiatric disorders

Adolescent Behaviour Checklist
Carey's Survey of Temperamental Characteristics
Child Behaviour Checklist
Child Psychiatric Interview
Children's Psychiatric Rating Scale
Children's Depression Inventory
Conners Parent Rating Scale
Conners Teacher Rating Scale
Development and Well-Being Assessment
Developmental Behaviour Checklist
Diagnostic Interview for Children and Adolescents
Dimensions of Temperament Survey
Emotional Disorders Rating Scale
Ghuman–Folstein Screen for Social Interaction
Nisonger Child Behaviour Rating Form
Rutter Parent (A) and Teacher (B) Scales
Schedule for Affective Disorders and Schizophrenia for School Age Children
Toddler Temperament Scale
Yale–Brown Obsessive Compulsive Scale

TABLE 3.3

Schedules for the assessment of problem behaviours

Aberrant Behavior Checklist
British Isles Survey Rett Syndrome Screening Questionnaire
Functional Independence Measure for Children
Leyton Obsessive Inventory
Matson Evaluation of Social Skills in Persons with Severe Retardation
Matson Evaluation of Social Skills with Youngsters
Motivational Assessment Scale
Night Time Behavior Questionnaire
Self-Injurious Behavior Questionnaire
Sleep Behavior Questionnaire
Society for the Study of Behavioural Phenotypes Postal Questionnaire
Stereotyped Behavior Scale
Vineland Adaptive Behavior Scales

APPENDIX 3.1
SCHEDULES FOR THE DETECTION, DIAGNOSIS AND ASSESSMENT OF AUTISTIC SPECTRUM DISORDER

Asperger Syndrome Screening Questionnaire (ASSQ)

The ASSQ is designed to screen for Asperger syndrome in children aged between 7 and 16 years. It is completed by teachers who rate behaviour on 27 items, using a three-point rating scale, producing a score within the range of 0–54. The suggested cut-off score for Asperger syndrome is 5 or above. However, using this cut-off score widens the screening to include other social abnormalities. Therefore the authors have suggested that a cut-off score of 13 should be used for parents and one of 22 for teachers.

REFERENCES

Ehlers S, Gillberg C (1993) 'The epidemiology of Asperger syndrome: A total population study.' *Journal of Child Psychology and Psychiatry and Allied Disciplines*, **34**, 1327–1350.
Ehlers S, Gillberg C, Wing L (1999) 'A screening questionnaire for Asperger syndrome and other high functioning autism spectrum disorders in school age children.' *Journal of Autism and Developmental Disorders*, **29**, 129–141.
Gillberg C, Nordin V, Ehlers S (1996) 'Early detection of autism: diagnostic instruments for clinicians.' *European Journal of Child and Adolescent Psychiatry*, **5**, 67–74.
Gillberg IC, Gillberg C (1989) 'Asperger syndrome: Some epidemiological considerations: a research note.' *Journal of Child Psychology and Psychiatry and Allied Disciplines*, **30**, 631–638.

Australian Scale for Asperger Syndrome

This schedule measures behaviour and abilities relative to Asperger syndrome in children. It is a 29-item parent/teacher questionnaire. The schedule covers social and emotional abilities, communication skills, cognitive skills, specific interests, movement skills and other characteristics (*e.g.* response to noise). Behaviours are rated on a seven-point scale of 0 to 6. A rating of 0 indicates that the child is functioning within the normal range. If the child receives consistent ratings between 2 and 6 this is indicative that they should be referred for further assessment. At time of press, there are no psychometric data available.

REFERENCE

Attwood T (1998) *Asperger's Syndrome: A Guide for Parents and Professionals.* London: Jessica Kingsley.

Autism Behavior Checklist

The Autism Behavior Checklist is a screening tool that was originally developed to aid in the process of educational placement of children. It was not intended as a diagnostic instrument. However, it is widely used and is a good screening instrument for the detection of potential cases of autism. The schedule consists of 57 items that are grouped into five domains: Sensory; Relating; Body and Object Use; Language; and Social and Self-help. The items require a dichotomous (Yes/No) forced response. The schedule is in checklist format and is carried out by any professional within the field of learning disability. Cut-off scores are provided with the schedule. A total score above 67 gives a "high probability of being autistic"; a total score within the range of 53–67 is indicative that the child "questionably" or probably does have autism; and a total score less than 53 signifies that the child is unlikely to have autism. The Autism Behaviour Checklist has generated a great deal of research. The psychometric properties of the schedule warrant further investigation.

REFERENCES

Eaves RC, Milner B (1993) 'The criterion-related validity of the Childhood Autism Rating Scale and the Autism Behavior Checklist.' *Journal of Abnormal Child Psychology*, **21**, 481–491.

Krug DA, Arick J, Almond P (1980) 'Behaviour checklist for identifying severely handicapped individuals with high levels of autistic behaviour.' *Journal of Child Psychology and Psychiatry and Allied Disciplines*, **21**, 221–229.

Krug DA, Arick JR, Almond PJ (1988) *The Autism Behavior Checklist*. Portland, OR: ASIEP Education Co.

Oswald DP, Volkmar FR (1991) 'Signal detection analysis of items from the Autism Behavior Checklist.' *Journal of Autism and Developmental Disorders*, **21**, 543–549.

Sturmey P, Matson JL, Sevin JA (1992) 'Analysis of the internal consistency of three autism scales.' *Journal of Autism and Developmental Disorders*, **22**, 321–328.

Volkmar FR, Cicchetti D (1988) 'An evaluation of the Autism Behaviour Checklist.' *Journal of Autism and Developmental Disorders*, **18**, 81–97.

Wadden NP, Bryson SE, Rodger RS (1991) 'A closer look at the Autism Behavior Checklist: Discriminant validity and factor structure.' *Journal of Autism and Developmental Disorders*, **21**, 529–541.

Yirmiya N, Sigman M, Freeman BJ (1994) 'Comparison between diagnostic instruments for identifying high-functioning children with autism.' *Journal of Autism and Developmental Disorders*, **24**, 281–291.

Autism Diagnostic Interview—Revised (ADI-R)

The ADI-R is a modified version of the ADI. It has been subject to revision, partly due to the increasing ability to diagnose autism at an early age and the importance in differentiating autism when it is accompanied by profound learning disability. The ADI-R is specifically tailored to these issues as it has been modified for use with children with a mental age of approximately 18 months upwards. Some of the schedule items are directly related to specific age periods and allow comparisons to be made in order to judge severity and abnormality of behaviours. A number of items have been modified. In the section on communication, items focus on autism-specific impairments. Other items, such as sensitivity to noise level, have been given a broader definition to include sensitivity to specific noises. Repetitive behaviour has been differentiated from compulsions and rituals.

The ADI-R focuses on developmental deviance and developmental delay. The schedule predominantly measures behaviour across three areas—communication and language; reciprocal social interaction; and restrictive, repetitive and stereotyped behaviour—but also includes opening questions and questions relating to general behavioural problems. It is a semistructured interview with primary caregivers. Behaviour is typically rated by the clinician on a four-point scale: (0) "no definite behaviour of the type is specified"; (1) "behaviour of the type specified probably present but defining criteria not fully met"; (2) "definite abnormal behaviour of the type described in the definition and coding"; and (3) "extreme severity". The ADI-R uses a scoring algorithm based on DSM-IV and ICD-10 criteria. In the communication section, a cut-off score of 8 is needed for verbal subjects and a score of 7 is required for nonverbal subjects. Within the social domain, a minimum score of 10 is the proposed cut-off score for all subjects. A cut-off score of 3 is required for restricted and repetitive behaviours. To reach a diagnosis of autism that is conducive to DSM-IV and ICD-10 guidelines, the subject must meet criteria in all three areas, and the symptomology must be present in at least one area by the age of 36 months.

REFERENCES

Cox A, Charman T, Baron-Cohen S, Drew A, Klein K, Baird G, Swettenham J, Wheelright S (1999) 'Autism spectrum disorders at 20 and 42 months of age: Stability of the clinical and ADI-R diagnosis.' *Journal of Child Psychology and Psychiatry*, **40**, 719–732.
le Couteur A, Rutter M, Lord C, Rios P, Robertson S, Holdgrafer M, McLennan J (1989) 'Autism Diagnostic Interview: A standardized investigator-based instrument.' *Journal of Autism and Developmental Disorders*, **19**, 363–387.
Lord C (1995) 'Follow-up of two-year-olds referred for possible autism.' *Journal of Child Psychology and Psychiatry*, **36**, 1365–1382.
Lord C, Rutter M, Goode S, Heemsbergen J, Jordan H, Mawhood L, Schopler E (1989) 'Autism Diagnostic Observation Schedule: A standardized observation of communicative and social behaviour.' *Journal of Autism and Developmental Disorders*, **19**, 185–212.
Lord C, Browder DM, le Couteur A (1994) 'Autism Diagnostic Interview—Revised: A revised version of a diagnostic interview for caregivers of individuals with possible pervasive developmental disorders.' *Journal of Autism and Developmental Disorders*, **24**, 659–685.
Lord C, Pickles A, McLennan J, Rutter M, Bregman J, Folstein S, Fombonne E, Leboyer M, Minshew N (1997) 'Diagnosing autism: Analyses of data from the Autism Diagnostic Interview.' *Journal of Autism and Developmental Disorders*, **27**, 501–517.
Pilowsky T, Yirmiya N, Shulman C, Dover R (1998) 'The Autism Diagnostic Interview—Revised and the Childhood Autism Rating Scale: Differences between diagnostic systems and comparison between genders.' *Journal of Autism and Developmental Disorders*, **28**, 143–151.

Autism Diagnostic Observation Schedule (Generic) (ADOS-G)

The ADOS-G measures the presence of symptoms and deficits associated with autism. The schedule consists of four modules, each being appropriate to the developmental level of the subject. In order to determine which module to use, it may be advisable to carry out a cognitive assessment of the individual prior to administration of the ADOS-G. Module 1 is for use with subjects who are "preverbal or have single words". Module 2 can be used in individuals with "phrase speech". Module 3 is suitable for use with a "child/adolescent with fluent speech" and Module 4 is for use with "adolescents/adults with fluent speech". Each module consists of standard situations (either task-based or social-based) in which the individual is assessed according to three broad areas: communication, social interaction, and play/imaginative use of objects. These situations use 'presses' that are designed to elicit specific behaviours. To administer the ADOS-G, the experimenter must have extensive training in its use.

Administration time of the ADOS-G is 30–45 minutes, after which the clinician's observations must be scored using standardized coding procedures. These scores can then be used to produce an algorithm. The psychometric properties are well researched and established.

REFERENCES

DiLavore PC, Lord C, MR (1995) 'The Pre-Linguistic Autism Diagnostic Observation Schedule.' *Journal of Autism and Developmental Disorders*, **25**, 355–379.

Lord C, Rutter M, Goode S, Heemsbergen J, Jordam H, Mawhood L, Schopler E (1989) 'Autism Diagnostic Observation Schedule: A standardized observation of communicative and social behaviour.' *Journal of Autism and Developmental Disorders*, **19**, 185–212.

Robertson JM, Tanguay PE, Lecuyer S, Sims A, Waltrip C (1999) 'Domains of social communication handicap in autism spectrum disorder.' *Journal of the American Academy of Child and Adolescent Psychiatry*, **38**, 738–745.

Autism Screening Questionnaire

This schedule is derived from the ADI-R and is used to detect the presence of pervasive developmental disorder in children and adults. It is relatively short in duration, and consists of 40 items relating to autism-specific behaviours, specifically: reciprocal social interaction; language and communication; and repetitive and stereotyped patterns of behaviour. A rating scale of 0 ("absence of abnormal behaviour") to 1 ("presence of abnormal behaviour") is used. For children with language, the scoring range is 0 to 39. However, for children who are nonverbal, the scoring range is 0 to 34 because the items relating to language are inapplicable.

The validity of the instrument has been established but at time of press there are no data pertaining to its reliability. There are two versions of the Autism Screening Questionnaire, one for children under the age of 6 years and another for individuals aged 6 years and over.

REFERENCE

Berument SK, Rutter M, Lord C, Pickles A, Bailey A (1999) 'Autism screening questionnaire.' *British Journal of Psychiatry*, **175**, 444–451.

Behavioral Summarized Evaluation Scale—Revised

The Behavioral Summarized Evaluation Scale—Revised is derived from the Infant Behavioral Summarized Evaluation. It is designed to evaluate the severity of autistic behaviours in children with developmental disabilities, and can also be used to record behaviour change over time. The original BSE scale has been used to measure treatment outcome. It consists of 29 items that are rated on a five-point scale: 0 if "the disorder is never observed"; 1 if "sometimes"; 2 if "often"; 3 if "very often"; and 4 if "always observed". Interrater reliability is very good. Criterion and convergent validity has been established in research. At present, a standardized version of the schedule is only available in French; the British version has yet to be standardized.

REFERENCES

Adrien JL, Barthelemy A, Perrot A, Roux S, Lenior P, Hameury L, Sauvage D (1992) 'Validity and reliability of the Infant Behavioral Summarized Evaluation (IBSE): A rating scale for the assessment of young children with autism and developmental disorders.' *Journal of Autism and Developmental Disorders*, **22**, 375–394.

Barthelemy C, Adrien J, Roux S, Garreau B, Perrot A, DeLord G (1992) 'Sensitivity and specificity of the Behavioral Summarized Evaluation (BSE) for the assessment of autistic behaviours.' *Journal of Autism and Developmental Disorders*, **22**, 23–31.

Barthelemy C, Roux S, Adrien JL, Hameury L, Guerin P, Garreau B, Fermanian J, LeLord G (1997) 'Validation of the Revised Behavior Summarized Evaluation Scale.' *Journal of Autism and Developmental Disorders*, **27**, 139–153.

Boiron M, Barthelemy C, Adrien JL, Martineau J, LeLord G (1992) 'The assessment of psychophysiological

73

dysfunction in children using the BSE scale before and during therapy.' *Acta Paedopsychiatrica. International Journal of Child and Adolescent Psychiatry*, **55**, 203–206.

Childhood Autism Rating Scale (CARS)

The CARS aids the clinician in the identification of autism in children. The CARS is sensitive to developmental changes in autistic symptomology, and can thus be useful in the periodic monitoring of symptomology. The schedule consists of 15 items and administration time is 20–30 minutes. The format is a parent/carer interview and direct observation of the child; the child's behaviour is rated on a Likert scale. The authors of the CARS maintain that it can be used with children and adults. Research proposes that a number of the items relating to language and communication may be inappropriate to adolescents and adults because often a trend of developmental improvement can be seen in people with autism as they age.

The psychometric properties are well documented. Reliability has been established for use of the CARS in the adolescent population. Test–retest reliability of the CARS has been demonstrated in children as young as 18 months. However, it has been suggested that the 'Inconsistencies in Intelligence' item should be removed when administering the CARS to adolescents with autism as it has been found to reduce the reliability of the instrument.

REFERENCES

Garfin DG, McCallon D, Cox R (1988) 'Validity and reliability of the Childhood Autism Rating Scale with autistic adolescents.' *Journal of Autism and Developmental Disorders*, **18**, 367–378.
Kurita H, Miyake Y, Katsuno K (1989) 'Reliability and validity of the Childhood Autism Rating Scale—Tokyo Version (CARS-TV).' *Journal of Autism and Developmental Disorders*, **19**, 389–396.
Kurita H, Kita M, Miyake Y (1992) 'A comparative study of development and symptoms among disintegrative psychosis and infantile autism with and without speech loss.' *Journal of Autism and Developmental Disorders*, **22**, 175–188.
Lord C (1995) 'Follow-up of two-year-olds referred for possible autism.' *Journal of Child Psychology and Psychiatry*, **36**, 1365–1382.
Morgan S (1988) 'Diagnostic assessment of autism: A review of objective scales.' *Journal of Psychoeducational Assessment*, **36**, 139–151.
Nordin V, Gillberg C, Nyden A (1998) 'The Swedish version of the Childhood Autism Rating Scale in a clinical setting.' *Journal of Autism and Developmental Disorders*, **28**, 69–75.
Pilowsky T, Yirmiya N, Shulman C, Dover R (1998) 'The Autism Diagnostic Interview—Revised and the Childhood Autism Rating Scale: Differences between diagnostic systems and comparison between genders.' *Journal of Autism and Developmental Disorders*, **28**, 143–151.
Schopler E, Reichler RJ, DeVellis RF, Daly K (1980) 'Towards objective classification of childhood autism: Childhood Autism Rating Scale (CARS).' *Journal of Autism and Developmental Disorders*, **19**, 91–103.
Stone WL, Lee EB, Ashford L, Brissie J, Hepburn SL, Coonrod EE, Weiss BH (1999) 'Can autism be diagnosed accurately in children under 3 years?' *Journal of Child Psychology and Psychiatry and Allied Disciplines*, **40**, 219–226.
Sturmey P, Matson JL, Sevin JA (1992) 'Analysis of the internal consistency of three autism scales.' *Journal of Autism and Developmental Disorders*, **22**, 321–328.

Checklist for Autism in Toddlers (CHAT)

The CHAT is a short screening schedule that aims to detect possible features of autism in toddlers as young as 18 months. It provides the first level of evaluation for GPs and health visitors in the early stages of a possible diagnosis. The CHAT consists of nine items that target autistic behaviours, including social play, joint attention, gesturing skills, motor development, and functional play. In addition to a parent interview, the CHAT also includes five observations of the interaction between parent and child, thus allowing the clinician to validate the child's behaviour with the parental reports. The schedule demonstrates a high degree of sensitivity in detecting autism in children aged 18 and 40 months.

REFERENCES

Baron-Cohen S, Allen J, Gillberg C (1992) 'Can autism be detected at 18 months? The needle, the haystack, and the CHAT.' *British Journal of Psychiatry*, **161**, 839–843.
Baron-Cohen S, Cox A, Baird G, Sweettenham J, Nighingale N, Morgan K, Drew A, Charman T (1996) 'Psychological markers in the detection of autism in infancy in a large population.' *British Journal of Psychiatry*, **168**, 158–163.
Baron-Cohen S, Wheelwright S, Cox A, Baird G, Charman T, Sweettenham J, Drew A, Doehring P (2000) 'Early identification of autism by the Checklist for Autism in Toddlers (CHAT).' *Journal of the Royal Society of Medicine*, **93**, 521–525.
Cox A, Charman T, Baron-Cohen S, Drew A, Klein K, Baird G, Swettenham J, Wheelright S (1999) 'Autism spectrum disorders at 20 and 42 months of age: Stability of the clinical and ADI-R diagnosis.' *Journal of Child Psychology and Psychiatry*, **40**, 719–732.

Diagnostic Instrument for Social and Communication Disorders (DISCO)

The DISCO is a new instrument and measures symptomatology relating to autistic spectrum disorders. It has been cited as an alternative to the ADI-R. The DISCO is used in research, but at time of press no publications are yet available.

REFERENCE

Wing L, Leekam S, Gould J, Larcombe M (1999) *The Diagnostic Interview for Social and Communication Disorders.* The Centre for Social and Communication Disorders, Elliott House, 113 Masons Hill, Bromley, Kent, England.

Handicaps, Behaviour and Skills (HBS)

The HBS is designed to provide clinicians with a framework in which to collate information about a child using a wide variety of resources. The HBS consists of 42 sections that examine developmental abilities and 21 sections that investigate abnormalities of behaviour. Ratings of behaviour are based on observations of the child's behaviour over the last month. The section on developmental skills uses a scoring system that is hierarchical in nature, according to steps in normal development. The higher the score, the higher the developmental level. The items relating to abnormalities of behaviour are ranked according to severity, the higher the rating, the more severe the behaviour is. The schedule can take from 45 minutes to 2.5 hours to complete, depending on the complexity of the child's behaviour. The psychometric properties of the schedule are established and demonstrate good reliability and validity.

REFERENCES

Aman MG (1991) 'Review and evaluation of instruments for assessing emotional and behavioural disorders.' *Australia and New Zealand Journal of Developmental Disabilities*, **17**, 127–145.

Sales J (1993) 'Angelman syndrome: understanding the behavioural phenotype.' Paper presented at the Scientific Meeting of The Society for the Study of Behavioural Phenotypes: Fragile X Syndrome: A Model for Behavioural Enquiry. Royal Society of Medicine, London, 8 December 1993.

Wing L (1982) *Schedule for the Assessment of Handicaps, Behaviour and Skills.* London: Institute of Psychiatry, MRC Social Psychiatry Unit.

Wing L, Gould J (1978) 'Systematic recording of behaviours and skills of retarded and psychotic children.' *Journal of Autism and Childhood Schizophrenia*, **8**, 79–97.

Wing L, Yeates SR, Brierly LM, Gould J (1976) 'The prevalence of early childhood autism: A comparison of administrative and epidemiological studies.' *Psychological Medicine*, **6**, 89–100.

Parent Interview for Autism (PIA)

The PIA is a semi-structured parent interview that measures autism in children at preschool level and below. The schedule covers 118 items that are grouped into 11 dimensions. Items were derived from existing diagnostic schedules including the Autism Behavior Checklist, Rimland's Diagnostic Checklist, the Autistic Descriptors Checklist and the Childhood Behaviour Schedule. Behaviour is rated for frequency, with scores ranging from (1) "almost never" to (5) "almost always". Reliability and validity have been established. However, research has found that not all of the PIA dimensions clearly differentiate between children with autism and those with learning disability.

REFERENCES

Filipek PA, Accardo PJ, Baranek GT, Cook EH, Dawson G, Gordon B, Gravel JS, Johnson CP, Kallen RJ, Levy SE, Minshew NJ, Ozonoff S, Prizant BM, Rapin I, Rogers SJ, Stone WL, Teplin S, Tuchman RF, Volkmar FR (1999) 'The screening and diagnosis of autistic spectrum disorders.' *Journal of Autism and Developmental Disorders*, **29**, 439–484.

Krug DA, Arick J, Almond P (1980) 'Behaviour checklist for identifying severely handicapped individuals with high levels of autistic behaviour.' *Journal of Child Psychology and Psychiatry and Allied Disciplines*, **21**, 221–229.

Stone WL, Hogan KL (1993) 'A structured parent interview for identifying young children with autism.' *Journal of Autism and Developmental Disorders*, **23**, 639–652.

Pre-Linguistic Autism Diagnostic Observation Schedule (PL-ADOS)

This schedule is derived from the ADOS, and is intended as a diagnostic tool for nonverbal children under the age of 6 years. It is a semi-structured assessment of play, interaction and social communication in relation to autism. Administration time is 30 minutes and the scoring algorithm is based on DSM-IV criteria. The schedule requires extensive training and may therefore be applicable only to certain clinical situations. The schedule would benefit from further research into its psychometric properties.

REFERENCES

DiLavore PC, Lord CMR (1995) 'The Pre-Linguistic Autism Diagnostic Observation Schedule.' *Journal of Autism and Developmental Disorders*, **25**, 355–379.

Lord C, Rutter M, Goode S, Heemsbergen J, Jordan H, Mawhood L, Schopler E (1989) 'Autism Diagnostic Observation Schedule: A standardised observation of communicative and social behaviour.' *Journal of Autism and Developmental Disorders*, **19**, 185–212.

Scale for Pervasive Developmental Disorder in Mentally Retarded Persons

This schedule measures a wide range of behaviours specific to autism. It has been developed for use in autistic adults with confounding learning disability. It can be used as a diagnostic tool as it is derived from ICD-10/DSM-IV criteria for PDD. It takes approximately 30 minutes to complete and is in interview format. So far there has been no independent investigation of its psychometric properties.

REFERENCE

Kraijer D (1997) *Autism and Autistic-Like Conditions in Mental Retardation.* Lisse: Swets & Zeitlinger.

APPENDIX 3.2
SCHEDULES DESIGNED FOR THE PURPOSE OF DETECTION, DIAGNOSIS AND ASSESSMENT OF PSYCHIATRIC DISORDERS

Adolescent Behaviour Checklist

This schedule screens for the presence of psychiatric disorders, based on DSM-III-R criteria, in adolescents with learning disability. It compromises eight scales, which cover a wide range of disorders. In addition the schedule has a 'Lie' scale to estimate the honesty of answers. The format is self-report, although the checklist is read aloud by a clinician to the individual, and employs a forced choice response (Yes/No). A Total score is calculated by summing all the 'Yes' responses. A Clinical score is calculated by subtracting the Lie score from the Total score. The authors propose using 11 as the cut-off score for the presence of psychiatric disorder.

REFERENCE

Demb HB, Brier N, Huron R, Tomor E (1994) 'The Adolescent Behaviour Checklist: Normative data and sensitivity and specificity of a screening tool for diagnosable psychiatric disorders in adolescents with mental retardation and other developmental disabilities.' *Research in Developmental Disabilities*, **15**, 151–165.

Carey's Survey of Temperamental Characteristics

This schedule measures temperamental characteristics in children between the ages of 4 and 8 months. It has been used in children with varying levels of learning disability and has also been used in research in Down syndrome.

REFERENCES

Carey WB (1973) 'Measurement of infant temperament in paediatric practice.' *In:* Westman JC (ed) *Individual Differences in Children.* New York: John Wiley, pp 188–194.

Carey WB (1981) 'Measuring infant temperament.' *Journal of Paediatrics*, **77**, 188.

O'Brien G (1992) 'Behavioural phenotypy in developmental psychiatry: Measuring behavioural phenotypes: A guide to existing schedules.' *European Child and Adolescent Psychiatry*, Suppl. 1, 1–61.

Child Behaviour Checklist (CBCL)

The CBCL was initially designed to assess psychopathology in children without learning disability, but it is now widely used in the field of learning disability. The schedule covers a wide range of psychopathology and divides behaviour into two broad factors—internalizing and externalizing behaviours. In addition, the CBCL covers a further eight narrow factors: Withdrawn; Somatic complaints; Anxious/depressed; Social problems; Thought problems; Attention problems; Delinquent behaviours; and 'Others'. The CBCL consists of 118 items on which a parent or carer rates the child's behaviour on a three-point rating scale of "not true" (0), "somewhat or sometimes true" (1), or "very true or often true" (2). Ratings of behaviour are based on the previous six months. The authors have suggested a cut-off score of 40 for boys and 37 for girls. These cut-off scores apply only to 6- to 11-year-old children.

The CBCL has been used with individuals with Prader–Willi syndrome. The psychometric properties of the CBCL are established for use in the normative population, but reliability is reduced when the schedule is used in learning disability.

There are five versions of the CBCL: Child Behaviour Checklist (2–3 years); Child Behaviour Checklist (4–18 years) (reported here); Teacher Report Form (6–18 years); Youth Self-Report (11–18 years); and Direct Observation Form (6–18 years).

REFERENCES

Achenbach TM (1991) *Manual for the Child Behaviour Checklist and 1991 Profile.* Burlington, VA: University of Vermont, Dept of Psychiatry.
Achenbach TM, Edelbrock CS (1983) *Manual for the Child Behaviour Checklist and Revised Profile.* Burlington, VT: University of Vermont, Dept of Psychiatry.
Emberts PJCM (2000) 'Reliability of the Child Behaviour Checklist for the assessment of behavioural problems of children and youths with mild mental retardation.' *Research in Developmental Disabilities,* **21,** 31–41.
Hodapp RM, Dykens EM, Masino LL (1997) 'Families of children with Prader–Willi syndrome: Stress-support and relations to child characteristics.' *Journal of Autism and Developmental Disorders,* **27,** 11–24.
Matson JL, Barrett RP, Helsel WJ (1988) 'Depression in mentally retarded children.' *Research in Developmental Disabilities,* **9,** 39–46.
Skuse D, Percy E, Stevenson J (1993) 'Psychosocial functioning in the Turner syndrome.' Paper presented at the Scientific Meeting of The Society for the Study of Behavioural Phenotypes: Fragile X Syndrome: A Model for Behavioural Enquiry. Royal Society of Medicine, London.

Child Psychiatric Interview

This schedule measures psychiatric disturbance in children. Although it has been succeeded by more modern schedules, it is one of the few interview schedules that provide psychometric data for children with mild to moderate learning disability.

REFERENCES

O'Brien G (1992) 'Behavioural phenotypy in developmental psychiatry: Measuring behavioural phenotypes: A guide to existing schedules.' *European Child and Adolescent Psychiatry,* Suppl. 1, 1–61.
Rutter M, Graham P, Yule W (1970) *A Neuropsychiatric Study in Childhood. Clinics in Developmental Medicine No. 35/36.* London: Spastics International Medical Publications.

Children's Depression Inventory (CDI)

The original CDI was designed as a measure of depression in children aged between 7 and 17 years. The schedule covers areas such as hedonic capacity, disturbed mood and vegetative functions. In its original form, the CDI consists of 27 items that are scored on a range of 0–2, in the direction of increasing severity, with responses being forced choice statements. It is scored by summing the total of all the individual items. The cut-off score for depression is set at 17. The psychometric properties are well established, although its factor structure may differ according to the population used.

The CDI has been modified for use in adults with learning disability. The structure and scoring technique are the same as for the original CDI but the modified version has only

24 items: three were deleted (these referred to regular attendance at school) as the applicability of these items to the learning disabled population was questionable. The scoring range is from 0 (normal) to 48 (severe depression). Research using the modified CDI has tended to focus on the informant version, thus allowing it to be applied to various levels of learning disability. The psychometric properties of the modified CDI have been reported; internal consistency and interrater reliability is reported to be adequate, but these would benefit from further research, as would the optimal cut-off score of the instrument.

REFERENCES

Helsel WJ, Matson JL (1984) 'The assessment of depression in children: the internal structure of the Child Depression Inventory (CDI).' *Behavioural Research and Therapy*, **22**, 289–298.
Hepperlin CM, Stewart GW, Rey JM (1990) 'Extraction of depression scores in adolescents from a general purpose behaviour checklist.' *Journal of Affective Disorders*, **18**, 105–112.
Kovacs M (1985) 'The Children's Depression Inventory (CDI).' *Psychopharmacology Bulletin*, **21**, 995–998.
Meins W (1993) 'Assessment of depression in mentally retarded adults: Reliability and validity of the Children's Depression Inventory.' *Research in Developmental Disabilities*, **14**, 299–312.

Children's Psychiatric Rating Scale

The original Children's Psychiatric Rating Scale was devised by the Psychopharmacology Research Branch of the NIMH. It was designed to assess psychiatric symptomatology in children. In total, the original schedule consists of 63 items. However, researchers have modified the Scale for use in children with autism. This modified version is shorter than the original and consists of 14 items, which focus on domains such as language, intonation, motor activity and social behaviour. Results of factor analysis yield four factors: autism, anger/uncooperativeness, hyperactivity, and speech deviance. The modified version has been used extensively in pharmacological studies.

REFERENCES

Campbell M, Palij M (1985) 'Behavioural and cognitive measures used in psychopharmacologic studies of infantile autism.' *Psychopharmacology Bulletin*, **21**, 1063–1082.
Fish B (1985) 'Children's Psychiatric Rating Scale (Scoring).' *Psychopharmacology Bulletin*, **21**, 753–764.
Guy W (1976) *ECDEU Assessment Manual for Psychopharmacology.* Kensington, MD: US Department of Health and Human Resources.
Overall JE, Campbell M (1988) 'Behavioural assessment of psychopathology in children: Infantile autism.' *Journal of Clinical Psychology*, **44**, 708–716.
Psychopharmacology Bulletin (1973) *Special Issue. Pharmacotherapy of Children.* Washington: NIMH.
Psychopharmacology Bulletin (1985) *Special Issue. Rating Scales and Assessment Instruments for Use in Pediatric Psychopharmacology Research.* Washington: NIMH.

Conners Parent Rating Scale

The original Conners Parent Rating Scale consisted of 93 items that measured behaviour problems in children and was a useful research tool for monitoring psychosocial and drug treatment outcomes. The schedule was revised because the author felt that the items covered in the schedule were too comprehensive and were not specific to the level of knowledge of behaviour disorders that exists today, especially in relation to ADHD.

The revised Scale contains fewer items, focuses on ADHD-related behaviour and has clearer definitions of items. It consists of 57 items, which are rated on a Likert scale of 0 ("not true at all") to 4 ("very much true"). It consists of seven subscales: Psychosomatic; Anxious–Shy; Perfectionism; Cognitive Problems; Hyperactivity; Oppositional Problems; and Social Problems. The Oppositional Problems domain measures behaviour that is consistent with oppositional defiant disorder and conduct disorder yet excludes behaviour associated with ADHD. The schedule has a 12-item subscale called the ADHD Diagnostic Index. Research has shown it to be validated, with good discriminatory power in distinguishing between ADHD patients and a control sample. It is also available as a teacher rating scale.

REFERENCES

Conners CK (1970) 'Symptom patterns in hyperkinetic, neurotic and normal children.' *Child Development*, **41**, 667–682.
Conners CK, Sitarenios G, Parker J, Epstein N (1998) 'The revised Conners Parent Rating scale (CPRS-R): Factor structure, reliability, and criterion validity.' *Journal of Abnormal Child Psychology*, **26**, 257–269.

Conners Teacher Rating Scale Revised (CTRS-R)

The original Conners Teacher Rating Scale was revised in 1998. The schedule assesses the behaviour of children in the classroom and can also be used to monitor treatment effects. Factor analysis derived six stable factors. The schedule has increased specificity and sensitivity to inattention/ADHD symptoms. This schedule is also available for use with parents (see above).

REFERENCES

Conners CK (1969) 'A teacher rating scale for use in drug studies.' *American Journal of Psychiatry*, **126**, 152–156.
Conners CK, Sitarenios G, Parker J, Epstein N (1998) 'Revision and re-standardization of the Conners Teacher Rating Scale (CTRS-R): Factor structure, reliability and criterion validity.' *Journal of Abnormal Child Psychology*, **26**, 279–292.

Development and Well-Being Assessment (DAWBA)

The DAWBA is a comprehensive assessment package that focuses upon child and adolescent psychopathology. It consists of four components: an interview for parents of 5- to 17-year-olds; a teacher questionnaire for 5- to 17-year-olds; an interview for children 11–17 years of age; and a computer program that produces a diagnostic rating based on information from the interviews and questionnaires. The DAWBA uses ICD-10 and DSM-IV criteria as a basis of diagnosis.

The Parent Interview covers, in detail, disorders such as: separation anxiety; specific and social phobias; post-traumatic stress disorder; obsessive–compulsive disorder; generalized anxiety; major depression; hyperkinesis/ADHD; and conduct–opposition disorders. Disorders covered in less detail include panic disorder, autistic disorders, eating disorders and tic disorders. The Interview for 11- to 17-year-olds is the same as the Parent Interview except that the sections on hyperactivity are shorter. The Teacher Questionnaire focuses on three domains: hyperactivity/inattention, oppositional/conduct disorders, and emotional symptoms. The interviews have a 'skip rule' that allows the interview to pass over sections that are not applicable.

Although not designed for use in learning disability, it could be used with informants with mild to moderate levels of learning disability. The DAWBA has good discriminant validity when comparing clinical and community samples, but further research is required regarding the reliability of the schedule.

The DAWBA can be downloaded from the www.dawba.com website.

REFERENCE

Goodman R, Ford T, Richards H, Gatwood R, Meltzer H (2000) 'The Development and Well-Being Assessment: Description and initial validation of an integrated assessment of child and adolescent psychopathology.' *Journal of Child Psychology and Psychiatry*, **41**, 645–655.

Developmental Behaviour Checklist (DBC)

The DBC is designed to assess behavioural and emotional problems in children and adolescents with developmental disabilities over a six-month period. It shares the same structure as the Child Behaviour Checklist. It consists of 96 items, which are rated on a 0–2 rating scale: 0 = "not true as far as you know", 1 = "somewhat or sometimes true", and 2 = "very true or often true". The DBC produces three levels of scoring: (i) a "total behaviour problem score" provides an overall measure of emotional and behavioural problems; (ii) subscale scores; and (iii) scores on individual items, which can be useful for assessing the severity of an individual problem. The DBC is epidemiologically derived from the medical files of 664 children with varying levels of learning disability. Norms are available for mild to profound learning disability.

The psychometric properties of the DBC are well documented. Reliability is well established, although this declines with parent–teacher ratings. Test–retest and internal consistencies are also high. With relation to validity, the DBC correlates highly with the Adaptive Behaviour Scale—School Edition. Two versions of the DBC are available, the Parent/Carer Version (DBC-P), and the Teacher Version (DBC-T).

REFERENCES

Einfeld SL, Tonge B (1991) 'Psychometric and clinical assessment of psychopathology in developmentally disabled children.' *Australia and New Zealand Journal of Developmental Disabilities*, **17**, 147–154.

Einfeld SL, Tonge BJ (1995) 'The Developmental Behaviour Checklist: The development and validation of an instrument to assess behavioural and emotional disturbance in children and adolescents with mental retardation.' *Journal of Autism and Developmental Disorders*, **25**, 81–104.

Einfeld SL, Tonge BJ. (1996) 'Population prevalence of psychopathology in children and adolescents with intellectual disability: I. Rationale and methods. II. Epidemiological findings.' *Journal of Intellectual Disability Research*, **40**, 91–98; 99–109.

Einfeld SL, Tonge BJ, Florio T (1994) 'Behavioural and emotional disturbance in fragile X syndrome.' *American Journal of Medical Genetics*, **51**, 386–391.

Einfeld SL, Tonge BJ, Florio T (1997) 'Behavioural and emotional disturbance in individuals with Williams syndrome.' *American Journal on Mental Retardation*, **102**, 45–53.

Einfeld SL, Smith A, Durvasula S, Florio T, Tonge BJ (1999) 'Behaviour and emotional disturbance in Prader–Willi syndrome.' *American Journal of Medical Genetics*, **82**, 123–127.

Mount R, Hastings R, Charman T, Reilly S, Cass H (1999) 'Behavioural and emotional features of Rett syndrome.' Paper presented at the Society for the Study of Behavioural Phenotypes 8th Annual Meeting: From Research to Clinical Practise in Behavioural Phenotypes. Beeches Management Centre, Birmingham, England, 16–19 November 1999.

Diagnostic Interview for Children and Adolescents (DICA)

The original DICA was revised in 1997. The schedule aims to provide clinicians with diagnoses using items based upon DSM-III-R criteria. It is a semi-structured interview that covers diagnoses such as ADHD, conduct disorder, hypomania, obsessive–compulsive disorder and eating disorders. In addition to diagnoses, the schedule covers items relating to psychosocial measures, and a section that measures the presence or absence of psychotic symptoms. Administration time is 1–2 hours, although the computer version takes less time. An extensive training period of 2–3 weeks has been suggested in order to be fully conversant with the DICA.

The DICA is available in three versions: the DICA for 6- to 12-year-olds; the DICA (Youth Version) for 13- to 18-year-olds; and a Parent Interview covering both age groups. Interestingly, within the Parent Version there is a Perinatal Section, which details items such as developmental milestones, developmental delay, temperament, and behaviour problems. In addition, it is available as a computer package.

REFERENCES

Ezpeleta L, de la Osa N, Domenech JB, Navarro JB, Losilla JM (1997) 'Diagnostic agreement between clinicians and the Diagnostic Interview for Children and Adolescents – DICA-R – in an outpatient sample.' *Journal of Child Psychology and Psychiatry*, **38**, 431–440.

Herjanic B, Reich W (1982) 'Development of a structured psychiatric interview for children: agreement between child and parent on individual symptoms.' *Journal of Abnormal Child Psychology*, **10**, 307–324.

Reich W (2000) 'Diagnostic Interview for Children and Adolescents (DICA).' *Journal of the American Academy of Child and Adolescent Psychiatry*, **39**, 59–66.

Reich W, Herjanic B, Welzer Z, Grandhy PR (1982) 'Development of a structured psychiatric interview for children: agreement on diagnosis comparing child and parent interviews.' *Journal of Abnormal Child Psychology*, **10**, 325–336.

Rojahn J, Warren VJ, Ohringer S (1994) 'A comparison of assessment methods for depression in mental retardation.' *Journal of Autism and Developmental Disorders*, **24**, 305–313.

Willekens D, Steyaert J, Umans S, De die-Smulders C, Goemans N, Legius E, Fryns JP (1996) 'Myotonic dystrophy in children and adolescents: neuropsychological and child psychiatric study.' Paper presented at the Society for the Study of Behavioural Phenotypes 4th International Symposium: Behavioural Phenotypes in Practice. Marino Institute of Education, Dublin, 14–16 November 1996.

Dimensions of Temperament Survey (DOTS)

The DOTS measures temperament in relation to psychosocial adaptation. It has been used extensively to assess age-related changes in temperament from early childhood to young adulthood. There are two adaptations of the DOTS: the original version consists of 89 items and the other has 34 items that are specific to age-related changes. Most research uses the full 89-item version. In addition to this, there are three versions that vary according to rater: child (self-report), child (parent rated), and adult (self-report). With regards to psychometrics, there are few data pertaining to the validity of the schedule and there is a need for further research. Reliability is cited as being low to moderate.

REFERENCES

Ireland M, Berney TP, Burn J (1991) 'Cornelia de Lange survey.' Paper presented at the Society for the Study of Behavioural Phenotypes Workshop, Kings Fund College, London.

Lerner RM, Palmero M (1982) 'Assessing the dimensions of temperamental individuality across the life span: The Dimensions of Temperament (DOTS).' *Child Development*, **53**, 149–159.

McDevitt SC, Carey WB (1978) 'The measurement of temperament in 3–7 year old children.' *Journal of Child Psychology and Psychiatry*, **19**, 245–253.

Merikangas KR, Swendsen JD, Preisig MA, Chazan RZ (1998) 'Psychopathology and temperament in parents and offspring: results of a family study.' *Journal of Affective Disorders*, **51**, 63–74.

Emotional Disorders Rating Scale for Developmental Disabilities (EDRS-DD)

The EDRS-DD is designed to assess emotional symptomology in children and adolescents with learning disability. The schedule consists of 59 items that are divided into seven subscales: irritability; hostility/anger; psychomotor retardation; depressive mood; somatic/ vegetative; elated/manic; and sleep disturbance. Items relating to depressive mood meet DSM-III criteria for anxiety disorder. The schedule is in checklist format and takes 15 minutes to administer. The informant can be anyone who knows the individual. Inter-rater reliability is high, but the validity of the schedule needs further research.

REFERENCES

Aman MG (1991) 'Review and evaluation of instruments for assessing emotional and behavioural disorders.' *Australia and New Zealand Journal of Developmental Disabilities*, **17**, 127–145.

Feinstein C, Kaminer Y, Barret RP, Tylenda B (1988) 'The assessment of mood and affect in developmentally disabled children and adolescents: The Emotional Disorders Rating Scale.' *Research in Developmental Disabilities*, **9**, 109–121.

Sturmey P, Reed J, Corbett J (1991) 'Psychometric assessment of psychiatric disorders in people with learning difficulties (mental handicap): A review of measures.' *Psychological Medicine*, **21**, 143–155.

Ghuman–Folstein Screen for Social Interacti\on

The Ghuman–Folstein Screen for Social Interaction measures social abilities in children between the ages of 6 months and 5 years. It contains 54 items that are rated on a scale of "almost never" to "almost all of the time". Because many of the items relate to social inter-action it has been used in autism. The psychometric properties of the schedule have been established, with moderate inter-rater reliability, and good test–retest reliability being reported. Validity is also good. The schedule can successfully differentiate between clinical cases and normal children and also between autistic and other PDD children.

REFERENCE

Ghuman JK, Freund L, Reiss A, Serwint J, Folstein S (1998) 'Early detection of social interaction problems: Development of a social interaction instrument in young children.' *Journal of Developmental and Behavioural Pediatrics*, **19**, 411–419.

Nisonger Child Behaviour Rating Form (CBRF)

The Nisonger CBRF was designed to measure psychopathology in children and adolescents. It was derived from the Child Behaviour Checklist. The schedule is divided into two sections: section one, Social Competence, consists of 10 items that describe adaptive and prosocial behaviour; and section two, Problem Behaviour, addresses maladaptive behaviours. The two sections differ in how the items are rated. The Social Competence section requires rating of items on a four-point Likert scale that ranges from 0 ("not true") to 3 ("completely or always true"). The Problem Behaviour section rates behaviour on a scale of 0 ("did not occur or was not a problem") to 3 ("occurred a lot or was a severe problem"). Informants are required to consider the frequency of the behaviour and severity of the behaviour when rating problem behaviour. The Nisonger CBRF contains an additional 11 items relating to the measurement of self-injury and stereotypic behaviour.

The Nisonger CBRF is available in two versions, parent and teacher. Factor analysis yielded different factors for the two versions. The Parent version yielded six items: conduct problems, insecure/anxious, hyperactive, self-injury/stereotypic, self-isolation/ritualistic, and overly sensitive. The Teacher version yielded these same factors, in addition to irritability. The psychometric properties of the Nisonger CBRF are established.

REFERENCES

Aman MG, Tasse MJ, Rojahn J, Hammer D (1996) 'The Nisonger CBRF: A child behaviour rating form for children with developmental disabilities.' *Research in Developmental Disabilities*, **17**, 41–57.
Tasse MJ, Aman MG, Hammer D, Rojahn J (1996) 'The Nisonger Child Behaviour Rating Form: Age and gender effects and norms.' *Research in Developmental Disabilities*, **17**, 59–75.

Rutter Parent (A) and Teacher (B) Scales

The Rutter Parent and Teacher Scales were initially developed of use in the Isle of Wight Studies. However, they have come to be widely used in research. The Rutter Scales measure emotional and behavioural disturbance in children between the ages of 9 and 13 years. The scales both take approximately six minutes to administer and they share the same scoring structure. Behaviour is rated on a three-point rating scale: 0 ("does not apply"), 1 ("applies somewhat") and 2 ("certainly applies"). The Parent Scale (Scale A) consists of 31 items that are divided into three broadly defined categories: conduct disorder, emotional disorder, and hyperactivity. A cut-off score of 13 is needed for the identification of a disorder, with the exception of the hyperactivity scale for which a cut-off score of 3 is needed. The Teacher Scale (Scale B) consists of 26 items, and has a cut-off score of 9. It shares the same subscales as the Parent Scale. Research has highlighted the need for caution when using the proposed cut-off scores. In addition, the hyperactivity subscale has been criticised for lacking clear and narrow definitions. The Rutter scales have been modified in research, the most popularized version being the Preschool Behaviour Questionnaire.

REFERENCES

Elander J, Rutter M (1996) 'Use and development of the Rutter Teacher Scales.' *International Journal of Methods in Psychiatric Research*, **6**, 63–78.
Fombonne E (1989) 'The Child Behaviour Checklist and the Rutter Parental Questionnaire: A comparison between two screening instruments.' *Psychological Medicine*, **19**, 777–785.
Rutter M, Tizard J, Yule W, Graham P, Whitmore K (1976) 'Research report: Isle of Wight studies.' *Psychological Medicine*, **6**, 313–332.

Schedule for Affective Disorders and Schizophrenia for School-Age Children (K-SADS)

The K-SADS measures psychiatric symptomatology in school-aged children and adolescents. The schedule covers affective, anxiety, behavioural, eating and psychotic disorders, as well as substance abuse, using DSM-III-R criteria. However, it is not designed to be mutually inclusive of all DSM disorders, and does not assess axis II diagnoses, pervasive developmental disorders or learning disorders. Two versions of the K-SADS are in use, the K-SADS-E (epidemiological), and the K-SADS-P (present state). The K-SADS-P measures behaviour occurring in the past 12 months and current state at time of interview. Although the K-SADS is intended for use in a normative sample, the parent interview could be used for children with a mild level of learning disability (P Ambrosini, personal communication 2001). In addition there is the K-SADS-PL (present and lifetime), although psychometric data are not available for this instrument. The K-SADS-E has a useful screening component, which allows the clinician to screen for potential diagnostic cases without having to conduct the entire interview. Symptoms are rated on severity.

The K-SADS-P was updated in 1996 to include the severity/improvement domain of the Clinical Global Impressions Scale. Items are scored on a scale of 0–4 or 0–6 for severity and frequency of behaviour. It has a streamlining feature, which allows clinicians to focus on specific disorders. Both are semi-structured interviews that take approximately 90 minutes to complete, the scoring taking a further hour. Interviews can be conducted with either the parent or the child. Generally, the parent interview is conducted first, in which the parent has to rate their child's behaviour when it was at its worst and also the child's current state. After the child interview the clinician then conducts a third rating of the child using the information from the two interviews to establish a clinical diagnosis. Reliability and validity has been established for both versions.

REFERENCES

Ambrosini PJ (2000) 'Historical development and the present status of the Schedule for Affective Disorders and Schizophrenia for School Age Children.' *Journal of the American Academy of Child and Adolescent Psychiatry*, **39**, 49–58.

Kaufman J, Birmaher B, Brent D, Rao U, Flynn C, Moreci P, Williamson D, Ryan N (1997) 'Schedule for Affective Disorders and Schizophrenia for School Age Children Present and Lifetime version (K-SADS-PL): Initial reliability and validity data.' *Journal of the American Academy of Child and Adolescent Psychiatry*, **36**, 980–988.

Toddler Temperament Scale

This schedule is a structured questionnaire for use in toddlers. It has been used in children with brain damage and also learning disabled children. This schedule should be used in conjunction with other developmental assessments. The language used in the schedule has been found by English researchers to be geared towards American use.

REFERENCES

Fullard W, McDevitt SC, Carey W. (1984) 'Assessing temperament in one- to three-year-old children.' *Journal of Pediatric Psychology*, **9**, 205–217.

O'Brien G (1992) 'Behavioural phenotypy in developmental psychiatry: Measuring behavioural phenotypes: A guide to existing schedules.' *European Child and Adolescent Psychiatry*, Suppl. 1, 1–61.

Yale–Brown Obsessive Compulsive Scale (YBOCS)

The Yale–Brown Obsessive Compulsive Scale (YBOCS) is designed to assess the severity of obsessive–compulsive symptoms in individuals with obsessive–compulsive disorder (OCD). It is not a diagnostic tool. The YBOCS is in the format of a semi-structured interview. The interview consists of three separate sections: a list of examples and definitions; and a symptom checklist and the YBOCS proper, both of which are clinician rated.

The YBOCS shows sensitivity to treatment effects, and research has demonstrated good convergent and construct validity. Discriminant validity varies according to findings. Research has shown that discriminant validity can be established only when patients with OCD are compared with patients with low levels of depression. Reliability of the YBOCS has been demonstrated in numerous research studies.

The YBOCS is user friendly, and each item is accompanied by a definition and example to make it explicit what is being measured. There are two versions of the YBOCS, the adult version and a version for use with children called the CY-BOCS. It differs from the adult version only in respect to modification of the language of the interview and the items to make it more accessible to children with OCD.

REFERENCES

Goodman WK, Price LH, Rasmussen SA, Mazure C, Fleischmann RL, Hill CL, Heninger GR, Charney DS (1989) 'The Yale–Brown Obsessive Compulsive Scale. I: Development, use and reliability.' *Archives of General Psychiatry*, **46**, 1006–1011.

Goodman WK, Price LH, Rasmussen SA, Mazure C, Delgado P, Heninger GR, Charney DS (1989) 'The Yale–Brown Obsessive Compulsive Scale. II: Validity.' *Archives of General Psychiatry*, **46**, 1012–1016.

Goodman WK, Rasmussen SA, Price LH, Mazure C, Heninger GR, Charney DS (1989) *Manual for the Yale–Brown Obsessive Compulsive Scale (Revised).* New Haven, CT: Connecticut Mental Health Centre.

Taylor S. (1995) 'Assessment of obsessions and compulsions: Reliability, validity and sensitivity to treatment effects.' *Clinical Psychology Review*, **15**, 261–296.

APPENDIX 3.3
SCHEDULES FOR THE ASSESSMENT OF PROBLEM BEHAVIOURS

Aberrant Behavior Checklist (ABC)

The ABC was initially designed to measure treatment effects and common behaviour problems in adults with learning disability. It consists of 58 items that are rated on a four-point Likert scale of 0 ("not a problem at all"), 1 ("a problem to a slight degree"); 2 ("moderately serious") and 3 ("severe"). The psychometric properties of the ABC are well established, with good reliability and validity consistently being reported. Factor analysis yields five factors: Irritability/agitation and crying; Lethargy/social withdrawal; Stereotypic behaviour; Hyperactivity/non-compliance; and Inappropriate speech. Recently, a version of the ABC has been devised for use in the community: the ABC-C. The factor structure of the ABC-C differs from the original ABC; the fifth factor of the ABC-C consisted of items pertaining to Hyperactivity/Compliance and self-injury, rather than Inappropriate speech.

The appropriateness of the ABC for use with children with a dual diagnosis of learning disability and another psychiatric disorder has been investigated. Research has shown that the factor structure and the internal consistency of the ABC were stable in this population. However, interrater reliability was reported to be low.

REFERENCES

Aman MG, Singh NN, Stewart AW, Field CJ. (1985) 'The Aberrant Behavior Checklist: A behavior rating scale for the assessment of treatment effects.' *American Journal of Mental Deficiency*, **89**, 485–491.

Aman MG, Singh NN, Stewart AW, Field CJ (1985) 'Psychometric characteristics of the Aberrant Behavior Checklist.' *American Journal of Mental Deficiency*, **89**, 492–502.

Aman MG, Burrow WH, Wolford PL. (1995) 'The Aberrant Behavior Checklist—Community: Factor validity and effect of subject variables for adults in group homes.' *American Journal on Mental Retardation*, **100**, 283–292.

Clarke D, Marston G (1997) 'Problem behaviours associated with Angelman syndrome: A comparative study using the Aberrant Behavior Checklist.' Paper presented at the Society for the Study of Behavioural Phenotypes 7th Annual Meeting: The Development of Research Strategies to Investigate Behavioural Phenotypes, The Moller Centre for Continuing Education, Cambridge, England, 13–14 November.

Marshburn EC, Aman MG (1992) 'Factor validity and norms for the Aberrant Behavior Checklist in a community sample of children with mental retardation.' *Journal of Autism and Developmental Disorders*, **22**, 357–373.

Rojahn J, Helsel WJ (1991) 'The Aberrant Behavior Checklist with children and adolescents with a dual diagnosis.' *Journal of Autism and Developmental Disorders*, **21**, 17–28.

British Isles Survey (BIS) Rett Syndrome Health Questionnaire

The schedule measures the course of Rett syndrome and evaluates the effects of treatment intervention by assessing health and skills in people who have Rett syndrome. It is derived from clinical research investigating Rett syndrome. It takes the form of a postal questionnaire and can be used in both children and adults. Although it has been used successfully in research there has been no formal investigation into the psychometric properties of the schedule.

REFERENCES

Corbett JA, Sansom DT (1990) 'Psychiatric features of Rett syndrome.' Paper presented at the Behavioural
Phenotypes Study Group Symposium, Welshpool, Wales, 22–24 November 1990.
Kerr A (1992) 'Rett syndrome British Longitudinal study (1982–1990) and 1990 survey.' *In:* Roosendaal JJ
(ed) *Mental Retardation and Medical Care.* Zeist: Uitgeverij Kerckbosch.
O'Brien G (1992) 'Behavioural phenotypy in developmental psychiatry: Measuring behavioural phenotypes:
A guide to existing schedules.' *European Child and Adolescent Psychiatry*, Suppl. 1, 1–61.

Functional Independence Measure for Children (WeeFIM®)

The WeeFIM® is derived from the Functional Independence Measure (FIM) for adults.
The aim of the schedule is the measurement of functional behaviour in children with physical
and learning disabilities, aged between 6 months and 7 years. It allows clinicians to record
changes in functional behaviour over time and is intended as an aid in the development of
individual treatment plans. The WeeFIM® consists of 18 items that are subdivided into six
domains: self-care, sphincter control, transfers, locomotion, communication, and social
cognition. Behaviour is rated on a seven-point ordinal scale that rates behaviour from
complete dependence (1) to complete independence (7). The minimum score is 18 and the
maximum is 126. Ratings of behaviour are determined from an interview with a primary
caregiver and/or direct observation of the child.

Reliability and inter-rater agreement for this schedule are established. In addition,
equivalence reliability has been established for the two methods of assessment used in the
schedule. However, the schedule would benefit from further research regarding its psychometric properties. The authors of the WeeFIM® are aware of this and propose that further
investigation into the psychometric properties regarding the sensitivity of the instrument
in measuring change is required.

REFERENCES

Msall ME, Rogers BT, Ripstein H, Lyon N, Wilczenski F (1997) 'Measurements of functional outcomes in
children with cerebral palsy.' *Mental Retardation and Developmental Disabilities Research Reviews*, **3**,
194–203.
Ottenbacher KJ, Taylor ET, Msall ME, Braun S, Lane SJ, Granger CV, Lyons N, Duffy C (1996) 'The stability
and equivalence reliability of the Functional Independence Measure for Children.' *Developmental Medicine
and Child Neurology*, **38**, 907–916.
Ottenbacher KJ, Msall ME, Lyon NR, Duffy LC, Granger CV, Braun S (1997) 'Interrater agreement and stability
of the Functional Independence Measure for Children (WeeFIM): use in children with developmental
disabilities.' *Archives of Physical Medicine and Rehabilitation*, **78**, 1309–1315.
WeeFIM (2000) *WeeFIM System^SM Clinical Guide: Version 5.01.* Buffalo, NY: University at Buffalo.

Leyton Obsessional Inventory

The Leyton Obsessional Inventory is designed to measure obsessive–compulsive symptoms
and traits and the impact they have on the person. It consists of 69 items, 46 that relate to
obsessive–compulsive symptoms and 23 that focus on obsessive–compulsive traits. It has
a self-report format, using forced responses (Yes/No). The schedule's psychometric properties
are well established. However, because the schedule was developed to measure cleanliness
and tidiness, it is restrictive in relation to the measurement of other types of obsessive–

compulsive behaviours. This schedule has been used as part of a battery of instruments to assess self-injurious behaviour in Tourette syndrome.

REFERENCES

Cooper, J (1970). 'The Leyton obsessional inventory.' *Psychological Medicine*, **1**, 48–64.
Robertson MM, Trimble MR, Lees AJ (1989) 'Self-injurious behaviour and the Gilles de la Tourette syndrome: a clinical study and review of the literature.' *Psychological Medicine*, **19**, 611–625.

Matson Evaluation of Social Skills with Youngsters (MESSY)

The MESSY is a teacher questionnaire designed to assess the development and decline of appropriate and inappropriate social skills (both verbal and nonverbal) in children. It can be used with children with borderline to mild levels of learning disability, and may have limited use in children with moderate learning disability. To measure social skills in children with severe to profound learning disability, the Matson Evaluation of Social Skills with Youngsters with Severe Retardation (MESSIER) should be employed. The MESSY has been used with children with autism; it can also be used to measure change during the treatment process.

The MESSY consists of 64 items, which are divided into two factors: Factor 1, "Inappropriate Assertiveness/Impulsiveness", and Factor 2, "Appropriate Social Skills". Behaviour is rated on a five-point Likert scale, with 1 being "not at all" and 5 being "very much". The reliability and validity of the MESSY have been established.

REFERENCES

Bell-Dolan DJ, Allan WD (1998) 'Assessing elementary school children's social skills: Evaluation of the parent version of the Matson Evaluation of Social Skills with Youngsters.' *Psychological Assessment*, **10**, 140–148.
Matson JL, Rotatori AF, Helsel WJ (1985) 'Development of a rating scale to measure social skills in children: The Matson Evaluation of Social Skills with Youngsters.' *Psychopharmacology Bulletin*, **21**, 855–896.
Matson JL, Compton LS, Sevin JA (1991) 'Comparison and item analysis of the MESSY for autistic and normal children.' *Research in Developmental Disabilities*, **12**, 361–369.
Matson JL, Carlsle CB, Bamburg JW (1998) 'The convergent validity of the Matson Evaluation of Social Skills for Individuals with Severe Retardation (MESSIER).' *Research in Developmental Disabilities*, **19**, 493–500.

Matson Evaluation of Social Skills in Persons with Severe Retardation (MESSIER)

The MESSIER is a relatively new schedule in the field of learning disability. It is designed to assess social strengths and weaknesses in people with severe to profound learning disability, providing the clinician with a profile of positive and negative social skills and maladaptive behaviour. The schedule consists of 85 items that are rated on a four-point Likert scale; 0 indicates "never", a score of 1 is "rarely", 2 is "sometimes", and 3 is "often". The items on the MESSIER are grouped into six subscales: (1) Positive Verbal; (2) Positive Non-verbal; (3) Positive General; (4) Negative Verbal; (5) Negative Non-verbal; and (6) General Negative.

The schedule is derived from clinical experience of working in developmental disabilities. The items were derived from lists formulated by professionals and also from a survey of common instruments used in the field. Reliability of the MESSIER has been established. It has good concurrent validity with the Socialization domain of the Vineland Adaptive Behavior Scales.

REFERENCES

Matson JL (1995) *Manual for the Matson Evaluation of Social Skills in Persons with Severe Retardation (MESSIER).* Baton Rouge, LA: Scientific Publishers.
Matson JL, Carlsle CB, Bamburg JW (1998) 'The convergent validity of the Matson Evaluation of Social Skills for Individuals with Severe Retardation (MESSIER).' *Research in Developmental Disabilities,* **19**, 493–500.

Motivational Assessment Scale (MAS)

The MAS is designed to measure the functions of self-injurious behaviour in adolescents and adults with moderate to profound levels of learning disability. The schedule has 16 items that measure sensory consequences, escape, attention and tangible consequences of self-injurious behaviour. Behaviour is rated by an informant on a seven-point Likert rating scale, ranging from 0 to 6. A high score on any of the subscales is indicative that the identified variables may be responsible for maintaining the self-injurious behaviour. Reliability and validity of the MAS are good, and research indicates that it has a robust factor structure, consistently yielding four factors, although using it to measure anything but self-injurious behaviour affects the psychometrics of the instrument.

REFERENCES

Durand VM, Crimmins DB (1992) *The Motivation Assessment Scale.* Topkepa, KS: Monaco & Associates.
Emerson E, Bromley J (1995) 'The form and function of challenging behaviours.' *Journal of Intellectual Disability Research,* **39**, 388–398.
Newton JT, Sturmey P (1991) 'The Motivation Assessment Scale: inter-rater reliability and internal consistency in a British sample.' *Journal of Mental Deficiency Research,* **35**, 472–474.
Singh NN, Donatelli LS, Best A, Williams DE, Barrera FJ, Lenz MW, Landrum TJ, Ellis CR, Moe TL (1993) 'Factor structure of the Motivation Assessment Scale.' *Journal of Intellectual Disability Research,* **37**, 65–74.
Sturmey P (1994) 'Assessing the functions of aberrant behaviours: A review of psychometric instruments.' *Journal of Autism and Developmental Disorders,* **24**, 293–304.

Night Time Behaviour Questionnaire

This schedule was designed to investigate sleep problems and daytime behaviour. The schedule is derived from Simonds and Parraga's Sleep Questionnaire. The schedule is divided into five parts: Parts I and II relate to general information about the person such as medical conditions, medication, weight and alcohol intake; Part III refers to bedtime routines and specific problems with sleep; Part IV has to be completed by someone other than the individual, typically a carer, and focuses on problems observed while the individual is asleep (talking in their sleep, restlessness); and Part V concentrates on daytime behaviour problems, and is also completed by a carer. The schedule covers a comprehensive range of behaviours and would be a useful tool in the investigation of the relationship between sleep problems and the negative affect on behaviour. However, the schedule would benefit from independent research into its psychometric properties.

REFERENCES

Brylewski JE, Wiggs L (1998) 'A questionnaire survey of sleep and night-time behaviour in a community-based sample of adults with intellectual disability.' *Journal of Intellectual Disability Research*, **42**, 154–162.

Brylewski JE, Wiggs L (1999) 'Sleep problems and daytime challenging behaviour in a community-based sample of adults with intellectual disability.' *Journal of Intellectual Disability*, **43**, 504–512.

Simonds JF, Parraga H (1982) 'Prevalence of sleep disorders and sleep behaviors in children and adolescents.' *Journal of American Academy of Child Psychiatry*, **21**, 383–388.

Self-Injurious Behavior Questionnaire (SIBQ)

The SIBQ has predominantly been used in studies measuring the effects of medication in reducing the frequency of self-injury in individuals with learning disability, although it was originally designed to be a behavioural schedule. It covers four main areas: severity and frequency of self-injury and the use of physical restraint and related injuries; problem behaviour such as aggression, sleep disturbance and stereotyped behaviour; attention and conduct problems; and emotional and mood problems. The psychometric properties of the schedule are yet to be established.

REFERENCE

Schroeder SR, Rojahn J, Reese RM (1997) 'Brief report: Reliability and validity of instruments for assessing psychotropic medication effects on self-injurious behaviour in mental retardation.' *Journal of Autism and Developmental Disorders*, **27**, 89–102.

Sleep Behavior Questionnaire

This questionnaire aims to measure sleep behaviour, with a focus on movement during sleep and behaviours exhibited prior to sleep and awakening. The structure of the schedule varies, and some questions require forced choice 'Yes/No' responses or frequency ratings. Items in Part II are rated for frequency from "more than 1x week but not daily" to "less than once a month".

REFERENCES

Brylewski J, Wiggs L (1999) 'Sleep problems and daytime challenging behaviour in a community-based sample of adults with intellectual disability.' *Journal of Intellectual Disability*, **43**, 504–512.

Simonds JF, Parraga H (1982) 'Prevalence of sleep disorders and sleep behaviours in children and adolescents.' *Journal of the American Academy of Child Psychiatry*, **21**, 383–388.

Society for the Study of Behavioural Phenotypes Postal Questionnaire (SSBP)

This schedule has been developed for use in detecting cross-syndrome differences in the behaviours of children with syndromes that include learning disorder. The questions relate to behaviour and development. The schedule is very much research led, as the majority of the questions are derived from recently published work. The schedule has been used in research investigating callosal agenesis, Apert syndrome and Crouzon syndrome.

REFERENCES

O'Brien G (1991) 'Discriminatory power of the SSBP postal questionnaire demonstrated by findings for children with different types of callosal agenesis.' Paper presented at the Society for the Study of Behavioural Phenotypes Workshop. Kings Fund College, London, 20 November 1991.

Sarimski K (1994) 'Behavioural patterns and family stress in families with Apert and Crouzon syndrome children.' Paper presented at the Scientific Meeting of the Society for the Study of Behavioural Phenotypes: Fragile X Syndrome: A Model for Behavioural Enquiry. Royal Society of Medicine, London, 23–26 November 1994.

Stereotyped Behavior Scale

The Stereotyped Behavior Scale is designed to assess the frequency and type of stereotyped behaviour. The schedule itself is short in duration, compromising only 26 items. Behaviour is rated on a six-point rating scale. The schedule has good interrater and test–retest reliability. However, validity is yet to be established and the instrument would benefit from further research upon this issue. Due to its frequency-based rating scale, researchers should be cautious if using this instrument to measure change.

REFERENCE

Rojahn J, Tasse MJ, Sturmey P (1997) 'The Stereotyped Behavior Scale for adolescents and adults with mental retardation.' *American Journal on Mental Retardation*, **102**, 137–146.

Vineland Adaptive Behavior Scales (VABS)

The VABS was designed as a measure of adaptive behaviour in children and adults. The VABS is available in Survey (for screening, placement and diagnostic purposes), Expanded (for developing education and treatment plans) and Classroom versions. Behaviour is measured across four domains (communication, daily living skills, socialization, motor skill). The Survey version of the VABS additionally contains a maladaptive behaviour domain, which can only be used in children aged 5 years and over. The VABS is in interview format, and administration time is 30–60 minutes. The informant can be any primary carer who knows the child (or adult) well. The interview is semi-structured and is informant-led.

Reliability and validity are well established. Supplementary norms for children with autism are now available. The data were normed from four groups comprising verbal and nonverbal children aged under 10 years and aged 10 years and over.

REFERENCES

Carter AS, Volkmar FR, Sparrow SS, Wang J, Lord C, Dawson G, Fombonne E, Loveland K, Mesibov G, Schopler E (1998) 'The Vineland Adaptive Behavior Scales: Supplementary norms for individuals with autism.' *Journal of Autism and Developmental Disorders*, **28**, 287–302.

Clarke D (1991) 'A clinical, psychological and genetic study of Prader–Willi syndrome.' Paper presented at the Society for the Study of Behavioural Phenotypes Workshop, Kings Fund College, London, 20 November 1991.

Sparrow S, Balla D, Cicchetti D (1984) *The Vineland Adaptive Behaviour Scales: Interview Edition, Expanded Form.* Circle Pines, MN: American Guidance Service.

Sparrow S, Balla D, Cicchetti D (1984) *The Vineland Adaptive Behaviour Scales: Interview Edition, Survey Form.* Circle Pines, MN: American Guidance Service.

Sparrow S, Balla D, Cicchetti D (1985) *The Vineland Adaptive Behaviour Scales: Classroom Edition.* Circle Pines, MN: American Guidance Service.

Sparrow SS, Cicchetti, CD (1985) 'Diagnostic uses of the Vineland Adaptive Behavior Scales.' *Pediatric Psychology*, **10**, 215–225.

APPENDIX 3.4
CLINICAL FEATURES OF THE PRINCIPLE GENETIC SYNDROMES OF DISABILITY

The following table summarizes the important clinical features of the principle genetic syndromes of disability, whose management is outlined in Chapter 8. The aim is to provide an *aide-mémoire* to clinical examination and investigation. The table therefore includes findings on direct clinical examination, together with those from some of the most important specialist investigations that inform clinical management. Details of behaviour and cognition are not included. Restrictions of space do not allow the table to include details of the frequency of the occurrence of findings in the given conditions—for these, consult text entries on the individual syndromes in Chapter 8.

Syndrome	Musculoskeletal	Typical facies/head size	Neurological/ neuromuscular
Aicardi syndrome	Abnormalities of the ribs and spine, kyphoscoliosis		Agenesis of the corpus callosum, infantile spasms, epilepsy
Angelman syndrome		Elongated face with prominent jaw, wide mouth with widely spaced teeth and thin upper lip, flat occiput, midfacial hypoplasia, deep-set eyes and microcephaly	Epilepsy, delayed psychomotor development, ataxic movement, speech delay
Cockayne syndrome	Progressive kyphosis	Microcephaly, striking prematurely aged appearance	Hydrocephalus, tremor
Coffin–Lowry syndrome	Scoliosis, hyperextensible hands with lax joints	Coarse facies that become more pronounced with age	Hypotonia, epilepsy
Coffin–Siris syndrome	Absent/underdeveloped terminal phalanx, delayed skeletal development and cranial malformations	Coarse facies, microcephaly, teeth abnormalities	Hypotonia
Cornelia de Lange syndrome	Limb abnormalities: short forearms and short hands and feet, shortening of the pre- and post-axial digits	Small, upturned nose, anteverted nostrils, neat well-defined arched eyebrows that meet in the middle and may fan out laterally, long curly eyelashes, thin lips and crescent-shaped mouth, long philtrum, high arched palate and micrognathia	

94

Cardiovascular	Genitourinary/ sexual	Respiratory	Gastro- intestinal	Sensory	Other
				Severe visual defects	
		Frequent upper respiratory tract infections		Otitis media	Obesity in adulthood
				Hearing and vision impairments	Severe photosensitivity, dwarfism
		Respiratory restriction and infections, due to spinal curvatures			Small stature, disorder of connective tissue
	Undescended testes		Gastro- oesophageal abnormalities	Vision and hearing abnormalities	Delayed growth
	Undescended testes	Recurrent respiratory infection, aspiration pneumonia	Gastro- oesophageal reflux	Eye abnormalities	Low birthweight, severe growth retardation, feeding difficulties

➡

95

Syndrome	Musculoskeletal	Typical facies/head size	Neurological/ neuromuscular
Cri du chat syndrome	Poor muscle development	Round face with hypertelorism, epicanthal folds, slanting palpebral fissures, posteriorly rotated low-set ears with preauricular tags, broad flat nose, microretrognathia and microcephaly. Facial features coarsen with age	
Crouzon syndrome	Fusion of limb joints in some cases	Craniostenosis leads to microcephaly; severe midfacial deformities, variety of dental abnormalities	Seizures in a minority of affected individuals
Down syndrome		Upward- and outward-slanting eyes, epicanthus and wide nasal bridge	Hyperflexia, hypotonia
Duchenne muscular dystrophy	Degenerative atrophy of voluntary muscles, spine curvatures, joint contractures		
Fragile X syndrome		Macrocephaly, large prominent ears and long face, dental crowding	Seizures
Galactosaemia*			Motor functional abnormalities, especially cerebellar ataxia and intentiontremor in older individuals
Hypomelanosis of Ito	Asymmetric frame, with scoliosis, joint contractures, unequal bone lengths and partial or entire hemihypertrophy	Possible malformations of facial bones, macrocephaly, cleft palate, conical teeth, partial adontia, dental hypoplasia or dysplasia and defective enamel	Early-onset epilepsy, often refractory to treatment
Joubert syndrome		Triangular-shaped mouth	Absent/underdeveloped cerebellar vermis, agenesis of corpus callosum, hypotonia, ataxia, abnormal tongue movements, unstable gait
Kallman syndrome	Osteoporosis	Cleft lip and palate	Paraplegia, agenesis of olfactory lobes, cerebellar ataxia
Lesch–Nyhan syndrome	Motor delay, poor muscle control, delayed bone age	Microcephaly	Dystonic posturing, variable involuntary movements, hypotonia, seizures

*If maintained on dietary treatment; otherwise, high mortality.

Cardiovascular	Genitourinary/ sexual	Respiratory	Gastro-intestinal	Sensory	Other
Septal defects and patent ductus arteriosus	Undescended testes	Frequent respiratory infections	Gastrointestinal complications, with chronic constipation in 50% of cases	Frequent ear infections, including otitis media	Low birthweight, short stature
			Feeding difficulties	Conductive hearing loss, deformity of the middle ear and absent ear canals, corneal damage and other vision involvement	
Congenital heart disease			Gastrointestinal complications, especially upper intestinal obstruction	Glue ear; early cataract formation	Short stature, hypothyroidism
Cardiac failure, often terminal by by second or third decade		Respiratory insufficiency, and failure, terminally			
Mitral valve prolapse and other anomalies			Gastro-oesophageal reflux in infancy		Connective tissue dysplasia, failure to thrive
	Delayed puberty, reduced fertility			Cataracts	Prolonged growth period
	Occasional genital abnormalities			Corneal opacity, microphthalmia, strabismus	Characteristic hypopigmentation of skin, mottling of hair, alopecia
	Renal defects and progressive renal degeneration	Hyperventilation, hypercapnoea, sleep apnoea		Visual defects, sensitivity to touch	
Congenital heart disease	Hypogonadism, absence of natural puberty, hyposmia, renal agenesis			Anosmia and hearing difficulties	Note variable presentation of types 1 to 3, as detailed in Chapter 8
	Urinary tract infections, renal failure			Variable visual impairments	Small stature, uricaemia, severe self-mutilation, haematuria, growth retardation

➡

Syndrome	Musculoskeletal	Typical facies/head size	Neurological/ neuromuscular
Lowe syndrome	Joint swelling and hypermobility, recurrent fractures, scoliosis, arthritis	Deep-set eyes, frontal bossing, progressive facial elongation	Infantile hypotonia, seizures
Mucopoly-saccharidoses* (MPS I: Hurler, Scheie; MPS II: Hunter; MPS III: Sanfilippo; MPS IV: Morquio; MPS VI: Maroteaux–Lamy; MPS VII: Sly)	Progressive musculoskeletal problems figure highly, varying in severity from stiff, hypermobile joints and carpal tunnel syndrome to widespread myelopathy, muscle deterioration, kyphosis, compression of cervical cord and quadriplegia	Facial coarsening and thickening of facial features, with enlarged tongue and hirsutism, especially in more severe types (Hurler, Hunter, Sanfilippo, and some variants of Morquio and Sly)	Neurological degeneration in more severe cases, often terminal in first decade in Hurler and Hunter syndromes
Myotonic dystrophy (congenital)	Muscle weakness and wasting leading to muscle atrophy, muscle contractures, and talipes deformity	Facial weakness and lack of expression are characteristic	
Neuro-fibromatosis type 1 (von Recklinghausen)	Macrocephaly, scoliosis, bowing and thinning of bones	Mild hypertelorism, ptosis, downward-slanting palpebral fissures, posteriorly rotated ears	Neurofibromas may result in pressure effects, with neurological deficits
Noonan syndrome	Chest deformities, delayed bone age, skeletal abnormalities including scoliosis and kyphosis	Hypertelorism with downward-slanting palpebral fissures, arched eyebrows, low-set posteriorly rotated ears with thick helix, deeply grooved philtrum with pronounced top lip	Hypotonia
Phenyl-ketonuria**		Widely spaced teeth, microcephaly	Hypertonia, movement disorders, seizures, spasticity
Prader–Willi syndrome	Scoliosis	Flat face, prominent forehead with bitemporal narrowing, almond-shaped eyes and triangular mouth	Hypotonia

*Multi-system disorders, presentation varying according to type and severity of disorder.
**Untreated or partially treated.

Cardiovascular	Genitourinary/ sexual	Respiratory	Gastro-intestinal	Sensory	Other
	Progressive renal dysfunction, cryptorchidism	Pneumonia in later stages		Congenital cataracts, glaucoma corneal keloid	Short stature
Mild variants often show aortic or other valvular involvement; cardiac failure presents early in severe cases		Obstructive abnormalities of upper and lower respiratory tract, with frequent refractory infections in severe cases, often terminal in second or third decade, notably in Sanfillipo and Maroteaux–Lamy syndromes	In more severe and progressed cases, hepato-splenomegaly, umbilical and other hernia formation; chronic diarrhoea and progressively marked swallowing difficulties figure highly; tube feeding required in later stages, notably in Sanfillipo syndrome	Corneal clouding (Hurler, Maroteaux–Lamy, Morquio, Scheie); progressive hearing loss (Hunter, Sanfillipo)	Small stature/ delayed growth, according to severity/disease progression (Hurler, Hunter, Morquio, Maroteaux–Lamy, Sly)
Cardiomyopathy		Progressive respiratory failure secondary to muscle wasting	Progressive swallowing difficulties secondary to muscle wasting		
Hypertension			Constipation		Café-au-lait spots, cutaneous neurofibromas, short stature
Congenital heart defects are common; atrial and septal defects; hypertrophic cardiomyopathy; pulmonary stenosis	Undescended testes, delayed puberty, infertility (all males, some females)		Gastrointestinal abnormalities	Ophthalmic abnormalities, otitis media	Short/webbed neck, short stature, bleeding abnormalities, lymphatic defects
					Reduced pigmentation leading to fair skin, blonde hair, blue eyes
Hypertension associated with obesity	Incomplete puberty, infertility, hypogenitalism	Respiratory difficulties associated with obesity	Feeding difficulties in infancy progress to later insatiable overeating	Various eye abnormalities	Short stature, growth hormone deficiency, obesity, diabetes

➡

Syndrome	Musculoskeletal	Typical facies/head size	Neurological/ neuromuscular
Rett syndrome	Spine curvatures, foot deformities, joint contractures	Head growth retardation	Hypotonia, involuntary jerking/tremors, poor muscular coordination, epilepsy, hand and facial stereotypies, increasing spasticity of lower limbs with progression
Rubinstein–Taybi syndrome	Broad thumbs and toes, abnormalities of lower vertebrae leading to abnormal gait, delay in skeletal maturation, frequent fractures, abnormalities of cervical spine, hyperextensible joints	Prominent beaked nose with broad fleshy bridge, slightly malformed ears, hypertelorism, downward-slanting palpebral fissures, ptosis, thickened eyelids, heavy or highly arched eyebrows, highly arched palate with small oral opening and pouting lower lip, crowded teeth, microcephaly	Hypotonia, seizures
Sex chromosome aneuploidies:			
• Turner syndrome	Osteoporosis	Webbed neck, low posterior hairline	
• Klinefelter syndrome: 47XXY, 48XXYY, 49XXXXY	Poor muscle development	47XXY—microcephaly 48XXYY—mild macrocephaly and craniofacial dysmorphism with brachycephaly and maxillary hypoplasia	Mild neuromotor deficiency, clumsiness, hypotonia
• 47XYY			Minor neuromotor deficit
• 47XXX, 48XXXX, 49XXXXX		Microcephaly	Motor incoordination especially of fine motor movements and balance, hypotonia
Smith–Lemli–Opitz syndrome*	Toe syndactyly	Cleft palate, small tongue and micrognathia; facial capillary haemangiomas; broad nasal bridge and epicanthal folds; ptosis, strabismus, cataracts; large low-set ears; microcephaly	Severe motor retardation, CNS involvement, hypertonia
Smith–Magenis syndrome	Scoliosis	Brachycephaly, broad face and nasal bridge, flat mid-face, downward-slanting corners of the mouth with cupid's bow shape to the upper lip and anomalies of ear shape/positioning	

*Multi-system disorder with wide phenotypic variability.

Cardiovascular	Genitourinary/ sexual	Respiratory	Gastro- intestinal	Sensory	Other
		Breathing abnormalities: hyperventilation and disrupted breathing	Feeding problems, constipation		Small stature; note progressive change of presentation over time
Congenital heart defects	Urinary tract abnormalities, undescended testes	Recurrent respiratory infections	Gastro- oesophageal reflux, vomiting, constipation	Visual problems due to eye infections, cataracts, refractive errors, glaucoma; hypersensitivity to loud noise	Short stature, hirsutism, obesity
Coarctation of the aorta, hypertension in adulthood	Failure of normal pubertal development, infertility, renal abnormalities			Premature ageing of the auditory system	Short stature, broad chest with widely spaced nipples, diabetes, thyroid dysfunction
	Microgenitalism, infertility, gynaecomastia				Increased growth, especially of the legs, tall stature, obesity
					Tall stature, acceleration of leg and body growth, acne
	Slight delay in onset of puberty				Underweight, tall stature
Endocardial cushion defect and tetralogy of Fallot	Severe to complete absence of male genitalia (varies according to severity); renal (hydroplasia and microcystic kidney disease) and urinary tract malformations	Structural defects of lungs: pulmonary hypertension and small lung volume, abnormal/absent pulmonary lobation	Malformations of gastro- intestinal tract, Hirschsprung's disease, dysmotility	Cataracts	Multiple congenital anomalies involving most organs; metabolic disorder; growth deficiency
Congenital heart defects	Genitourinary abnormalities			Recurrent otitis; various eye abnormalities, predisposition to retinal detachment	Multiple congenital abnormalities, hypothyroidism, immunoglobin deficiency

➡

Syndrome	Musculoskeletal	Typical facies/head size	Neurological/ neuromuscular
Sotos syndrome	Joint laxity, foot abnormalities, advanced bone age	Round face and round high forehead, frontal bossing, prominent jaw, anteverted nares, high arched palate, antemongoloid slant of the palpebral fissures, premature eruption of the teeth and sparseness of hair	Delayed motor development, clumsiness, hypotonia
Tuberous sclerosis*		Distinctive facial angiofibromas	Epilepsy, brain involvement, sclerotic brain tumours in advanced cases
Velocardio-facial syndrome		Distinct facial dysmorphism, velopharyngeal insufficiency	Hypotonia
Williams syndrome	Skeletal anomalies including radioulnar synostosis, joint contractures, laxity and progressive impairment, gait abnormalities	Distinct 'elfin-like' face with prominent cheeks, wide and long philtrum, retroussé nose with flat nasal bridge, heavy orbital ridges, medial eyebrow flair and stellate iris pattern. Dental abnormalities including microdontia, missing teeth and enamel hypoplasia	Hypotonia in childhood, hypertonia later
Wolf–Hirschhorn syndrome	Skeletal gait abnormalities, deformities of the feet, scoliosis	Severe microcephaly, hypertelorism, highly arched eyebrows, epicanthal folds, beaked nose with a broad base, carp-shaped mouth with downturned corners, micrognathia, prominent glabella and short philtrum with cleft lip and palate, large and simple low-set ears and scalp defects	Seizures, hydrocephalus, cortical atrophy, agenesis of corpus callosum, hypotonia

*Multi-system disorder with wide phenotypic variability, according to site and extent of hamartomas.

Cardiovascular	Genitourinary/ sexual	Respiratory	Gastro- intestinal	Sensory	Other
	Delayed puberty in males	Upper respiratory tract infections, asthma	Feeding difficulties, constipation		Accelerated prenatal and infantile growth, sialorrhoea, allergies
Cardiac involvement common: rhabdomyomas	Renal involvement, especially in teenage years	Pulmonary lymphangio-leiomyomatosis		Eye involvement	Progressive degeneration not typical, but possibly reduced lifespan depending on site and extent of hamartomas
Congenital heart anomalies		Respiratory infections		Ear infections	Immune disorders, hypocalcaemia, absent/partially absent thymus gland
Cardiovascular abnormalities, cardiac murmurs, hypertension	Urinary tract abnormalities		Feeding difficulties, vomiting and constipation in early life, other gastrointestinal problems later		Short stature, hoarse voice, raised blood calcium
Cardiovascular involvement, congenital heart defects including septal defects	Dysplasia of the kidneys, simple hypoplasia and polycytosis	Respiratory complications and infections		Eye and hearing disorders including squints, conductive hearing defects, preauricular/ auricular abnormalities	Multiple congenital abnormalities, severe prenatal growth retardation and profound postnatal growth retardation

103

4

BEHAVIOURAL APPROACHES TO THE MANAGEMENT OF CHALLENGING BEHAVIOUR IN CHILDREN WITH BEHAVIOURAL PHENOTYPES OF GENETIC SYNDROMES

Kirsty R Lowe and Kirk Zimbelman

Traditionally behavioural approaches to the management of challenging behaviour have focused on its environmental associations. However, understanding challenging behaviour in persons with phenotypic expression of genetic and chromosomal syndromes often requires more of clinicians and carers* than a simple understanding of the environmental contingencies that maintain the behaviour. As O'Brien and Gillberg (2000) have observed, the majority of these syndromes produce physical distress, neurologically mediated emotional dyscontrol, sensory and perceptual impairment, distorted drives and motivation, or responses from the child's social environment that have a profound and enduring impact on behaviour. Consequently, we can understand the causes of challenging behaviour only by considering factors both internal and external to the child.

In this chapter, we provide an overview of applied behaviour analysis, focusing specifically on behaviour change techniques that can be used with children, such as those with severe learning disability and physical disabilities, who lack the linguistic or conceptual ability to benefit from cognitive behavioural therapy and similar interventions. The literature in the field of behaviour analysis is vast, and the theories and techniques of applied behaviour analysis have been developing for almost a century (*e.g.* Thorndike 1932, Skinner 1938). Readers who are interested in expanding their skills and knowledge in this field are advised to read any of a number of detailed guides to the evaluation and treatment of behaviour disorders, including those by Martin and Pear (1996) and Donnellan *et al.* (1988). Obviously, behaviour modification is but one component of a multi-element treatment model. In light of the complex and frequently resolute nature of the challenging behaviour encountered in children with genetic disorders, we outline an assessment and intervention process that takes into consideration the biological, psychological and social dimensions of challenging behaviour.

---

*For the sake of simplicity, in this chapter we use the term 'carer' to refer to anyone who routinely assists the child in meeting the demands of their environment, or anyone who mediates the child's access to reinforcement. Such people would include staff of residential facilities, teachers and parents.

Basic terminology and behaviour change

The central principle of learning theory is that we are active in our interchanges with the world. Behaviour enables us to effect changes in the environment, and the environment effects changes in our behaviour. We wake up to the sound of the alarm clock and are reinforced for working by the money we earn. We are polite to the person we want to see more of, because experience or observation of others has taught us that this will increase our level of contact with them. A child learns, in part by chance, that they gain sympathy and attention when they are injured. Thereafter, they may inflict injury on themselves to achieve this goal. A review of the basic components of learning theory will facilitate understanding of the interventions we describe subsequently in this chapter.

POSITIVE AND NEGATIVE REINFORCEMENT

Reinforcement is any event that increases the frequency of the behaviour that it follows. We emphasize that determining whether something is a reinforcer is largely an empirical endeavour. Reinforcement is defined solely with respect to its effects on behaviour. Consequently, events that would not seem reinforcing, such as being shouted at by a parent, or (as indicated above) self-injury, frequently function as reinforcement.

Positive reinforcement is an event that increases the probability of occurrence of the behaviour that it follows. Money, praise and stimulation are common examples of positive reinforcement. Money is often called a *secondary reinforcer*, because, rather than being intrinsically reinforcing, it mediates access to other reinforcers.

Negative reinforcement (sometimes confused with *punishment*) occurs when the behaviour we engage in results in the cessation or reduction of an annoying or unpleasant stimulus. Thus, we slap a mosquito bite to reduce an uncomfortable itch. Our slapping behaviour is then negatively reinforced. We raise our voice to our child or partner to gain a bit of peace and quiet. Our aggressive behaviour is negatively reinforced.

Some behaviour can at the same time be both negatively and positively reinforcing. In the example above, in addition to having shouted at a family member negatively reinforced by the ensuing removal of irritating noise, a father may find reading the sports section without distraction positively reinforcing.

CURRENT VIEWS ON PUNISHMENT

Here 'punishment' is defined as any event that decreases the probability of occurrence of the behaviour it follows (Donnellan *et al.* 1988, Martin and Pear 1996). In the 1960s and '70s punishment was frequently employed in procedures like response cost (removal of a specified amount of reinforcer following a challenging behaviour) (Weiner 1962) or time out (transferring a child from a more reinforcing to less reinforcing setting) (White *et al.* 1972). More recently, however, despite its effectiveness in some situations, punishment as a behaviour modification technique has fallen into disrepute. While still a mainstay of the criminal justice system, and a frequently employed method of behaviour modification in the majority of human relationships, punishment has unacceptable side-effects. For example, as Donnellan *et al.* (1988) note, punishment can produce social withdrawal, aggression, and emotional side-effects such as shyness. Punishment can become addictive to the

A specific and detailed *description of the problem behaviour* is essential. The carer's statement that "Julie is dreadful in the mornings!" does little to aid our understanding of what Julie is doing that is "dreadful". Our task in the interview is to encourage the carer to pinpoint and describe in some detail specific behaviours. Frequently we are faced with a variety of challenging behaviours that might be maintained by different factors. Equally often, several seemingly different challenging behaviours are maintained by the same set of factors. The following questions (adapted from Donnellan *et al.* 1988) may assist the carer in specifying the nature of the challenging behaviour.

- What does the behaviour look or sound like?
- Can the behaviour occur at a lower intensity and be OK?
- Are the episodes ongoing or discreet?
- How long does an episode last?
- Does the behaviour start at high intensity or build up?
- How does the behaviour differ from similar but non-problematic behaviour?
- When do you know that the challenging behaviour has stopped?
- How often does the behaviour occur?
- How much harm does the child's challenging behaviour cause to the child or to others?
- How much assistance is needed and by whom to control the behaviour?

The *antecedent analysis* involves a consideration of all aspects of the child's internal and external environment that might be related to the challenging behaviour. Because our learning history, and the attitudes, beliefs and expectations that result from it, affect our behaviour, the antecedent analysis will already have begun with a careful review of the child's history. A carer's perplexity regarding the antecedents of challenging behaviour is frequently reflected in statements like, "I just can't work out why she does it." Often careful questioning about possible antecedents will resolve this mystery. In some instances, the questions below will prompt the carer subsequently to observe the behaviour more carefully. We invite carers to consider possible antecedents with questions such as the following.

- What in the physical environment might be causing the behaviour?
- Where does the behaviour occur? Are there places where it does not occur?
- Are the task demands that are made on the child too difficult, or perhaps boring or irrelevant?
- Do the same things regularly occur before the behaviour (*e.g.* crying, pacing or hand wringing)?
- Can you tell when the behaviour is about to begin, or whether it will begin shortly?
- Are there possible internal causes (such as illness, sleep problems or medication changes)?
- Is the behaviour better or worse around certain carers or peers?
- Do specific types of interactions, such as criticism or requests, make the problem worse?
- Are there activities during which the behaviour is more or less likely to occur?
- Does the behaviour occur during transitions from one activity to another?

The detailed consideration of antecedents is followed by an *analysis of consequences*. Exploring what happens because of the challenging behaviour may provide insight into the *contingencies* (the relationship between the behaviour and its consequences) that maintain the behaviour. What happens because of the behaviour also provides information on the function of the behaviour. This portion of the interview needs to be conducted with considerable sensitivity. Carers, out of desperation, may have adopted punitive approaches to dealing with challenging behaviour. An empathetic, non-judgemental approach will go a long way in establishing an honest open consideration of consequences. Questions like the following can be used to structure this inquiry.

- Is the child using the behaviour to communicate something?
- What environmental changes occur because of the behaviour?
- What do others do in response to the behaviour?
- Does the challenging behaviour result in the removal of something the child does not like?
- Does the challenging behaviour result in something that the child might find rewarding?
- Might the person be engaging in the behaviour for fun?
- Does the behaviour happen during relatively quiet times (suggesting it is a form of self-stimulation)?
- Does the behaviour happen when the child believes that no one is watching?
- How have people reacted to the behaviour in the past?

A review of available records may provide some history of the challenging behaviour. Invariably, however, it is useful to discuss the *history of the behaviour* during the interview. We often pose questions like the following.

- Did the challenging behaviour begin around a significant event?
- Have there been medication changes?
- Have there been changes in the carers' lives?
- Has the behaviour been improving or getting worse?
- Does the behaviour show any predictable variation (for example cycling) over time?

As was the case when we reviewed the child's records, it is useful during the interview to *review in considerable detail previous interventions*—what has worked in the past and what has not worked? Often carers will have implemented management strategies with varying degrees of success. This 'track record' of interventions can often point the way to useful approaches to addressing the challenging behaviour. Often previous efforts may have been implemented in an inconsistent, haphazard manner, or not tried for a sufficient amount of time. You may find yourself in a position of advocating an intervention that, while superficially similar to something that the carer has tried before, is implemented more thoroughly. If you are to gain the compliance of the carer in your effort, you need to address with them how things might vary from their previous attempt at the intervention. Often you can frame such an explanation with encouragement and praise, such as "It sounds as though you were on the right track. Let's give it another go, with a few changes."

In anticipation of implementing a behavioural programme that uses positive reinforcement, you may wish to undertake a *motivational analysis*. This involves discussing with the carer, or in some instances the child, potential reinforcers. A motivational analysis might also entail determining what sort of reinforcement is currently being delivered non-contingently.

It is likely that observation, recording and administration of reinforcement will be accomplished not by the clinician, but by parents, carers or teachers. Before implementing an intervention, you will need to assess the skills and motivation of the person or persons who will in fact mediate the relationship between the child's behaviour and the reinforcement received. This *mediator analysis* is a critical component of most behavioural interventions (Martin and Pear 1996).

FACILITATING COMPLIANCE—THE MEDIATOR ANALYSIS

The literature on patient compliance with medical advice paints a dismal picture (Meichenbaum and Turk 1987). Even in the case of simple procedures like filling a prescription and taking medication as prescribed, a minority of patients comply. Compliance rates improve only marginally in the case of life-threatening illnesses. It follows that our task as clinicians is daunting. Seldom will we request assistance of carers with a task as simple as giving the child a pill, and in most cases the challenging behaviour we address will not be life-threatening.

We cannot assume compliance. Our behavioural programmes and various recommendations will probably make substantial and sustained demands on carers. We must construct our intervention programmes and present them in is such a way as to ensure that they will be followed.

In discussing the implementation of behavioural programmes in various service settings, Hastings and Remmington (1993) cite these factors that militate against compliance:
• use by programme consultants of unnecessarily technical language
• staff lacking the background knowledge and skills necessary to implement programmes
• lack of available resources
• shortages of equipment
• lack of appropriate reinforcement
• high staff turnover
• lack of support and encouragement from management to pursue programmes
• competition and contention between staff groups
• poor or absent communication between those implementing the programme.
• behaviour changes being too slow to maintain carers' enthusiasm for the programme.

A mediator analysis involves examining characteristics of the carer or their situation that will influence compliance with our recommendations and the provisions of the intervention programme. Questions to be asked or issues to consider will likely include:
• Does the carer find the challenging behaviour sufficiently irritating to be motivated to assist us in changing it?
• How much social support does the carer have?
• Are there major disruptions in the carer's life that might divert their attention from following our recommendations?
• What sort of experience has the carer had with previous professionals? Are there trust issues that need to be addressed before we offer a behavioural programme?
• Are the reinforcement schemas we propose within the carer's means?
• Can recording procedures or other facets of the programme be simplified in order to insure compliance?
• Are the recommendations we make consistent with the carer's view of the challenging behaviour? If not, have we negotiated these differences of opinion with the carer?

- Is our formulation of the challenging behaviour and the intervention we advocate consistent with the carer's cultural or religious beliefs?
- Is the carer demoralized or 'burnt out' due to the severity or chronicity of the challenging behaviour, lack of social support, or other factors?
- If a child has sufficient self-awareness and conceptual ability, might we consult them in designing the behavioural programme?

PSYCHOMETRIC TESTING

Psychometric testing might be useful in quantifying the child's level of cognitive functioning. The child's level of intellectual functioning will have implications for the nature of the re-inforcement selected, and whether the child can comprehend and be motivated by secondary reinforcers like tokens or money. Because challenging behaviour is often the result of children's inability to communicate their needs, it is imperative that we have accurate information on their level of expressive and receptive language. Consequently, an evaluation by a speech and language therapist is often indicated. Speech and language therapists can offer useful recommendations on facilitating communication, which are often sufficient to resolve the challenging behaviour.

RECORDING INFORMATION ABOUT THE CHALLENGING BEHAVIOUR

Not all information needed about the challenging behaviour can be ascertained retrospectively via interviews. Carers may be biased in their observations or recollections. When the challenging behaviour occurs frequently, or reliably, in particular settings (e.g. at mealtimes) the evaluator will likely have the opportunity to observe it directly. It might be useful for one's observations to 'sample' a range of situations in a child's life. Time sampling, for example, involves conducting observation during varying time intervals. Sampling can also occur across physical settings. Often it is useful to observe the child at times or in situations where the challenging behaviour does not occur, or occurs at a markedly lower rate.

When challenging behaviour occurs at a very low frequency, the evaluator may not have the opportunity to observe it directly. In such instances, it is more practical to employ event sampling where carers record observations of the behaviour, using a mechanism such as an *ABC chart*. ABC charts are often presented as a grid, in which the carer records information about the antecedents (A), further specifics of the challenging behaviour (B), and the consequences (C) of the behaviour. Specific questions to guide the carer's observation of the challenging behaviour can be added to the chart. For example, the clinician may suspect that the presence of a certain peer is an antecedent to the challenging behaviour, and may therefore invite carers to record whether the peer was present during an occurrence of the behaviour.

Carers invariably need some orientation to the use of an ABC chart. We have devised a handout to accompany our ABC charts that includes many of the points about antecedents, behaviour and consequences presented above. We discuss this handout with the carers before they begin to fill in the ABC chart.

Sometimes it is useful to set up a *diary* that stipulates specific antecedents, behaviours and consequences that need to be observed and recorded. One of the most widespread and useful applications of diary recording in clinical practice with children affected by genetic disorders of learning disability lies in the management of sleep disturbance. Disturbed sleep is frequently such a distressing issue in the life of the child and family that motivated and detailed compliance in recording can be anticipated. In Angelman syndrome, where there is commonly a reduction in overall sleep time, and frequent night-time awakening, a detailed sleep diary will give a clear description of the extent and nature of the problem, in terms of time spent asleep/awake. Such a record may demonstrate just how severe the index sleep problem is. In addition, however, consideration of any child's sleep should go beyond timed recording of night-time sleep. Additional information to be recorded may include: mood on waking; the time and duration of any daytime naps; activities prior to bed; and the carer's responses to night-time wakening episodes. When enlisting the cooperation of the carer in recording sleep behaviour in such a child, it is imperative that the demands on them are kept to a reasonable level. The carers also need to be informed that they are not being viewed as the cause of the child's poor sleep. Rather, the clinician should emphasize that children with this condition are predisposed to disturbed sleep. It is helpful to explore all avenues toward establishing more settled sleep, and on that basis a clinician will look for any means of optimizing the child's sleep rhythm, while also evaluating the extent to which the child is being adversely affected by lack of sleep.

Analogue assessment (confusingly referred to as *functional analysis* in some sources— *e.g.* see Martin and Pear 1996) is another technique that can be used to highlight in particular the antecedents of challenging behaviour. In analogue assessment, the evaluator creates a series of stimulus conditions, at least some of which are thought to be related to the challenging behaviour. In a series of studies, Iwata *et al.* (1990) used analogue assessment to highlight the environmental correlates of self-injurious behaviour in seven developmentally disabled children. In one condition, investigators responded to self-injury with attention (positive reinforcement). In a second condition, they withdrew from the child's presence in response to self-injury (negative reinforcement). A third condition evaluated rates of self-injury when the children were alone (positive reinforcement via self-stimulation), and in a fourth condition, the rate of self-injury was recorded during free play (control condition). Interestingly, the study indicated that self-injury occurred more frequently in the negative reinforcement condition.

Analogue assessment can be used with behaviours of lesser severity. Suppose, for example, a nonverbal child throws his shoes when his mother asks him to put them on. Analogue assessment might entail framing the request in several different ways. The evaluator might suspect that he dislikes physical contact. Consequently, his mother could be directed to request him to put on his shoes with and without physical prompting. A speech and language therapy evaluation might have indicated that he responds better to visual than to verbal instructions, so the mother could be asked to frame the request on some occasions verbally, and on other occasions by motioning for him to put on his shoes. The results may, for example, support the hypothesis that physical contact and frequent verbal commands increase the rate of aggressive behaviour.

Analogue assessment provides a degree of experimental control similar to other experimental and quasi-experimental designs. When carefully planned, this procedure can eliminate nuisance variables, thereby providing unambiguous information on the antecedents of challenging behaviour. Unfortunately, analogue assessment, like other experimental procedures, is prone to problems with external validity. Specifically, the sets of stimulus conditions we create, and the way we juxtapose them, may fail to represent the salient conditions in the child's environment. Like many experimental procedures, analogue assessment poses ethical concerns. We may find ourselves creating a set of stimulus conditions that cause distress to the child and to carers who participate in the assessment. Obviously, in planning such an assessment, careful consideration needs to be given to the child's rights, their safety, and whether the information sought can be obtained in a less intrusive manner.

Intervention strategies

Careful assessment of the chain of events associated with challenging behaviour will likely suggest the most humane and expedient method of intervention. Frequently, initial interventions will be 'reactive' in nature—their primary aim being to get the challenging behaviour under some measure of control. Subsequent interventions might then focus on more substantial and enduring changes, such as major alterations in the child's physical or social environment, or the teaching of coping skills.

MODIFICATION OF ANTECEDENTS

Often a careful assessment will reveal features of the child's physical or interpersonal environment that give rise to challenging behaviour. As we indicated previously, it is frequently more expedient and more humane to attempt to alter the environment, rather than focusing exclusively on the child's behaviour. We seek, through *environmental or ecological interventions* to change the environment to better suit the child's characteristics, needs and preferences.

Physical surroundings

Physical surroundings are a commonly overlooked antecedent to challenging behaviour. Their impact is often greatest with children who are unable to verbally communicate their needs. Carers sometimes forget that physically or learning disabled children lack the ability to alter their physical surroundings the way the rest of us do. Moreover, at times we encounter a 'one size fits all' attitude toward physical surroundings—in essence a conviction on the part of the carer that "the more stimulation the better". Often children with neurological impairment are averse to intense or changing levels of stimulation. Children with autistic features are particularly sensitive to stimulation from a variety of sources (Aarons and Gittens 1999). They derive a sense of comfort and predictability from unchanging physical surroundings, and consequently might experience changes in their physical surroundings as distracting and distressing.

An assessment may have indicated that a child with disturbed sleep wakes less during the winter than summer months. The parents may examine this further, leaving the window open on a hot summer evening and then further adapt the physical surroundings, such as placing a thermometer near the child's bed. For another child exhibiting hyperactivity, the number of toys or sources of excitement should be monitored for excess stimulation. The physical surroundings may be adapted to have a 'quiet/chill out' area/corner

Interpersonal surroundings

Most children and adults have, at least to some extent, the ability to avoid people whom they dislike and to associate with those they like. We have the ability to terminate interactions when we "need our own space". A child with intellectual and/or physical limitations frequently lacks the ability to structure their interpersonal world. Sometimes the child's challenging behaviour is a product of the child not liking the carer (or vice versa). Often the most expedient intervention involves working with carers to change their way of interacting with the child. Carers may be frustrated and demoralized by the child's challenging behaviour, and tension in their relationship with the child is a product of this frustration. In such instances, the support and structure provided by a behavioural programme can result in improvement in this critical relationship. Our efforts to change the carer's attitude toward the child might include a consideration of issues such as the following.

Expressed emotion. The adverse effect of a high degree of expressed emotion on people with psychiatric disorders is well established (Goldstein 1985, Strachan *et al.* 1986), and seems to be no less relevant in considering the adjustment of children with intellectual disability (Dossetor *et al.* 1994). A high level of negative expressed emotion is generally experienced by the child as punishment, and has all of the inherent pitfalls of punishment described above. A child sitting in a room with parents vigorously arguing can become catastrophically distressed. A child being shouted at when they struggle with a task will become agitated and less able to learn. It is useful to remind carers repeatedly to maintain a calm, matter of fact tone with children. Often efforts to assist them with the stresses of caring for an intellectually or physically disabled child will have a beneficial impact on their level of expressed emotion.

Active listening. The practice of active listening (Gordon 1970) is well integrated into literature of parenting and teaching, and is highly applicable to children with physical and intellectual limitations. When we advocate that carers use active listening we encourage them to actively infer how the child is feeling based on what s/he says or does, and to communicate this understanding to the child. Active listening accomplishes several things:
- It demonstrates to the child that their thoughts and feelings are being accepted—thereby increasing self-esteem, and decreasing their sense of isolation.
- It helps the child learn to 'own' both positive and negative emotions—rather than to deny and discount them.
- Children with a learning disability frequently lack the vocabulary to label their emotions. Active listening increases their ability to recognize and label an increasing range of emotions.

For example, a child who is overeating may respond with challenging behaviour when refused a second helping. Rather than simply be told, "You're getting no more and stop moaning!" the carer could state, "I am sorry that you are feeling hungry. You must be feeling angry that you can't get another yogurt.

'I messages'. 'I messages' are another frequently discussed communication tool in the

literature of parenting (Gordon 1970). Assuming the child has the capacity for empathy (unfortunately, not a given for many children with learning disabilities), 'I messages' focus on the effects of the child's challenging behaviour on the carer. In effect, it is left to the child to decide how to respond to that new information. 'I messages' (often contrasted with 'You messages') avoid common pitfalls in communication between carers and children such as:

- unconstructive criticism or shaming—"You ought to know better!"
- name calling—"You spoilt brat!"
- diagnosing—"You're doing that to make me angry."
- teaching—"Nice people don't do that!"

'You messages' make the child feel inadequate, reduce self-esteem and inhibit communication. 'I messages' (*e.g.* "Ouch! That really hurt me. I don't like being hit.") enable the child to see that you trust them to assume responsibility for their own behaviour.

Programmatic factors

Many of us have experienced the disillusionment, anger and frustration of working in a job that is too demanding, unrewarding or not sufficiently challenging. Unfortunately, the services we offer children with intellectual or physical limitations, whether through lack of ingenuity or lack of resources, frequently fail to provide an *optimal* amount of challenge or the opportunity for growth and development. On the one hand, children with special educational and recreational needs frequently have little if any choice of their day-to-day activities. Consequently, they may feel bored, despondent or otherwise distressed by their routine. Often, offering a child a range of meaningful choices regarding activities can diminish challenging behaviour.

On the other hand, carers at times might go overboard with providing an unrelenting array of activities. In such instances, the child can become overwhelmed with having too many choices. For example, a child with Angelman syndrome, phenotypically predisposed to a high level of arousal, will need careful attention paid to the programmatic factors that can elicit overactivity and limited attention span. It may be useful to remind carers that:

- Children with intellectual limitations have difficulty choosing between more than two alternatives.
- The very act of repeatedly making choices can be taxing on children with a learning disability.
- Children may occasionally benefit from the sort of 'down time' that many of us enjoy.

Activities schedules

It seems appropriate, when considering the issue of activities, to examine the role of an activities schedule in affording the severely learning disabled child a sense of predictability and control. Many children with learning disabilities have difficulty ordering events in time, or remembering what is coming next in their lives. Consequently, the immediate future becomes an anxiety provoking 'flight into the unknown'. Encouraging carers to formulate a simple schedule and review it frequently with the child can provide substantial security and reassurance. Particularly when the child has significant communication difficulties, speech and language therapists might provide assistance in formulating a pictorial schedule. There are a variety of icons available for illustrating pictorial schedules. With the advent of affordable digital photography, pictures of the child engaging in an activity can be used. We emphasize again that it is not incumbent on frequently overworked and under-resourced carers and parents to provide an unrelenting barrage of activities, but merely to more carefully plan, organize, and illustrate existing activities to the child. Activities schedules are integral to effective programmes for children with autism who require predictability, structure and routine.

SKILLS TEACHING

In advocating skills teaching as a method for addressing challenging behaviour, we consider a different set of antecedents. The intervention strategies discussed above target external antecedents—factors in the child's physical or interpersonal environment that give rise to challenging behaviour. With skills teaching we shift our focus to the internal antecedents of challenging behaviour—the anxiety, frustration or other distressing internal stimulation the child experiences when confronted with various events. We cannot control or modify all aspects of a child's environment; consequently, our task in part is to equip the child to deal with the world as it is. Even children with severe physical and intellectual limitations are not helpless pawns of the antecedents and consequences of their physical environment. They, like us, are often capable of acquiring skills and abilities that help them cope with the demands of living.

Shaping new behaviours

Behaviour modification technology such as forward and backward chaining (Donnellan *et al.* 1988) can be employed to teach the child a variety of functional skills. Cheseldine and Stansfield (1993) remind us how anxious children with a learning disability can be when learning a new task: "It must be like sitting your driving test every day of your life, and only having to guess whether the Highway Code has been changed but nobody had told you!" Cheseldine and Stansfield make several recommendations for teaching new skills to a child, including:

- Look for an 'entry point'—examine carefully what the child is already doing and build on existing skills and competencies.
- Teach one small step at a time.
- Give encouragement frequently.
- 'Share the task' with the child.
- Praise any approximation to the skill or behaviour you desire.

For example, a child presenting with hyperactivity may be resistant to a teacher's attempts to engage him in class work. An analogue assessment may have indicated that he has difficulty grasping a writing istrument, and his hyperactivity is more prevalent when he is engaged in tasks involving the use of a pencil. The entry point could be use of a large broad pencil, with frequent reinforcement for maintaining grip. He could be engaged in potentially intrinsically reinforcing 'games' such as writing in sand, with the teacher playing the 'game' alongside the child. The skills teaching process then continues gradually towards the development of meaningful written prose.

Functional communication training

We have already emphasized the necessity of determining the function of challenging behaviour and pointed out that often challenging behaviour is an attempt by the child to communicate their needs or preferences. Functional communication training involves teaching the child more appropriate and efficient ways of communicating their needs. Suppose a child finds the task too demanding and consequently strikes a teacher to escape the task. The child could be taught, for example, to raise a red card when they find things too difficult. Teaching communication skills has been repeatedly demonstrated to lead to reductions in challenging behaviour (Carr *et al.* 1994, Emerson 1995).

Self-regulation strategies

Skills teaching may also consist of self-regulation strategies such as anxiety management, anger management or learning how to undertake problem solving. The child with severe physical disability who becomes frustrated when they cannot open their drinks can because of fine manipulation difficulties may be taught to put the can down, use relaxation techniques, and seek assistance from a carer. The child who becomes anxious at bedtime when the carer leaves the room may learn to relax with soothing music. The carer can fade (gradually reduce) their presence while the soothing music plays so the child learns to associate the music with relaxation and calmness.

Benson (1994) describes an *anger management* training programme for people with a learning disability as having four components: *identification of feelings*, *relaxation training*, *self-instructional training* and *problem-solving skills*. In this simplified approach to anger management, three feeling states are identified: happy, sad and angry. A pictorial mood check form is used to assist in self-monitoring. A tension-release method of relaxation is taught, and following this, self-instructional coping statements are practised via role-play. Basic problem-solving skills are taught, often via role-play.

The child may be taught *tolerance skills* to enable them to cope with unpleasant tasks. Consider, for example, a child who dislikes having her hair washed and engages in self-injury and bites her mother when taken to the bathroom. First water could be associated with the idea of fun. The child could, for example, be invited to her favourite room, with her toys around her and her favourite music or video playing, and there be encouraged to explore the use of a small bucket or bowl of water. Gradually this vessel could be moved closer to the environment where the child has her hair washed and stimuli such as toys, music or video could then be faded. Clinicians familiar with behaviour therapy will recognize this approach as a variant of systematic desensitization or counter-conditioning.

Some children might benefit from being taught to use symbols, pictures or basic words as *self-help aids and prompts*. Children with intellectual limitations are to varying degrees able to engage in rule-governed behaviour. They simply have difficulty recalling the rules. Suppose, for example, a child has difficulty coping with situations that arouse anger, this being related to hyperactivity. A small pictorial wallet card could be provided illustrating the various steps in coping with anger arousing situations. Prompts can also be on audio tape. Again, this is discreet and creates a sense of novelty.

A 'solutions book' is a more elaborate version of a self-help aid or prompt. Each time the child experiences a difficult situation, what has been learned can be recorded pictorially or in writing. The child can then be encouraged to consult this collection of solutions as the need arises. One of us (KZ) developed a collection of 'solutions' for a teenager with autism of unknown aetiology. The young man was distressed by a variety of situations, mostly dealing with loud noises or unpredictable and unscheduled events in his daily routine. A separate sheet was developed to deal with each of these many circumstances. Each sheet directed him to engage in a self-calming response (deep breathing) and calming self-statements. The sheet then provided a rational for the occurrence of the unanticipated event, and suggested two or three ways that he could cope with the frustration. He had an extraordinary ability to memorize information, and therefore did not require having a book on his person. His mother reported that she could at times, when he was confronted with anxiety-arousing circumstances, hear him whispering verbatim the solutions provided. The collection of solutions resulted in a substantial reduction of anxiety-related outbursts. He also experienced a sense of increased self-esteem because of having controlled his behaviour through his own efforts.

MODIFICATION OF CONSEQUENCES—REINFORCEMENT

Having reviewed methods of reducing the occurrence of challenging behaviour by modifying antecedents, both internal and external, we now shift our focus to interventions directed at the consequences of behaviour. In this section, we summarize how reinforcement contingencies can be altered to address challenging behaviour.

The nature of reinforcement

The *reinforcement schedules* espoused by BF Skinner in the middle of the last century were discovered in research primarily with non-human species (Ferster and Skinner 1957). However, the collective experience of researchers and clinicians over the past 50 years suggests that these schedules of reinforcement are equally applicable to humans. Knowledge of the dynamics of reinforcement, including schedules of reinforcement, is imperative in understanding the development of challenging behaviour, the factors that maintain it, and the extent to which the behaviour is amenable to change. We summarize briefly the schedules of reinforcement and their implications in intervening with challenging behaviour. Donnellan *et al.* (1988) and Martin and Pear (1996) provide extensive discussion of the topic.

Reinforcement schedules can be continuous or intermittent. If we engage in *continuous reinforcement* of behaviour, we reinforce every response of the desired behaviour. Continuous reinforcement is most useful when you are trying to teach a child a new behaviour. A disadvantage of continuous reinforcement is that the sheer frequency with which it must be administered may make it too demanding in terms of time, effort or cost. In addition, behaviours that are elicited as a result of continuous reinforcement are more prone to extinction. That is to say, the child quickly ceases to engage in newly learned behaviours if reinforcement is not forthcoming.

In situations where reinforcement is being used to teach or increase behaviour, one ultimately 'thins' the reinforcement schedule, and gravitates to *intermittent reinforcement*.

Behaviour that is reinforced intermittently is more resistant to extinction. In addition, intermittent reinforcement schedules more closely resemble naturally occurring reinforcement schedules. For example, we are not paid every time we finish teaching a class, or writing a report or a letter.

Intermittent reinforcement schedules can be further divided into:

- *Ratio schedules*, where a reinforcer is given upon completion of a specified number of responses—piece workers in a factory are on a ratio schedule, reinforcement is contingent on the volume of production
- *Interval schedules*, where reinforcement is gained after a certain interval of time—most salaried employees are on an interval schedule, and provided we engage in some work during the month or fortnight, we gain monetary reinforcement at the end of the interval.

We previously indicated that determining what constitutes reinforcement for a particular child is a purely empirical endeavour. All things being equal, if the contingent presentation of a reward does not affect the target behaviour, then it is probably not a reinforcer. Consequently, relying on stock reinforcement schemas like star charts may be ineffective. The challenge to clinicians and carers is to engineer consequences for behaviour change that are reinforcing to the child. Moreover, to be effective, these consequences must be more reinforcing than those that the child currently gains by engaging in the challenging behaviour. Star charts and other intrinsically interesting recording systems have their place, but they must often be backed up by more potent primary reinforcers. Fortunately, we find in many instances that freely available responses like praise and positive attention function as potent reinforcers. Activity reinforcers are also frequently effective. They have an advantage over material reinforcers (discussed below) in that the activities can be engineered to provide useful social contacts, and enhance the child's leisure skills.

It is worth noting that interventions based on modification of antecedents and modification of consequences are not mutually exclusive. Consider, for example, a child who continually calls for her parents as she is falling asleep. Our functional analysis may have identified antecedents that can be readily modified, such as closing the window to reduce noise levels, covering with a sheet rather than a duvet in hot weather, a night light, and avoiding over-stimulation and caffeinated beverages close to bedtime. These environmental changes can be combined with providing reinforcement for the child the next morning for reducing the number of times she calls out to her parents.

In particular, children with severe intellectual disability often require immediate reinforcement. In contrast to the above examples, severely intellectually impaired children might be unable to make the connection between, for example, a change in their behaviour at bedtime, and a reward the next day. Moreover, activities and secondary reinforcers such as money might be of little value to children with severe intellectual disability. They may require positive physical contact, effusive praise, and even edible reinforcers as soon as the non-occurrence of the target behaviour is observed.

In many instances when working with a child with a severe learning disability, we may need to opt for material reinforcers. Material reinforcers will be reinforcing only if what is offered is not already freely available to the child. A 60 g bag of chocolates at the end of the week will not be rewarding if granny brings the child a 500 g bag when she visits.

A child can experience *satiation* if the same reinforcer is used for a long time. Going out for pizza on Friday night because you achieved a behavioural target may initially be reinforcing. However, children can even tire of pizza after a time. Satiation can frequently be avoided by allowing the child to choose from a menu of reinforcers. The menu can be illustrated in a variety of ways to engage the interest of the child. For example, the child could be encouraged to pick items that they have chosen to depict favourite activities, or intrinsically valuable items out of a bag. The 'grab bag' could, for example, contain a new fancy hair tie, a piece of a board game to indicate an activity that evening, a new set of paints or a favourite singalong tape.

Often it is useful to establish a token system, wherein the child can 'bank' their reinforcer and spend it on different priced items from the menu of reinforcers. Token systems tend to work best with children who have sufficient abstraction ability to grasp the connection between the token and subsequent reinforcement. However, such systems can be engineered to have increased relevance to the child. In the foregoing example, the girl having difficulty falling to sleep could be rewarded at breakfast the next morning, for falling to sleep reasonably promptly, with a picture of a Barbie doll. A specified number of these could be exchanged for Barbie items on the next weekend shopping trip.

REINFORCEMENT-BASED BEHAVIOUR CHANGE STRATEGIES

Differential Reinforcement of Other Behaviour (DRO) is a type of interval schedule, and is perhaps the most widely used reinforcement-based technique for addressing challenging behaviour. This protocol involves reinforcing the child for not engaging in the target behaviour for a specified interval, regardless of what other responses occur or do not occur during this period. Donnellan *et al.* (1988) provide the following examples:

- Sue was allowed to have a video of her choice on Saturday if she did not cut any classes the entire week.
- Tom received extra juice and time with the teacher each morning and afternoon when he did not have a tantrum.
- Alison, who responded to teasing from peers by throwing stones, could get a comic for each three days in a row without such behaviour.

A further example relates to a boy engaging in overeating. He could receive a token for each meal that he kept his intake within certain limits. On a Friday, the boy could exchange these for varyious reinforcers dependent on the number of tokens obtained. Should he be a football fan the tokens could be in the shape of a football and stuck on a chart depicting a football field with each of his favourite players being 'given' a football. The aim could be to have footballs for the entire team.

Often, challenging behaviour occurs with such frequency that it is unrealistic to expect that the child can be free of engaging in it for a specified time period. Under such circumstances, *reinforcement of low rates of the target behaviour* may be the most effective strategy. This protocol involves reinforcing the child if they keep the occurrence of the challenging behaviour below a specified frequency. For example, a child may throw his pencil case off the desk 20 times every hour. In the first instance, he may gain reinforcement for throwing the pencil case 10 times or less per hour. Gradually the criterion for reinforcement is made more stringent, to the point where the programme is converted to a DRO schedule. A child who attempts to bite his thumb every 10 seconds could be reinforced for absence of biting for 15 seconds, with this length of time to achieve reinforcement increasing.

The *reinforcement of alternative behaviours* involves the selective reinforcement of those behaviours that are topographically different from the target behaviour (Donnellan *et al.* 1988). Donnellan and her co-authors give examples of biting one's fingernails versus knitting; running around the classroom versus sitting at one's desk; and grabbing items off a shop shelf versus walking the aisles while pushing a cart with both hands. Successful learning of skills that are incompatible with the challenging behaviour should be reinforced. An example is teaching a child to finger paint as opposed to using her hands to hit her head and using the social activity and praise as reinforcers.

Extinction is another reinforcement-based procedure for decreasing challenging behaviour. Extinction involves withholding whatever reinforcement the challenging behaviour is achieving. Some practitioners discourage the use of extinction (Donnellan *et al.* 1988). Upon implementation of the procedure, there is often an extinction burst—an increase in the behaviour that is no longer being reinforced. Many carers find it difficult to tolerate this extinction burst, and therefore revert to the original pattern of reinforcement. This reversion to reinforcing the challenging behaviour in essence constitutes an intermittent reinforcement schedule. Consequently, the challenging behaviour becomes increasingly resistant to change in the future. Moreover, extinction in itself does not teach new, more appropriate behaviour. It can, however, have a dramatic effect on behaviour when paired with reinforcement of appropriate replacement behaviour. Lovaas and Simmons (1969) were able, for example, to reduce the self-injurious behaviour of three children from more than 2000 acts during the first session to no self-injurious acts in the tenth session.

Conclusions

Undertaking the assessment of and designing interventions to address challenging behaviour in children with learning disabilities, who may have a concomitant physical disability, demands more of the clinician than unreflective application of behaviour modification principles. For such children, challenging behaviour often represents a desperate plea for help. To 'hear' this plea and respond to it in the most humane (and often most expedient) fashion requires that we understand the nature of the injury or syndrome that causes the child's physical or learning disability. As indicated elsewhere in this volume, genetic syndromes often have behavioural phenotypes. Understanding these phenotypes will not only alert us to both environmental and internal causes of the child's challenging behaviour, it will also allow us to interpret these to the carer, and frame reasonable expectations about the outcome of our interventions. However, no child's behaviour can be explained completely in terms of biology. Consequently, factors we would consider important in producing challenging behaviour in any child require thorough examination. We need to assess the child's learning history, their needs and preferences, their physical environment, and the pattern of reinforcement provided by significant others. Finally, we must be realistic in terms of the demands we place on carers.

REFERENCES

Aarons M, Gittens T (1999) *The Handbook of Autism, 2nd Edn.* London: Routledge.

Benson BA, (1994) 'Anger management training: A self-control programme for persons with mild mental retardation.' *In:* Bouras N (ed) *Mental Health in Mental Retardation.* Cambridge: Cambridge University Press, pp 224–232.

Carr EG, Levin L, McConnachie G, Carlson JI, Kemp DC, Smith CE, (1994) *Communication-based Intervention for Problem Behaviour: A User's Guide for Producing Positive Change.* Baltimore: Brookes.

Chesledine S. Stansfield J (1993) *Gentle Teaching, A Guide for Carers.* University of Strathclyde, Jordanhill Campus.

Donnellan AM, LaVigna GW, Negri-Shoultz N, Fassbender LL (1988) *Progress Without Punishment: Effective Approaches for Learners with Behaviour Problems.* New York: Teachers College, Columbia University.

Dossetor DR, Nichol AR, Stretch DD, Rajkhowa SJ (1994) 'A study of expressed emotion in the parental primary carers of adolescents with intellectual impairment.' *Journal of Intellectual Disability Research,* **38,** 487–499.

Emerson E (1995) *Challenging Behaviour: Analysis and Intervention in People with Learning Disabilities.* Cambridge: Cambridge University Press.

Ferster CB, Skinner BF (1957) *Schedules of Reinforcement.* New York: Appleton-Century-Crofts.

Goldstein MJ (1985) 'Family factors that antedate the onset of schizophrenia and related disorders: The result of a fifteen year prospective longitudinal study.' *Acta Psychiatrica Scandinavica Supplement,* **319,** 7–18.

Gordon T (1970) *Parent Effectiveness Training: The No-Lose Program for Raising Responsible Children.* New York: PH Wyden.

Hastings R, Remington B (1993) 'Is there anything on? Why 'good' behavioural programmes fail. A brief review.' *Clinical Psychology Forum,* **55,** 9–11.

Iwata BA, Pace GM, Klasher MJ, Cowdery GE, Cataldo MF (1990) 'Experimental analysis, and extinction of self-injurious escape behaviour.' *Journal of Applied Behavioural Analysis,* **23,** 11–27.

Lovaas IO, Simmons JQ (1969) 'Manipulation of self-destruction in three mentally retarded children.' *Journal of Applied Behaviour Analysis,* **2,** 143–157.

Martin G, Pear J (1996) *Behaviour Modification: What It Is and How to Do It. 5th Edn.* Upper Saddle River, NJ: Prentice Hall.

Meichenbaum D, Turk DC (1987) *Facilitating Treatment Adherence: A Practitioner's Guidebook.* New York: Plenum Press.

O'Brien G, Gillberg C (2000) 'Introduction: Different disabilities, different behaviours—same management?' *In:* Gillberg C, O'Brien G (eds) *Developmental Disability and Behaviour. Clinics in Developmental Medicine No.149.* London: Mac Keith Press, pp 1–11.

Pavlov I (1927) *Conditioned Reflexes: An Investigation of the Physiological Activity of the Cerebral Cortex.* (GV Anrep, trans.) London: Oxford University Press.

Skinner BF (1938) *The Behavior of Organisms: An Experimental Analysis.* New York: Appleton-Century-Crofts.

Strachan AM, Leff JP, Goldstein MJ, Doane JA, Burtt C (1986) 'Emotional attitudes and direct communication in the families of schizophrenics: A cross-national replication.' *British Journal of Psychiatry,* **149,** 279–287.

Thonrdike EL (1932) *The Fundamentals of Learning.* New York: Teachers College, Columbia University.

Watson JB, Raynor R (1920) 'Conditioned emotional reactions.' *Journal of Experimental Psychology,* **3,** 1–14.

Weiner H (1962) 'Some effects of response-cost on human operant behaviour.' *Journal of the Experimental Analysis of Behavior,* **5,** 201–208.

White GD, Nielsen G, Johnson SM (1972) 'Timeout duration and the suppression of deviant behavior in children.' *Journal of Applied Behavior Analysis,* **5,** 111–120.

5
PHARMACOLOGICAL INTERVENTIONS

Gregory O'Brien

The clinical management of children affected by major genetic conditions of disability often entails drug therapy. This is, of course, instigated only as one part of the treatment programme, in conjunction with the other key elements of the multimodal plan. The syndrome-based accounts of management and therapy featured in Chapter 8 show how this can work in the context of the range of individual genetic conditions reviewed. As can be seen there, in clinical practice with children affected by these conditions, the clinician is often required to focus on aspects of physical and general health, rather than primarily on behaviour. Further pointers towards the incorporation of general medical and surgical interventions into cases referred for behavioural problems are also given in Chapter 8.

The present chapter is concerned with the drug treatment of behavioural phenotypes and in particular the use of those pharmacological agents that are in widespread use in psychiatric practice. These include drugs used in the treatment of a range of conditions encountered in this area of clinical practice, including pharmacotherapy for: anxiety, depression and other mood disorders; attention deficit hyperactivity disorder (ADHD); schizophrenia and related paranoid psychoses; sleep disorder; aggression; and self-injurious behaviour. The treatment of major physical problems with behavioural consequences is not within the scope of the chapter—drug therapy for epilepsy, hormone problems and other somatic problems are therefore not included here.

Applied psychopharmacology in behavioural phenotypes
Psychopharmacology is the study and application of pharmacological interventions to psychiatric disorders, including the treatment of behaviour disorders. The application of psychopharmacological agents to the treatment of children affected by behavioural phenotypes is a highly specialized endeavour, with its own set of special considerations.

1. Psychiatric Diagnosis
As emphasized throughout the present text, many of the behavioural constellations encountered in clinical practice with behavioural phenotypes do not constitute classical diagnosable psychiatric disorders. Consequently, the clinician will rightly consider whether standard approaches to drug treatment for recognized psychiatric disorders such as depression or ADHD, etc., may be readily applicable to children affected by behavioural phenotypes. However, diagnosable psychiatric disorder is relatively common among people affected by the major genetic syndromes of disability, and so there is some scope for the empirical use of those pharmacological approaches in general use in the wider population.

2. LEARNING DISABILITY

In most of the conditions with which one is concerned in this area of clinical practice, some degree of learning disability is present. This has major implications for the use of drug therapy. At a basic level, there is the pathoplastic effect of the level, or severity, of learning disability on psychiatric disorder. This effect is mediated through the individual's cognitive level, because so much of the expression of psychopathology is determined by overall intelligence and cognition. The more severely intellectually delayed is the child, the greater will be the divergence from more familiar presentations of any psychiatric disorders, and this effect operates *in addition to* the proneness of a certain condition to have its own, unique, behavioural phenotype. Clearly, as emphasized repeatedly throughout the present text, standardized testing of intellectual functioning is a fundamental element of clinical assessment, and indeed is a prerequisite to planning for drug treatment.

3. EVIDENCE-BASE

Until recently, there has been little or no evidence-base for the use of psychopharmacological agents in children affected by behavioural phenotypes. The issues cited above (1, 2) are important key considerations here. On the one hand, all of the amassed evidence for the use of pharmacology in psychiatric and behaviour disorders can be informative, giving the clinician some indicators of which agents may be useful in the treatment of such children. On the other hand, in this area of clinical practice we are frequently dealing with behaviour disorders that do not constitute diagnosable psychiatric disorders. This therefore substantially affects the relevance of the former evidence-base to the clinical management of children affected by behavioural phenotypes. Fortunately, there is now published evidence on the drug treatment of behavioural phenotypes. This recently accumulated evidence-base forms a substantial proportion of the present chapter.

4. DOSAGE

Here, the rules are simple: start low, go slow. Throughout psychopharmacological treatment of people with learning disability, the starting dose should be lower than with other patients: in most cases, half the usual recommended dose. This is done in order to minimize unwanted side-effects, particularly any sedation, movement problems, or any CNS side-effects—all of which are particularly undesirable in children with disabilities. For the same reason, incremental increases of dose should be done more slowly, increasing dose to maximal effect over twice the time that would apply in mainstream practice.

5. POLYPHARMACY

It is particularly important to avoid polypharmacy in the management of these children, especially where dealing with longer-term problems. In this respect, the clinician's first duty is to take a thorough *drug history*. This serves many purposes. At one level, issues such as the positive or negative impact of any medication used in treatment of other health problems will be identified. Drug interactions can also be minimized. In addition, a good impression will be gained of the child/family's attitude to drug treatment, which can be invaluable where one is dealing with difficult behaviour. Now and again, however, the clinician will be faced with requests to use more and more medication, especially where there has been some initial positive effect, which has subsequently apparently dissipated. In this common scenario, it is important to reappraise the child's whole situation, rather than add additional medication.

6. FORMULATION

For the most part, orthodox formulations, whether of oral or parenteral medication, will apply. However, especially where any compliance issues have arisen—and also where there are physical factors interfering with, for example, swallowing—it is occasionally necessary to explore less orthodox preparations or methods of administration. This may be something as simple as rendering the treatment more pleasurable, whether by attention to colour or taste. Any such considerations may be best worked through in close collaboration with a pharmacist.

7. COMPLIANCE

Throughout the present text, it is emphasized that the clinical management of children affected by behavioural phenotypes is most effectively carried out in the context of a partnership with the child's family and carers. This has substantial bearings on compliance, and an understanding of these issues may assist the clinician in maximizing compliance. Firstly, even more than elsewhere in practice in child health care, it can be safely assumed that drug therapy will be under adult supervision. The issue then becomes one of offering the relevant parents/carers every possible assistance and support in this endeavour, for their efforts will be the main determinants of compliance. In turn, their efforts will be all the more determined if they are fully informed of the effects of the medication in question, including side-effects. This can be quite a challenge, especially where unwanted effects have been experienced from any previous medication used. However, only a full and informed account of any likely problems will be accepted now by most parents. In doing so, it is helpful also to give detailed advice on the anticipated desirable, or positive, effects of the drug also—and especially the timing of effects. For example, careful explanation of the early effects of many antidepressants (where some mild sedation and the promotion of sleep is common within a few days) complemented by an account of the longer time taken for full effects to be apparent, will be most welcome to the informed parent, whose diligent observation and interest in the therapy will be enhanced.

8. CONSENT

In the treatment of children, consent to treatment is essentially the province of the parent/carer. However, many of the behavioural and psychiatric problems encountered in this area of practice persist into adulthood—where, also, new problems often appear. Careful consideration of the emergence or non-emergence of the capacity to consent to treatment should be given, because on the attainment of adulthood the legal structures that exist in most countries are different for children and adults who lack the capacity to consent. Essentially, the consent of parents does not carry the same force in respect of adults who cannot give consent, as it does in respect of children. Others can give their *assent*, but not consent. This places the clinician in the position of having to make therapeutic decisions on the child's behalf. Clearly, this must be done not in isolation, but in consultation. The clinician treating the growing child with learning disability does well to bear this in mind, and to explore the matter with the parents/carers and other members of the clinical management team, especially towards the transition period to adult services.

9. DECISION-MAKING: INCORPORATING DRUG TREATMENT INTO THE MULTIMODAL TREATMENT PROGRAMME

The application of psychopharmacology to the treatment of behavioural phenotypes needs to be carried out in context of the wider clinical management programme. Key issues include: when/at which point in progress to introduce drug treatment; duration of treatment/when to withdraw therapy; as well as general considerations such as selection of drug, dosage and formulation/mechanism of drug delivery. These matters are considered in greater detail in the section following.

Incorporating drug treatment into the multimodal treatment programme

INITIATING TREATMENT

The decision whether to incorporate drug treatment into a multimodal programme of management in clinical practice with children affected by behavioural phenotypes relies on a clear understanding of the nature and circumstances of the presenting problem. In general, a conservative approach to the use of medication should prevail—of course, many of the behavioural problems encountered in this area of practice do not merit treatment with psychopharmacological agents, especially problems that are brief, self-limiting, a reflection of intercurrent physical health problems, or due to some identifiable environmental or personal stressor in the child's life. On the other hand, the decision whether to commence drug treatment may sometimes be taken too late, on the basis that all other avenues should be explored first of all. It would be preferable if it were routinely possible to identify early in the clinical course just which problems would be more specifically responsive to drug treatment. Here, where a diagnosable psychiatric disorder presents, which has clear treatment implications (*e.g.* depression), then the decision to adopt psychopharmacology may be taken more readily. Also, where there presents a severe and florid behaviour that is known to be often responsive to pharmacological intervention (*e.g.* self-injury), then it is often appropriate to commence rational drug therapy promptly, rather than merely regarding psychopharmacology as a last resort. However, given the limited evidence-base in this field, and the concomitant need for a conservative approach to drug treatment to prevail, there is no simple answer to this problem.

CHOICE OF DRUG

Where pharmacological intervention in the clinical management of behavioural phenotypes focuses on a diagnosable psychiatric disorder, the choice of drug will obviously be guided by the diagnosis in question. Within many classes of drug—particularly antidepressants, neuroleptics, anxiolytics and hypnotics—wide choices of medications are now available. The individual drug selected will depend in part on the precise symptom profile of the child's disorder. For example, some antidepressants are more sedative than others, while some are more stimulating, allowing tailoring of drug according to the presence of either agitation or retardation in the presenting case. Also, among all tranquillizing drugs, including neuroleptics, anxiolytics and hypnotics, great variation in potency is apparent. This is most helpful to the clinician faced with the full range of situations in which some degree of tranquillization is warranted. This can be as mild as the tranquillization required in the treatment of children in whom some brief period of a moderate degree of calming attained by chemical means can be of immense assistance, paving the way for better performance through cooperation in some behavioural programme, towards overall clinical improvement. Such cases require only low potency mildly tranquillizing drugs. In more severe cases, such as in the treatment of aggression, more powerful preparations, particularly some of the more tranquillizing neuroleptics, are sometimes required. In all cases, drug choice will be governed substantially by side-effect profile, and more specifically by the presence in the child of any medical factors that might increase the predisposition to the latter. Overall, it is found that many of the newer psychotropics that have attained widespread use are less toxic in symptom profile, and are rapidly replacing many of the traditionally used preparations. Consequently, the more selective serotonergic reuptake inhibitors for the treatment of depression, and the atypical antipsychotics for serious psychoses and other cases requiring substantial tranquillization, are in the view of the present writer preferable to the previous generations of psychopharmacological agents, particularly in the index population, where great care has to be taken regarding side-effects.

DURATION OF TREATMENT

The duration of drug treatment will depend on various factors, not all of which will be determined by the clinician—treatment may often need to be curtailed due to any serious side-effects experienced, as well as to any issues regarding compliance in general. In addition, the type of clinical situation in which drug treatment is used will substantially inform a rational approach to duration of drug treatment, and especially decisions to withdraw medication. In general, there are three situations in which drug treatment is often incorporated into the multimodal treatment of children affected by behavioural phenotypes. Firstly, there is treatment of a diagnosable *psychiatric disorder*. Knowledge of the natural history of these disorders is a prerequisite for any clinician embarking on their treatment. Some are periodic, notably depression. The natural course of these disorders can therefore serve as the basis of attempted withdrawal of drug treatment after a period of a few months of a stable clinical picture. Other disorders, notably ADHD, are persistent. Here, treatment will be required for a period of some years; most clinicians will await the onset of puberty in the child before attempting withdrawal of stimulant medication for treatment of ADHD in a child with learning disability. Secondly, there is the treatment of *intermittent behaviour problems*, not amounting to diagnosable psychiatric disorder. This often occurs over the course of managing a child affected by, for example, autistic spectrum disorder. Periods of intense anxiety, panic or sleeplessness are not uncommon in such children. A variety of medications are commonly employed, largely empirically based. Withdrawal of any medication used for this purpose—whether an anxiolytic or hypnotic—should be initially attempted after a course of, say, around two to three weeks, indicating the close degree of active contact and follow-up required in this kind of intervention. In many cases, graded withdrawal of medication will suggest the need for a longer drug course, through some degree of relapse. But this should always be decided on the basis of demonstrable benefit, and following such attempted withdrawal. Thirdly, there are those cases where the behavioural phenotype includes some severe *persistent behaviour disorder*, such as merits longer-term drug therapy. Self-injury, sleep disturbance and aggression figure highly here, all being common problems in this area of clinical practice, having massive impact on the life of the child and family. In these situations drug treatment will, as a rule, be started only after at least one attempt has been made to apply some other intervention, most notably through behavioural approaches. It is often when these behaviours prove refractory to such interventions that drug treatment is employed. Also, in many cases, it is the detailed behavioural analysis of the problem that suggests the need for psychopharmacological intervention (see Chapter 5). In either scenario, once some degree of clinical or symptomatic improvement has been attained, it is often appropriate to reconsider the initiating of some behavioural intervention, as, once the child is in a more settled state, such approaches are likely to be more effective. The effective implementation of such a behavioural programme may then exert such sustained generalized change that an attempted withdrawal of drug treatment may be instigated.

Prescribing pharmacological treatment for behavioural phenotypes of individual syndromes

The selection and introduction of psychopharmacological agents for the treatment of behavioural phenotypes of individual genetic disorders depends on the nature of the presenting disorders. As such, much of the clinician's choice of therapy will be empirically based, derived from accumulated knowledge from general psychiatric and paediatric practice. In addition, there is now some published evidence on the rational drug treatment of some of the common and prominent problems encountered in the clinical management of behavioural phenotypes. The section following reviews the psychopharmacological treatment of some of the most common and important psychiatric and behavioural problems encountered in this area of practice. The entries are arranged according to the type of presenting psychiatric or behavioural problem. For each type of clinical problem (anxiety, ADHD, etc.) there is a brief account of the application of psychopharmacological treatment to some of the key syndromes in question.

Much of the material presented in this section is based on the collective experience of clinicians within the Society for the Study of Behavioural Phenotypes. Also, where published data have been identified on the application of specific pharmacological agents to the syndromes in question, this is referenced. For each heading, the syndromes on which published information or other prescribing guidance is available are considered separately, arranged in alphabetical order. However, once again, it is emphasized that these notes should be regarded as supplementary to diagnosis-based, empirically driven prescribing practice, which depends on the nature of the psychiatric diagnosis or behavioural problem presenting.

ANXIETY, DEPRESSION AND OTHER MOOD DISORDERS

Most cases of anxiety, depression and other mood problems encountered in clinical practice with behavioural phenotypes neither warrant nor require pharmacological intervention. However, some of the more severe cases encountered do benefit substantially from drug treatment. Importantly, prompt treatment of depression, especially, may prevent the disorder becoming persistent, and ultimately refractory to all intervention efforts. Where antidepressant medication is to be used, the newer, more selective serotonin reuptake inhibitors (SSRIs) are to be recommended, on the grounds of preferable side-effect profile, especially in this population, where any drug-induced problems in concentration, continence or coordination of movement are particularly problematic. These drugs are also helpful in the treatment of refractory anxiety, and related obsessional and phobic conditions.

Down syndrome

There is a strong suggestion in the literature that people affected by Down syndrome are prone to depression (Collacott 1993, Cooper and Collacott 1996). It has also been reported that depression may present atypically in this population, in that the clinical picture is often not one of classical depression. Obsessional behaviour in particular often figures prominently, but responds to the usual treatment modalities (Harris 1998).

Duchenne muscular dystrophy

Depression and anxiety often present over the course of this debilitating disease. Diagnosis is not always straightforward, because the motor slowing that characterizes the condition can easily result in depression being overlooked. A 'high index of suspicion' approach to diagnosing depression in this disorder is recommended. Rather than merely explaining away the individual's low mood or personal anxieties as 'understandable' reactions (which, of course, they are), it is found that appropriate antidepressant medication can, at times, be beneficial, in addition to personal and family supportive work and education regarding the future and its challenges.

Fragile X syndrome

One of the core features of the phenotype of fragile X syndrome is social anxiety, of such a degree as has been likened to autism, particularly when accompanied by marked obsessionality. In this context, a trial of SSRI antidepressant medication is warranted. When used in this context—unlike most uses of SSRI for depression, which will usually be time limited—longer-term medication may be warranted, always following a trial of withdrawal of medication. Similarly, there are reports in the literature of drug treatment of people with fragile X syndrome who have suffered from major disorders of mood stability, and who have benefitted from mood stabilizers, such as lithium carbonate or carbamazepine—again, longer-term drug treatment is indicated in such cases (Hagerman *et al.* 1994).

Phenylketonuria (PKU)

Severe anxiety and depression are among the serious psychiatric problems which present among untreated cases of PKU. Drug treatment with SSRIs may alleviate such symptoms, but any damage caused to the brain by poor dietary control cannot be reversed. However, its effects can be ameliorated by stricter dietary control. More commonly—as dietary management of PKU is the norm—it is found that even among those who do follow a strict phenylalanine-free diet, emotional difficulties such as depression and anxiety often arise, and may require either intermittent or longer-term drug therapy (Harris 1998).

Prader–Willi syndrome
Depression and major anxiety problems become more prevalent with increasing age in Prader–Willi syndrome, and respond well to SSRI medication (Harris 1998). However, the overeating in Prader–Willi syndrome is less responsive to SSRIs. This is disappointing, for in mainstream psychiatric practice the coincident overeating and mood problems that present in bulimia respond well to a combination of SSRI drug treatment and psychological therapy.

Williams syndrome
In individuals with Williams syndrome, a number of problems in social interaction occur. Poor peer relationship forming is common in affected children, but this often progresses to depression in adulthood (Davies *et al.* 1998). Any increase in proneness toward social isolation, particularly where accompanied by reduction in talk (among these characteristically loquacious individuals), and/or pronounced obsessionality, should prompt a trial of SSRI antidepressant medication, once other causes have been excluded.

ATTENTION DEFICIT HYPERACTIVITY DISORDER (ADHD)
Children with learning disability are at high risk of ADHD. Where symptoms are situation-specific or transient, drug treatment is usually not warranted. Also, it is crucial to consider carefully the concept of developmental equivalance before embarking on drug treatment—in other words, to consider whether what is being observed is a reflection of overall developmental level, and not a disorder as such. The issue here is that children with learning disability are more prone to be overactive, and to have poor concentration, and that such a picture will usually neither warrant nor benefit from medical intervention. However, in those classical cases of ADHD where the symptom profile of flitting and fleeting attention, impulsivity, restlessness, recklessness and overactive behaviour is apparent in different settings (typically, at home, at school and at play), a trial of stimulant medication is warranted.

Down syndrome
Pharmacological treatment of ADHD among children with Down syndrome figures prominently in clinical practice in behavioural phenotypes. This is to be expected: Down syndrome is the most prevalent genetic cause of learning disability, and ADHD in turn is very common among children with learning disability. Fortunately, ADHD in Down syndrome seems to be responsive to pharmaceutical intervention. For example, methylphenidate, in the usual dose range, is beneficial.

Fragile X syndrome

ADHD may require pharmacological attention in young people with fragile X syndrome, especially during adolescence when ADHD is reported to be more pronounced (Goldson and Hagerman 1992). The conventional CNS stimulants can be useful in the management of impaired attention and hyperactivity. In one series, it was found that methylphenidate had been prescribed to two-thirds of children with the syndrome (Goldson and Hagerman 1992).

Turner syndrome

In Turner syndrome, mild and specific learning problems are often complicated by attentional problems. Affected individuals often respond to a highly structured environment, with limited distractions, in order to maximize educational attainment. In some, pharmacological agents may be used: CNS stimulants such as methylphenidate are appropriate here (Harris 1998).

Velocardiofacial syndrome

The wide variety of psychiatric and behavioural symptoms that commonly present in individuals with velocardiofacial syndrome include inattention, poor socialization and concentration difficulties. This picture may often resemble ADHD. However, it is important that stimulant medications, such as methylphenidate, are *not* prescribed as these can cause particularly severe adverse reactions in velocardiofacial syndrome (Murphy *et al.* 1999, Wang *et al.* 2000).

SCHIZOPHRENIA AND RELATED PARANOID PSYCHOTIC DISORDERS

Schizophrenia and related paranoid psychotic illnesses are mainly encountered in adult practice. These disorders are not, in general, common, but they are around twice as frequent among people with learning disability than in the general population. Also, most notably where the disorder is secondary to some central neurological problem or lesion—such as occurs occasionally in tuberous sclerosis—onset in adolescence is not infrequent. Clinicians treating children affected by behavioural phenotypes should be aware of the potential development of these severe illnesses, especially perhaps in those conditions considered below (Prader–Willi, velocardiofacial syndromes). In contemporary practice, the mainstays of drug treatment of these conditions when presenting among people with learning disabilities are the newer 'atypical' antipsychotic drugs, such as amisulpride, clozapine, olanzapine, quetiapine, risperidone and sertindole, and the mood stabilizers, including lithium carbonate, carbamazepine and sodium valproate.

Prader–Willi syndrome

In common with other major psychiatric disorders such as anxiety, depression and numerous behavioural problems, paranoid psychosis becomes more prevalent with increasing age in Prader–Willi syndrome. There is good accumulated evidence of a high rate of a relatively specific psychotic illness in the syndrome, taking the form of a *cycloid psychosis* (Clarke *et al.* 1995, Boer and Clarke 1999). This unusual disorder presents with intermittent bouts of overactivity, irritability, and paranoid thinking with occasional aggressive outbursts, interspersed with periods of a withdrawn, apathetic and at times frankly depressed presentation. A trial of a mood stabilizer such as carabamazepine or valproate is probably the first line choice, as lithium is more liable to promote weight gain, which is already such a prominent problem in this condition.

Velocardiofacial syndrome
There is a high incidence of paranoid psychotic illness in velocardiofacial syndrome. The disorder typically presents in early adulthood, although careful clinical history taking often reveals that the disorder may have arisen earlier in development (Murphy *et al.* 1999). The characteristic behavioural phenotype of velocardiofacial syndrome is one in which extremes of behaviour figure highly—either withdrawn and shy, or highly disinhibited and impulsive (Wang *et al.* 2000). Given this baseline, the development of paranoid psychosis may be overlooked, until full-blown illness is present. The disorder is prone to persistence, but may respond favourably to some of the more recently introduced 'atypical' antipsychotic drugs, such as olanzapine or risperidone.

Aggression
Drug treatment of aggression is one of the most difficult and controversial issues in psychopharmacological practice. Most aggression does not warrant, let alone benefit from, drug treatment. As in the general population, aggressive acts may occur for a wide variety of reasons, including communication of anger, dislike and personal upset. In addition, there are special considerations that apply to the understanding of aggression among people with learning disabilities, such as the confusion that arises from their difficulties in understanding some of the niceties of everyday social interactions. This often results in personal upset on their part, and a coincident desire to exert their own control over situations, at times through aggressive acts. Such aggressive acts are unlikely to respond to drug treatment. It is those individuals who have some underlying treatable predisposition to aggression who are more likely to benefit from drug treatment, including those with mood problems and, in some cases, those who have such severe anger control difficulties, so much so that some element of calming through medication may be beneficial. Throughout any such endeavours, active partnership working with parents and carers is mandatory, given the controversial nature of the drug treatment of aggression.

Fragile X syndrome
People affected by fragile X syndrome are not characteristically aggressive. However, their high rates of ADHD, social anxiety and mood problems do occasionally lead to aggressive episodes. Also, as fragile X is such a common syndrome, such scenarios figure quite prominently in clinical practice in this area—as many colleagues of the present writer can attest, from bruising experience! Clearly, where ADHD underlies aggression, the problem may well be unresponsive to psychological and behavioural interventions alone, and stimulant medication may be indicated (Goldson and Hagerman 1992). SSRIs may be useful in the prevention of aggression, through the treatment of anxiety and impulsivity (Hagerman *et al.* 1994). Where aggression presents as in the context of a (bipolar type)

mood disorder, mood stabilizers, such as lithium carbonate or carbamazepine, can also be helpful. Although there are few published studies looking at the benefits of atypical antipsychotics in treating aggression in this group, anecdotal evidence suggests that they are of use. As always in this complex area of clinical practice, the use of medication should be carefully monitored, weighing up any symptomatic improvement with the various side-effects that may present—particularly where substantial doses of tranquillizing medication may be used to treat aggression.

Prader–Willi syndrome
Aggression is not a characteristic of individuals with Prader–Willi syndrome, but it does frequently present in certain situations. Many of these are food-centred, arising from the conflicts which may result from the insatiable drive to binge eating that characterizes this debilitating condition. Such scenarios will not regularly warrant psychopharmacological intervention. However, where aggression is one symptom of a more general psychiatric disorder, as is not uncommon in Prader–Willi syndrome, SSRIs, stimulants, neuroleptics and anticonvulsants have been used with some success (Harris 1998).

SELF-INJURY
Self-injury is one of the most difficult problems encountered in clinical practice with people affected by behavioural phenotypes. The disturbing and debilitating nature of this high-impact problem, and the proneness to recurrence and chronicity which is seen among some of the key syndromes of disability, regularly result in requests for medical intervention. Before embarking on any drug treatment for self-injury, careful consideration must be given to the precise type of self-injury, and any determinants discernible in the child's immediate environment (see Chapter 3). Objective measurement is important, especially in monitoring progress over the course of therapy. It is equally important to be frank and realistic in setting treatment targets, especially where the behaviour has already become persistent, or may even be entrenched. Most clinicians use a wide variety of psychopharmacological agents in their attempts to alleviate or reduce self-injury, which should always be carried out in association with other therapeutic inputs. Consideration of the site, nature, severity, topography, determinants and previous treatment history of self-injury in the individual case will guide the clinician's prescribing. One of the most widely used drugs in this area is the opiate antagonist, naltrexone, a trial of which is always warranted in more severe or refractory cases. One attraction of this drug is that, rather as in stimulant drug treatment of ADHD, an early response will be seen in those cases that do respond favourably. Other drug treatment of self-injury aims to reduce the behaviour by alleviating underlying anxiety, mood problems or other psychiatric symptoms, or by general calming effects: it is consequently important in such cases to avoid oversedation.

Cornelia de Lange syndrome
The self-injury of Cornelia de Lange syndrome can be severe and refractory, requiring careful multimodal management (see Chapter 8). Unfortunately, pharmacological intervention does not appear to be useful in most cases, although a substantial minority (reported in one

published series to be one-third) seem to respond favourably to naltrexone, SSRIs and atypical antipsychotics (Berney *et al.* 1999).

Lesch–Nyhan syndrome
Self-injurious behaviour is a primary feature of this syndrome: self-mutilation particularly affects the fingers and mouth. Vigorous concerted efforts are required by all concerned to reduce self-inflicted injuries, including behavioural therapy and restraint in addition to psychopharmacology. The most widely used pharmacological interventions are naltrexone and benzodiazapines (Saito and Takashima 2000), although SSRIs have also been found to be beneficial.

Prader–Willi syndrome
The most commonly observed pattern of self-injury in individuals with Prader–Willi syndrome has a characteristic quality, most aptly described as 'skin-picking'. There is no specific drug treatment known to be particularly helpful in alleviating this variant of self-injury; SSRI antidepressant drugs, stimulants, neuroleptics and anticonvulsants are all routinely used, the actual choice of drug depending largely on any coincident psychiatric or behavioural symptoms, and of course physician choice (Harris 1998).

SLEEP DISORDER
Clinicians who maintain regular contact with children who suffer from sleep disorder become keenly aware of the enormous impact of disrupted sleep on the whole family, and on the child's development. Requests for drug treatment of sleep problems are therefore common in clinical practice with children affected by a wide range of disabling conditions. In addressing such requests, the clinician is well-advised to consider carefully the need or relevance of drug treatment. In some cases, simple measures such as close attention to parental limit-setting may suffice. However, often, in the cases referred for disrupted sleep in this area of practice, drug treatment may be warranted, if only for the sake of an exhausted family. Drug treatment of disrupted sleep may concentrate on an underlying cause, such as epilepsy or a mood or anxiety problem: in any of these situations the drug of choice will depend on the underlying disorder. Where the sleep disorder is more circumscribed, melatonin is emerging as a most useful medication to promote sleep. Often, a short course (two weeks) may be sufficient to establish sleep pattern, after which the drug may be withdrawn.

Caution is to be exercised in the use of more conventional hypnotics, particularly benzodiazepines. In general, these drugs are rarely preferable to melatonin for the promotion if sleep, in the opinion of the present writer. Side-effects are common, and habituation—with the resultant well-recognized spiral of ever-increasing dosage—is a major drawback in their use. Some children may respond well to benzodiazepine hypnotics, but drug withdrawal is a major problem. For these reasons, melatonin is emerging as the hypnotic of choice in this area of clinical practice.

Angelman syndrome
Attention to sleep disorder in children with Angelman syndrome requires close attention

to epilepsy control. In addition, a characteristic pattern of sleep disturbance is seen, consisting of difficulty in the initiation and maintenance of sleep. Unfortunately (for the parents and carers concerned) it does seem that children with Angelman syndrome require less sleep than do other children. This has led to trials of intervention on a behavioural and pharmacological basis. While the prime pharmacological consideration is attention to epilepsy, there is evidence that melatonin treatment is of benefit in Angelman syndrome (Zhdanova *et al.* 1999).

Mucopolysaccharidoses
A variety of sleep problems present among children affected by the mucopolysaccharidoses, including night-time awakening due to sleep apnoea in Hurler and Hunter syndromes, and a range of disruptive night-time behaviours such as chewing the bedclothes, crying out during the night, and, more rarely, wandering around the family home at night, in children with Sanfilippo syndrome. Any underlying causes, including breathing difficulties, may be the focus of treatment. Unfortunately, medication to induce sleep is reported to have inconsistent effects among children with these disorders (Colville and Bax 2001).

Smith–Lemli–Opitz syndrome
Around 70% of individuals with Smith–Lemli–Opitz syndrome have sleep disturbances. Sleep disorders in this condition are reported to be particularly difficult to treat, and appear not to respond to sedatives (Tierney *et al.* 2001).

Smith–Magenis syndrome
Sleep disturbance is common in Smith–Magenis syndrome, and takes a number of forms including difficulty getting to sleep, frequent awakenings, early rising and reduced rapid eye movement sleep. Melatonin has been successfully used to treat sleep disturbance in Smith–Magenis syndrome (Potocki *et al.* 2000)

Conclusion
In some respects, the most rational conclusion regarding the application of psychopharmacology to children affected by behavioural phenotypes might be, "when in doubt, don't do it." The lack of a clear evidence-base, justifiable concerns over side-effects and the unconvincing experience of many—clinicians and families alike—serve as cautions to the clinician considering the use of drug treatment in many of these situations and conditions. That being said, there are few more rewarding experiences in clinical practice than witnessing a case 'turn around' and dramatically improve, through the alleviation of some crippling severe behaviour disorder. On that basis, and given a family motivated to embark on a course of therapy, "when in doubt, don't do it" should be tempered with "when encouraged, do."

REFERENCES

Colville G, Bax M (2001) 'Sleep disorders in children with mucopolysaccharidosis.' *In:*.Stores G (ed) *Sleep Disturbance in Children and Adolescents with Disorders of Development. Clinics in Developmental Medicine No. 155.* London: Mac Keith Press, pp 73–79.

Berney TP, Ireland M, Burn J (1999) 'Behavioural phenotype of Cornelia de Lange syndrome.' *Archives of Disease in Childhood*, **81**, 333–336.

Boer H, Clarke D (1999) 'Development and behaviour in genetic syndromes: Prader–Willi syndrome.' *Journal of Applied Research in Intellectual Disabilities*, **12**, 296–301.

Clarke DJ, Boer H, Webb T (1995) 'Genetic and behavioural aspects of Prader–Willi syndrome: A review with a translation of the original paper.' *Mental Handicap Research*, **8**, 38–53.

Collacott RA (1993) 'Down's syndrome.' *Current Opinion in Psychiatry*, **6**, 650–654.

Cooper SA, Collacott RA (1996) 'Depression in adults with learning disabilities: a critical review.' *Irish Journal of Psychological Medicine*, **13**, 105–113.

Davies M, Udwin O, Howlin P (1998) 'Adults with Williams syndrome. Preliminary study of social, emotional and behavioural difficulties.' *British Journal of Psychiatry*, **172**, 273–276.

Harris JC (1998) *Developmental Neuropsychiatry, Vol. II: Assessment, Diagnosis and Treatment of Developmental Disorders.* Oxford: Oxford University Press.

Goldson E., Hagerman RJ (1992) 'The fragile X syndrome.' *Developmental Medicine and Child Neurology*, **34**, 826–832.

Hagerman RJ, Wilson P, Staley LW, Lang KA, Fan T, Uhlhorn C, Jewell-Smart S, Hull C, Drisko J, Flom K (1994) 'Evaluation of school children at high risk for fragile X syndrome utilizing buccal cell FMR-1 testing.' *American Journal of Medical Genetics*, **51**, 474–481.

Murphy KC, Jones LA, Owen MJ (1999) 'High rates of schizophrenia in adults with velo-cardio-facial syndrome.' *Archives of General Psychiatry*, **56**, 940–945.

Potocki L, Glaze D, Tan DX, Park SS, Kashork CD, Shaffer LG, Reiter RJ, Lupski JR (2000) 'Circadian rhythm abnormalities of melatonin in Smith–Magenis syndrome.' *Journal of Medical Genetics*, **37**, 428–433.

Saito Y, Takashima S (2000) 'Neurotransmitter changes in the pathophysiology of Lesch–Nyhan syndrome.' Brain and Development, **22**, S122–S131.

Tierney E, Nwokoro NA, Porter FD, Freund LS, Ghuman JK, Kelley RI (2001) 'Behavior phenotype in the RSH/Smith–Lemli–Opitz syndrome.' *American Journal of Medical Genetics*, **98**, 191–200.

Wang PP, Woodin MF, Kreps-Falk R, Moss EM (2000) 'Research on behavioral phenotypes: velocardiofacial syndrome (deletion 22q11.2).' *Developmental Medicine and Child Neurology*, **42**, 422–427.

Zhdanova IV, Wurtman RJ, Wagstaff J (1999) 'Effects of a low dose of melatonin on sleep in children with Angelman syndrome.' *Journal of Pediatric Endocrinology and Metabolism*, **12**, 57–67.

6
BEHAVIORAL PHENOTYPES AND EDUCATIONAL PRACTICE: THE UNREALIZED CONNECTION

Robert M Hodapp and Leila A Ricci

To paraphrase Charles Dickens, now is both the best of times and the worst of times concerning interest in behavioral phenotypes.

It is the best of times in that researchers are increasingly appreciating that different genetic mental retardation disorders might differentially affect behavior. Such growing awareness has resulted in etiology-related books (this volume; O'Brien and Yule 1995, Dykens *et al.* 2000), societies (Society for the Study of Behavioural Phenotypes), conferences (1996 Gatlinburg conference on "Genetics and Developmental Disabilities"), and special journal issues (Dykens 2001).

However, now could also be considered the worst of times for interest in behavioral phenotypes. Despite better understanding of the behavioral outcomes of different genetic disorders, such knowledge has yet to reach most practitioners who work every day with children and adults with developmental disabilities. Nowhere is this researcher–practitioner divide more pronounced than within special education. Surveying the past five years of *Exceptional Children* and the *Journal of Special Education*, the USA's two main special education journals, only one research article (Powell *et al.* 1997) compared behavior in different etiological groups (see Hodapp and Fidler 1999). Although British-based journals may be slightly better (Hodapp and Dykens 1994), in both countries few behavioral articles examine behavior in children with different genetic mental retardation disorders.

Similarly, when asked directly, few special educators have knowledge of any genetic disorder apart from Down syndrome. In two studies, only about 50% of teachers were familiar with fragile X syndrome (Wilson and Mazzocco 1993, York *et al.* 1999). In addition, only about 5% of teachers had even heard of Williams syndrome (Wilson and Mazzocco 1993). Although this lack of knowledge may be changing slowly, most special educators still know little about the behavioral aspects of most genetic mental retardation disorders.

Why don't special educators know more about the behaviors of these children? Our sense is that such inattention to etiology is due to certain factors both within and outside of special education itself. This chapter thus focuses mainly on examples of etiology-related educational interventions, issues involved in using such "aptitude by treatment" approaches, and five principles involved in using etiology-based educational interventions. Before discussing such issues, however, we first examine factors that might be causing this "best of times, worst of times" situation within the field of special education.

Factors causing special education's knowledge–practice divide
Despite current publicity about the revolutionary advances in human genetics, most special educators are wary of the implications of genetic disorders for the children that they teach. Their concerns arise from three sources.

UNDERLYING PHILOSOPHY
Although overly simplistic, human development can be divided into factors related to "nature" versus "nurture"; in terms of their basic philosophical orientation, those studying human development can be similarly divided. By choice, teachers are "nurture people". That is, their concerns are with how one can make a portion of the environment—educational practice—better for all children. Indeed, the teaching profession essentially involves manipulating the environments in which children learn.

In addition to this more general philosophical orientation, one must also consider certain historical—and recent—portrayals of genetics. Historically, the field of genetics has been associated with conservative, social Darwinian views of human development. The most extreme cases involved the early 20th century reports of the Jukes and the Kallikaks, with their ideas that genes totally determine intelligence over successive generations (see Scheerenberger, 1983). Recent books such as *The Bell Curve* (Herrnstein and Murray 1994) have again asserted that genes determine intelligence. Such strongly held views of genetic determinism contradict everything that the teaching profession stands for.

Ironically, modern day behavior geneticists repudiate such views. Their studies find that approximately 50% of the variation in human intelligence is due to genetics and 50% is due to the environment (Plomin 1999). In addition, intelligence may consist of several (somewhat interrelated) skills and to say that a human characteristic is "genetic" does not mean that it is unchangeable (Plomin 1999). Although each of these lessons is obvious to today's behavior geneticists, their importance is underappreciated by many special educators.

THE SPECIAL EDUCATION FIELD
A second reason for the research–practice divide directly concerns special education itself. Although in most Western countries a child must be diagnosed with an identified problem to receive special education services, most special educators are apprehensive about labeling students. In recent years, this de-emphasis on labeling has led to non-categorical programming, the practice of teaching together children with many different types of disabilities (Reynolds 1990). The idea is that a "category"—or label—is rarely helpful in the educational process and that different types of children can therefore be educated together. Forness and Kavale (1994) have worried that, even if several disabilities do benefit from distinct educational approaches, we could approach the unwieldy situation of many groups requiring their own, specialized classrooms. Such a "Balkanization" of special education services would cause administrative nightmares for schools, teachers and districts.

Although we too are against unnecessary labeling or the Balkanization of special education, we argue that it may often help to intervene differently with children who have a particular etiology. To understand this argument, however, we must first address the ways in which genetic disorders affect behavior.

Particularly when discussing genetic mental retardation disorders, how do genes affect behavior? Although this issue is neither simple nor settled, several principles now seem certain. First, genetic disorders seem probabilistic, not determinative, in their effects (Dykens 1995). It will therefore rarely be the case that every person with a particular genetic disorder will show that disorder's "characteristic" behavior(s). Many more persons with, say, Prader–Willi syndrome, will show severe overeating (hyperphagia), but even here some exceptional individuals do exist.

Similarly, not every genetic disorder will result in a unique behavior or behaviors. Granted, certain genetic disorders do result in unique behaviors in most individuals. Prader–Willi syndrome is the sole disorder characterized by extreme hyperphagia; Lesch–Nyhan syndrome the sole disorder in which individuals are predisposed to such extreme self-injurious behaviors. More commonly, however, several different genetic disorders lead to a single outcome (Hodapp 1997). Among genetic mental retardation disorders, this pattern of "several roads to a single endpoint" is illustrated when boys with fragile X syndrome and children with 5p– syndrome both show higher-than-usual rates of hyperactivity (Dykens *et al.* 1994; Dykens and Clarke 1997). Summarizing this idea, Opitz (1985) notes that "The causes are many, but the final common developmental pathways are few."

Given these two principles, how should we define the term "behavioral phenotype"? We here follow Dykens' (1995) definition, noting that a behavioral phenotype involves "the heightened *probability* or *likelihood* that people with a given syndrome will exhibit certain behavioral and developmental sequelae relative to those without the syndrome." Compared to others with mental retardation, children with 5p– syndrome (or fragile X syndrome) are more likely to be hyperactive, those with Prader–Willi syndrome are more likely to show hyperphagia. A behavior may be either unique to one syndrome (*e.g.* hyperphagia in Prader–Willi syndrome) or shared with one or more additional syndromes (hyperactivity in 5p– and fragile X syndromes). In either case, though, the behavior in question is more often demonstrated in those with a particular syndrome versus groups with mental retardation in general.

Using behavioral phenotypes in special education

As interventions for maladaptive behavior/psychopathology are discussed elsewhere (Chapters 4, 5; see also Dykens and Hodapp 1997, Dykens *et al.* 2000), we therefore focus only on the educational implications of etiology-related cognitive–linguistic profiles. Our coverage is also limited to such highly researched disorders as Down, Prader–Willi, fragile X and Williams syndromes. We present below, then, merely a blueprint for how certain specific intellectual strengths/weaknesses might be used in intervention efforts.

Even as the nature of human intelligence continues to be debated, today's IQ tests have advanced greatly from earlier measures. Modern-day intelligence tests use various theories to determine a child's specific intellectual strengths and weaknesses; indeed, theory-based intelligence tests may constitute the greatest development within intelligence tests of the past two decades (Sparrow and Davis 2000).

Prominent among these theory-based tests is the Kaufman Assessment Battery for Children, or K-ABC (Kaufman and Kaufman 1983). Derived from Luria's (1980) neuropsychological perspective on intelligence, the K-ABC distinguishes between cognitive tasks involving simultaneous processing versus those requiring sequential processing. Simultaneous processing involves integration and synthesis of stimuli as a unified whole, and sequential processing involves consecutive, step-by-step order in problem solving (Das *et al.* 1975, Kaufman *et al.* 1984). Using this distinction, the K-ABC test is designed for children aged 2.5–12.5 years, but can also be used with older children with mental retardation.

In several studies, K-ABC profiles of children with fragile X syndrome and with Prader–Willi syndrome show that these individuals have a particular weakness in sequential processing and a relative strength in simultaneous processing (Dykens *et al.* 1987, 1992; Kemper *et al.* 1988; Powell *et al.* 1997). Thus, teens and young adults with Prader–Willi syndrome (and boys with fragile X syndrome) have special difficulties with sequential tasks such as imitating in order a series of hand movements and recalling a series of spoken digits. In contrast, these individuals do reasonably well on tasks requiring them to identify an entire picture from an incomplete drawing. Moreover, this relative weakness in sequential versus simultaneous processing is not shown by children with Down syndrome (Pueschel *et al.* 1986, Hodapp *et al.* 1992), nor by children with heterogeneous causes for their mental retardation (Naglieri 1985, Obrzut *et al.* 1987).

In differentiating between simultaneous and sequential learners, teachers first must be aware that the sequential processing deficits may lead to difficulties in specific areas. Thus, children with fragile X or Prader–Willi syndromes are likely to have difficulty with phonics and decoding words; breaking down math or science problems into their component parts; interpreting the parts or features of a design or drawing; understanding the rules of a game; following oral instructions; and remembering specific details and the sequence of a story. As extreme cases of "simultaneous learners", children with fragile X and Prader–Willi syndromes should find difficult any such task that involves dealing with information presented in a temporal or step-by-step manner.

In contrast, simultaneous learners should show relative strengths when dealing with a different set of tasks. Presenting different interventions based upon whether a student is a "simultaneous learner" or a "sequential learner", the *Kaufman Sequential or Simultaneous? (K-SOS)* (Kaufman *et al.* 1984) notes that simultaneous processing strengths may result in better sight word recognition; understanding overall math or science principles using concrete, hands-on materials; and using diagrams, maps or charts. Whenever the material is presented all at once, in a single, Gestalt-like manner, performance should be relatively high.

Kaufman *et al.* (1984) suggest three general guidelines for teaching "simultaneous learners" such as children with fragile X or Prader–Willi syndromes. First, teachers should present the overall concept or question before asking the child to solve a problem or engage in a task. Second, teachers should help children to visualize what is to be learned through the use of visual cues, directions, and memory strategies. And third, teachers should attempt to make tasks as concrete as possible, with manipulative materials, pictures, models,

TABLE 6.1
Examples of "simultaneous" teaching approaches

	Instructional objective	
Phonics	*Practicing subtraction*	*Learning a memory strategy*
• Students trace letters with fingers on paper and in air • Students close eyes and picture letters • Students think of things shaped like letters • Teacher moves to linguistic patterns, such as "at"; asks students to find patterns in words (cat, bat, hat) • Teacher focuses on sight words by placing them on cards; students make words with manipulatives	• Teacher presents concept of subtraction visually and concretely • Teacher gives students set of cubes on colored paper; students count and write down number of cubes • Teacher calls out numbers, asks children to remove number of cubes from their set and count remaining cubes • Students create subtraction sentences • Students close eyes and teacher removes a certain number of cubes from their sets; students open eyes and create more subtraction sentences	• Teacher introduces visualization as a memory strategy • Teacher asks students to close their eyes, tells a short story, and students try to visualize scene • Teacher asks about what students pictured in their minds, has students draw pictures or use props to represent the scene they imagined • Teacher tells students to try to "see" information in their minds as a way of remembering it

*Based on information provided by Kaukman *et al.* (1984).

diagrams and graphs. Table 6.1 gives examples of possible educational interventions for simultaneous learners. By emphasizing the relative simultaneous processing strength of children with fragile X and Prader–Willi syndromes, special educators may maximize student learning, and avoid the frustration students may experience when presented with instruction requiring high levels of sequential processing.

VISUAL OVER AUDITORY PROCESSING IN DOWN SYNDROME

A second example concerns Down syndrome. Children with Down syndrome display a different cognitive–linguistic profile, one that can also be linked to promising educational interventions. First, these children tend to have weak language skills. Grammatically, they often have difficulty using sentences with relative clauses, embedded clauses, and other sophisticated structures (Fowler 1990). Children with Down syndrome often display poor articulation, with most parents (95%) reporting that their child has some trouble being understood by others when speaking (Kumin 1994). Weaker expressive versus receptive language abilities are also often seen in children with Down syndrome, who generally comprehend more language than they can produce (Miller 1999).

Additionally, children with Down syndrome display relative strengths in visual versus auditory short-term memory (McDade and Adler 1980, Marcell and Armstrong 1982). Children with Down syndrome perform much better on the visual than the auditory subtests of the K-ABC (Pueschel *et al.* 1987, Hodapp *et al.* 1992), and this visual-over-auditory pattern is also seen on short-term memory subtests of the Stanford–Binet IV (Hodapp *et al.* 1999).

Rather than relying on their weaker auditory channel, children with Down syndrome might benefit most when information is presented visually. By pairing auditory input with visual cues (pictures, graphs), teachers can ensure that children with Down syndrome comprehend more content and circumvent their auditory processing and memory deficits (Laws *et al.* 1995).

Given both their weak expressive language skills and visual processing strengths, Sue Buckley (1995, 1999) and her colleagues have for many years promoted reading instruction for children with Down syndrome. In a study comparing 24 children with Down syndrome to a group of typical children who were average readers, Byrne *et al.* (1995) found that the children with Down syndrome had uneven cognitive profiles, with relatively advanced reading skills. In contrast, typically developing children scored significantly higher on all assessments except for reading, showing that children with Down syndrome can sometimes read at close to age-appropriate levels. Compared to non-readers with the syndrome, children with Down syndrome who were readers performed better on tests of receptive vocabulary, receptive grammar, auditory memory, and visual memory (Buckley 1999).

During the preschool years, reading instruction may even constitute a "way in" to language for children with Down syndrome (Buckley 1995). In following the progress of 15 preschool children for three years, Buckley (1985) found that the majority of children with Down syndrome could read single words by 3 or 4 years of age and sometimes earlier. This early reading instruction also had several benefits for the children's speech and language. Specifically, Buckley (1985) argued that (a) the new words learned from flashcards soon emerged in the children's speech; (b) two- or three-word utterances in reading helped accelerate similar utterances in speech; (c) reading proper sentences led to the use of function words and correct grammar and syntax in speech; (d) early reading instruction resulted in literacy attainments close to the children's chronological age; and (e) reading practice improved phonology and articulation in children with Down syndrome. Although each of these conclusions must be considered as tentative, it does appear that reading instruction is promising for children with Down syndrome.

In teaching reading to young children with Down syndrome, Buckley begins teaching a small sight vocabulary of familiar words printed in lower case on flashcards (Laws *et al.* 1995). Children learn to match words and pictures by playing matching games with flashcards, then to select the appropriate card when the word is spoken, and finally to "name" or read the word on the card (Buckley 1995). Because children are introduced to short written sentences early in this reading process, they practice using sentences in everyday speech to improve their grammar and expressive language skills.

Once children can read about 50 words through this whole-word approach, the teacher begins to point out letter–sound correspondences in the words the children can already read. By teaching letter–sound relationships and the phonetic components of words in this manner, educators can begin to develop phonological knowledge in children with Down syndrome.

LINGUISTIC OVER VISUOSPATIAL PROCESSING IN WILLIAMS SYNDROME

In contrast to children with Down syndrome, children with Williams syndrome often show high levels of such linguistic skills as vocabulary, grammar and storytelling (Bellugi *et al.* 1994). Although some early reports hinted that such skills were even at age-appropriate levels, such does not appear to be the case for most children (Mervis *et al.* 1999). Nevertheless, linguistic abilities remain a relative strength compared to other areas for most children with Williams syndrome.

In contrast to their relative strengths in language, children with Williams syndrome perform particularly poorly on tasks involving visuospatial abilities (Udwin *et al.* 1987, Udwin and Yule 1990). They seem unable to draw integrated figures, and such low-level performance may involve either dissociation ("seeing either the forest or the trees"—Bihrle *et al.* 1989) or extreme delays in acquiring visuospatial abilities (Dykens *et al.* 2001). In either case, visuospatial tasks seem particularly difficult for these children.

Educationally, it may prove beneficial to use verbal language to teach a wide variety of tasks to these children (for teaching methods for "linguistically intelligent" children, see Armstrong 1994). These children should benefit from educational tasks involving telling stories and playing word and rhyming games. Tasks such as "show and tell", group discussions, and other public, verbal tasks should also prove useful (Dykens and Hodapp 1997). In contrast to children with, say, Down syndrome, those with Williams syndrome may respond best to phonetic approaches to reading; an emphasis on letter–sound correspondences may be easier for these children than whole-word (*i.e.* primarily visual) approaches (Dykens *et al.* 2001). Given the musical strengths of many children with Williams syndrome (Lenhoff 1998), it may also be possible to use music in many educational interventions.

In addition to pronounced linguistic strengths and visuospatial weaknesses, children with Williams syndrome have also been described as friendly and outgoing. Dykens and Rosner (1999) report that parents considered almost all (100%) of their children with Williams syndrome as "kindspirited", 94% were caring, and 90% sought the company of others. At the same time, however, 76% had few friends, 67% were highly sensitive to rejection (Dykens and Rosner 1999), and 73–79% were considered to be unreserved or overly friendly with strangers (Udwin 1990, Gosch and Pankau 1994). Although such a "hypersocial" and indiscriminately friendly orientation can be problematic (Davies *et al.* 1990), teachers can capitalize on such personality traits by having children participate in cooperative learning groups, role playing, and "acting out" academic content. Using linguistic, musical and social interventions, many school-related tasks can be taught to the child with Williams syndrome.

THEORETICAL ISSUES IN APTITUDE–TREATMENT INTERACTIONS

Although etiology-based educational approaches seem promising, several issues remain unexplored. The first involves the very idea that the child's existing strengths and weaknesses can be linked to one or more specific intervention approaches. Indeed, throughout our discussions so far, we have implicitly advocated this so-called "aptitude × treatment interaction (ATI) approach. Common in medicine and psychiatry, the ATI approach holds that individuals with a particular aptitude respond better to one treatment, while those with a different aptitude will respond better to a second therapy (Smith and Sechrest 1991). Aptitudes can consist of one's age, gender, IQ, specifics of personality or psychopathology, or general reaction to medications. In the case of the education of children with genetic mental retardation syndromes, aptitudes consist of etiology-related cognitive–linguistic profiles.

Although appealing, ATIs have not always been easy to document in clinical psychology (Smith and Sechrest 1991), education (Braden and Kratochwill, 1997), or special education (Gresham and Witt 1997). Many workers have referred to ATIs as "elusive", something often searched for—but only occasionally found—in the relevant studies. As Gresham and Witt (1997) note, "Although the ATI approach has almost undeniable logical attractiveness, there is little evidence for the existence of significant ATIs in the school psychology and special education literatures."

Do ATIs not exist, or do we not yet know how to find them? A host of factors may mitigate against seeing ATIs that in fact exist. ATIs might be missed because we know too little about how to assess student cognitive abilities, or because tests have inadequate technical characteristics (Fuchs and Fuchs 1986). We may not know enough about the actual interactions that take place between students and teachers within any intervention program, or even whether teachers followed the intervention program as specified (*i.e.* treatment fidelity). In many ATI studies, the link between profile (*i.e.* the child's aptitude) and specific treatment is also unclear; in others, "groups" have so much within-group heterogeneity that it seems unlikely that a single specified intervention could be beneficial for the entire group. As Speece (1990) asks, are ATIs a bad idea or have they simply been given a bad rap?

Although controversial, we feel that ATIs may nevertheless constitute a promising approach when intervening with children with several different genetic syndromes. In addition to more specific, targeted interventions arising from etiology-related profiles, two aspects of aptitude in several genetic syndromes seem instructive.

PREVALENCE AND MAGNITUDE OF PROFILES IN CERTAIN SYNDROMES
In contrast to the profiles described above for fragile X and Prader–Willi syndromes, typically developing children less frequently show large discrepancies between sequential and simultaneous abilities. In examining ATIs in 117 first- and second-grade typically developing children, Ayres *et al.* (1988) found that only 24 (20.5%) were considered to be "sequential learners" (*i.e.* >12 point difference across domains) and 20 (17%) were defined as "simultaneous learners". Similarly, Good *et al.* (1993) reported that non-retarded "sequential learners" showed average standard scores of 135 in Sequential Processing, but also averaged 116 in their Simultaneous Processing scores. Conversely, simultaneous learners, though higher in Simultaneous Processing (X = 134), also exhibited fairly good Sequential Processing skills (X = 109). Although Good *et al.* (1993) showed no benefits in matching the child's aptitude (sequential *vs* simultaneous learner) to a specific treatment (sequential *vs* simultaneous), each group already performed well on *both* sequential and simultaneous processing tasks.

Similar issues arise when one examines children with mental retardation due to mixed or heterogeneous causes. In two studies, groups of school-aged children with heterogeneous mental retardation showed almost identical scores on K-ABC Sequential Processing and

Simultaneous Processing domains. In Naglieri (1985), children's standard scores on Sequential Processing averaged 67.2, while the average standard score in Simultaneous Processing was 67.7. In Obrzut *et al.* (1987), Sequential Processing and Simultaneous Processing scale scores were 72.38 and 72.79, respectively. Although neither study mentioned the percentage of simultaneous or sequential learners, it seems that few children showed extreme discrepancies in either direction.

In contrast, etiology-related profiles seem much more common and the profiles themselves are often more pronounced. In examining the K-ABC profiles of boys and young men with fragile X syndrome, Dykens *et al.* (1987) found that all 14 subjects showed advantages of one year or more in Simultaneous over Sequential Processing age-equivalent scores. On average, Simultaneous Processing age-equivalent scores were over two years higher than Sequential Processing age-equivalents (5.60 versus 3.31 years, respectively). Similarly, among teens and young adults with Prader–Willi syndrome, average age-equivalent scores were almost two years advanced in Simultaneous Processing versus Sequential Processing (7.10 years *vs* 5.29 years) (Dykens *et al.* 1992).

Similarly large discrepancies (affecting most children) are also found in etiology-related intellectual profiles of both Down syndrome and Williams syndrome. Using the K-ABC with children with Down syndrome, Hodapp *et al.* (1992) noted average differences of about two years between visual subtests such as Hand Movements (X = 5.58 years) and Gestalt Closure (5.40 years) compared to auditory subtests such as Number Recall (3.18 years) and Word Order (3.75 years). Similar results for children with Down syndrome were found for visual versus auditory subtests of the Stanford–Binet IV (Hodapp *et al.* 1999). In children with Williams syndrome, weaknesses—especially in visuospatial processing—are also particularly weak relative to linguistic strengths (Bellugi *et al.* 1999).

INTENSIFICATION OF PROFILES WITH INCREASING AGE

Within several genetic syndromes, cognitive–linguistic profiles seem to intensify with increasing chronological age, such that pre-existing strengths become more pronounced relative to weaknesses. Given the salience and intensification with age of these cognitive–linguistic profiles, one might definitely consider "playing to the child's strengths" in any educational intervention.

To date, examples of intensifying profiles can be found in fragile X, Down and Williams syndromes. In males with fragile X syndrome, Hodapp *et al.* (1991) noted that, among children below age 11, K-ABC age-equivalent scores in Sequential Processing were already below those of both Simultaneous Processing and Achievement. After age 11, such discrepancies widened even further. As shown in Figure 6.1, if one makes a "V" with the age-equivalent scores of Simultaneous Processing (a relative strength in this group), Sequential Processing (a relative weakness), and Achievement (a relative strength), the V becomes more "V-like" in older compared to younger males. Longitudinal analyses showed similar findings, with some younger—and no older—children showing Sequential Processing advances over a one-year span.

A similar phenomenon can be seen in the visual over auditory advantage in Down syndrome. Comparing older versus younger children with Down syndrome, average scores of

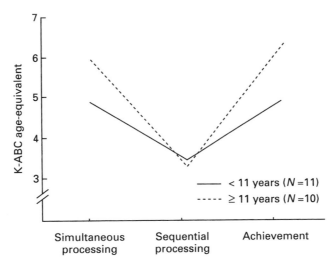

Fig. 6.1. Average levels of simultaneous processing, sequential processing and achievement for younger (up to 11 years) vs older (over 11 years) males with fragile X syndrome. (Reproduced by permission from Hodapp *et al.* 1991.)

TABLE 6.2
Intellectual profile in Down syndrome: changes with age*

| Age-group | N | Age-equivalents | | Average difference (years) | Individuals with ≥0.5 year difference |
		Bead memory (years)	Sentence memory (years)		
5 to <10	11	3.04	2.73	0.31	4/11
10 to <15	20	3.74	3.08	0.66	12/20
15 to 21	12	4.94	3.42	1.52	9/12

*Data from Hodapp *et al.* (1999).

the visual memory task on the Stanford–Binet IV (Bead Memory) become increasingly advanced over scores on the auditory memory task (Memory for Sentences). Also with increasing age, greater percentages of the Down syndrome group showed extreme (*i.e.* six months or more) advantages of visual over auditory abilities (Table 6.2). Similar findings have recently been reported for linguistic versus visuospatial skills in children with Williams syndrome (Bellugi *et al.* 1999). In each syndrome, as the child gets older strengths continue developing, weaknesses stay the same or develop less rapidly, and the contrast between strengths and weaknesses becomes increasingly pronounced.

We realize that, as children get older, educational or other interventions could be causing these more pronounced profiles. But since teachers generally lack knowledge about etiology-related behaviors (Wilson and Mazzocco 1993. York *et al.* 1999), it seems unlikely that more pronounced profiles with age are primarily due to environmental influences.

Such intensifying profiles do, however, highlight the strong predisposition of many children to their syndrome's etiology-related profiles and the possibilities of using such strong (and growing) predispositions in etiology-oriented educational interventions.

Five principles of etiology-based educational interventions

So far, we have argued that certain genetic disorders do indeed show etiology-related intellectual strengths and weaknesses. In addition, we have acknowledged the entire ATI issue, arguing that, in the case of genetic syndromes, such an approach at least deserves a try in the field of special education. We now end this chapter by presenting five general guidelines for etiology-based educational interventions.

1. PLAY TO THE CHILD'S STRENGTHS

When considering how cognitive–linguistic profiles might be used in educational practice, one might either try to ameliorate the weak areas or capitalize on the strong ones. Our sense is that one does better by playing to the child's strengths, thereby avoiding the use of strategies that conflict with what may be most natural for children with a particular disorder.

Playing to the child's strengths might also be wise because many cognitive–linguistic strengths transcend particular contents per se. For example, using the distinction between simultaneous and sequential processing, Kaufman *et al.* (1984) have devised strategies to teach phonics, math, memory and other content domains. Similarly, visual abilities would generally seem to be "all-purpose" in their application, and to some extent the same could be said of linguistic versus visuospatial skills. Granted, certain skills or modalities will be easier to use for some tasks than for others. Still, using the general guideline of playing to the child's strengths, creative teachers should be able to match etiology-based strengths to specific educational interventions.

2. CAPITALIZE ON ATI LINKS THOUGHT TO HOLD FOR TYPICALLY DEVELOPING CHILDREN

Throughout this chapter, we have relied on existing, proposed links between children's aptitudes and those treatments that should work best. Educational techniques that should help any simultaneous learner have been applied to boys with fragile X syndrome and to children with Prader–Willi syndrome. Similarly, we have looked for examples of teaching strategies employing visual or language-based interventions for typically developing children.

Our approach has therefore had little to do with mental retardation per se. Instead, we have assumed that most children with Prader–Willi syndrome or fragile X syndrome will learn in the same way as any typically developing child who is a simultaneous learner. Similarly, children with Down syndrome should be similar educationally to any visual learner, and children with Williams syndrome will be similar to any linguistic learner. Obviously, the level of instruction may need to be lower and certain modifications may at times be necessary. Generally, however, those ATI links proposed for typical children should work well for children with each of these genetic disorders.

3. Consider Etiology-Oriented ATI Connections as General, not Individual, Guides

Because genetic disorders are probabilistic in their behavioral effects (Dykens 1995), only some children will show any disorder's "characteristic" behaviors. Thus, not every child with Down syndrome will prove to be a visual learner, not every child with Prader–Willi or fragile X syndrome will show the simultaneous over sequential pattern, and not every child with Williams syndrome will show linguistic strengths.

For our purposes, within-group variation shows the limits of current etiology-oriented educational approaches. On a practical level, within-group variation lends a cautionary note to special educators: Even though a child has a genetic etiology that is usually linked to specific strengths or weaknesses, one still needs to examine the individual child to determine that child's profile. Etiology-based approaches therefore provide general educational guidelines, a set of activities and ways of looking at teaching that should be useful for most—not all—children with a specific genetic disorder.

4. Consider an Intervention as Useful for Children with any Syndrome Showing the Profile

Since there are many genetic causes but few behavioral outcomes (Opitz 1985, Hodapp 1997), children with several genetic etiologies may benefit from a single intervention approach. Most children with Prader–Willi syndrome may benefit from the K-SOS recommendations for simultaneous learners, but so too should such recommendations apply to boys with fragile X syndrome. Since children in each group show evidence of being simultaneous learners, for these educational approaches the two groups should be considered identically.

Inevitably, teachers will be forced to mix-and-match their educational strategies when working with children with different etiologies. To take the example of Prader–Willi and fragile X syndromes, educational techniques focusing on simultaneous processing should be useful for both groups, but recommendations will diverge when issues arise concerning food and temper tantrums (for Prader–Willi syndrome) or eye contact (for boys with fragile X syndrome). Etiology-based educational recommendations will thus involve combining various strategies to address the issues at hand.

5. Examine Whether Etiology-Based ATIs Exist in Specific Genetic Etiologies

Although we present examples of etiology-related cognitive–linguistic profiles and how such profiles might relate to targeted intervention efforts, we realize just how little we know about educating children with different genetic mental retardation syndromes. Even more troubling are the findings that, with typically developing children, ATIs using the K-ABC have often not been found, and such potential ATIs as those involving visual or linguistic strengths have never even been examined.

Conclusion

The job ahead, then, is to test whether seemingly reasonable educational interventions are, in fact, efficacious. Movement from "it should work" to "it does work" is gaining ground in such fields as medicine, clinical psychology, psychiatry and school psychology (Stoiber and Kratochwill 2000). Following this drive toward "empirically supported interventions", etiology-based workers in special education must do their part to determine whether these seemingly reasonable educational interventions are indeed more effective for children with specific etiologies. Granted, such intervention studies are labor-intensive, time-consuming and difficult to design, but only by performing such studies will we be able to effectively help children with different mental retardation syndromes. Only then will we have realized the potential connection between etiology and education, thereby moving our education of children with genetic disorders from the worst of times to the best of times.

ACKNOWLEDGEMENT

We would like to thank Elisabeth Dykens for her helpful comments on earlier versions of this chapter.

REFERENCES

Armstrong T (1994) *Multiple Intelligences in the Classroom.* Alexandria, VA: Association for Supervision and Curriculum Development.

Ayres RR, Cooley EJ, Severson HH (1988) 'Educational translation of the Kaufman Assessment Battery for Children: A construct validity study.' *School Psychology Review*, **17**, 113–124.

Bellugi U, Wang P, Jernigan TL (1994) 'Williams syndrome: An unusual neuropsychological profile.' *In:* Browman SH, Grafram J (eds) *Atypical Cognitive Deficits in Developmental Disorders.* Hillsdale, NJ: Erlbaum, pp 23–56.

Bellugi U, Mills D, Jernigan T, Hickok G, Galaburda A (1999) 'Linking cognition, brain structure, and brain function in Williams syndrome.' *In:* Tager-Flusberg H (ed) *Neurodevelopmental Disorders.* Cambridge, MA: MIT Press, pp 111–136.

Bihrle AM, Bellugi U, Delis D, Marks S (1989) 'Seeing either the forest or the trees: Dissociation in visuospatial processing.' *Brain Cognition*, **11**, 37–49.

Braden JP, Kratochwill TR (1997) 'Treatment utility of assessment: Myths and realities.' *School Psychology Review*, **26**, 475–485.

Buckley S (1985) 'Attaining basic educational skills: Reading, writing, and number.' *In:* Lane D, Stratford B (eds) *Current Approaches to Down's Syndrome: Life for the Teenager and for the Family.* London: Hot, Rinehart & Winston, pp 315–333.

Buckley S (1995) 'Teaching children with Down syndrome to read and write.' *In:* Nadel L, Rosenthal D (eds) *Down Syndrome: Living and Learning in the Community.* New York: Wiley-Liss, pp 158–169.

Buckley S (1999) 'Promoting the cognitive development of children with Down syndrome: The practical implications of recent psychological research.' *In:* Rondal JA, Perera J, Nadel L (eds) *Down's Syndrome: A Review of Current Knowledge.* London: Whurr, pp 99–110.

Byrne EA, Buckley S, MacDonald J, Bird G (1995) 'Investigating the literacy, language, and memory skills of children with Down's syndrome.' *Down's Syndrome: Research and Practice*, **3**, 53–58.

Das JP, Kirby J, Jarman RF (1975) 'Simultaneous and successive synthesis: An alternative model for cognitive abilities.' *Psychological Bulletin*, **82**, 87–103.

Davies M, Udwin O, Howlin P (1998) 'Adults with Williams syndrome: preliminary study of social, emotional and behavioural difficulties.' *British Journal of Psychiatry*, **172**, 273–276.

Dykens EM (1995) 'Measuring behavioral phenotypes: Provocations from the "new genetics".' *American Journal on Mental Retardation*, **99**, 522–532.

Dykens EM (ed) (2001) *American Journal on Mental Retardation. Special Issue: Behavioral Phenotypes of Genetic Mental Retardation Disorders*, **106** (1).

Dykens EM, Clarke DJ (1997) 'Correlates of maladaptive behavior in individuals with 5p– (cri-du-chat) syndrome.' *Developmental Medicine and Child Neurology*, **39**, 752–756.

Dykens EM, Hodapp RM (1997) 'Treatment issues in genetic mental retardation syndromes.' *Professional Psychology: Research and Practice*, **28**, 263–270.

7

COUNSELLING PARENTS AND CARERS OF INDIVIDUALS WITH BEHAVIOURAL PHENOTYPES

Jeremy Turk and Gregory O'Brien

In this chapter, we highlight some of the key principles and themes that guide our clinical work with families of people (mainly children) who are affected by behavioural phenotypes of genetic syndromes of disability.

Counselling can take many forms in clinical practice (see Turk 1996b). It may be psychoeducational, as in genetic counselling, where efforts are made to raise recipients' knowledge and understanding such that more valid and informed choices can be made regarding current and future conceptions. Much psychoeducational counselling can also now take the form of information on the nature of developmental and behavioural challenges likely to be faced by families who have a member with a genetically determined learning disability syndrome with associated characteristic behavioural features. Conversely, counselling can be psychotherapeutic as in the non-directive approaches taken when a therapist tries to facilitate the client's self-directed exploration of important yet often painful issues in order to assimilate them into a plan for future functioning and adaptation. However, psychotherapeutic counselling should also be directive, helping with problem-solving and other cognitive and behavioural approaches to developmental and behavioural challenges (Turk 1998). Some guides and literature focus on specific conditions (Contact-a-family 2002) and in so doing go into detail on specific associations. Others adopt a lifespan approach, in which they go through the various clinical problems and developmental hurdles, which might appear over the course of an individual's development, highlighting intervention needs at various key transition times and advising on specific developmental and behavioural tasks (Carr 1980, Douglas and Richman 1984). Here we have endeavoured to highlight some key principles that we find to be important in counselling families who have members with behavioural phenotypes.

Given the varying developmental and behavioural profiles and trajectories that are seen across the wide variety of syndromes under consideration, this subject does not lend itself easily to a lifespan/developmental task approach. We have therefore opted for an approach consisting of overview with examples. In this way principles and themes reviewed do not present themselves in a necessarily logical, conceptually coherent order, but more as a set of themes that inter-relate and overlap in many ways. The ideas and themes herein are therefore as varied and changing as the problems we encounter in clinical practice in behavioural phenotypes (O'Brien 2000).

What is counselling?

Counselling is a frequently used yet much misunderstood term. It can mean many different things to different people. Broadly speaking counselling can be *educational* or *psychotherapeutic*. It can be argued that in reality counselling should always contain components of both these essentials. Educational counselling can be about the cause or risk of a disorder in question as in *genetic counselling*. Increasingly, educational counselling comprises sharing of information on the developmental trends and emotional and behavioural challenges likely to be faced by individuals with a genetic condition relating to a recognized behavioural phenotype and their families. This is really one of the foundation stones of good clinical practice in the field of behavioural phenotype work. Individuals and their families are justified in wanting sympathy but are entitled to more besides, in the form of education and information about the relevant condition, its cause, recurrence risk, natural history, prognosis and therapies.

Psychotherapeutic counselling is also often referred to as *supportive psychotherapy*. This term is used to describe a 'non-directive' approach whereby the therapist tries to facilitate the client's self-exploration without imposing any direction or suggestions—a process far more difficult in reality than giving straight instruction! A number of critical 'therapist variables' have been identified which define those who are most adept at such work. These comprise emotional warmth, empathy (not just sympathy), genuineness and unconditional positive regard for the client. The development of useful, beneficial, therapeutic and non-directive reflectiveness takes training, time, effort and practice. However, awareness of the important 'nonspecific' therapeutic attributes will be useful to all clinicians.

Directive psychotherapeutic counselling requires application of more specific psychotherapeutic principles relating to one or other school of therapy, usually cognitive or behavioural, and often a combination of the two. These therapies are unashamedly directive, concerned with current problems, precipitants and perpetuating factors rather than the dim and distant past, and objective describable happenings such as punching, screaming, self-scratching, crying or mutism rather than interpretations about internal mental states such as fantasies and psychic conflicts. The cognitive components relate to ways we think about ourselves, the world, those about us and the future. Such cognitive 'schemata' or 'constructs' are crucial in dictating our appraisal of things that happen to and around us and hence our responses. This attention to often maladaptive or negative thoughts ('cognitions') can make a real difference to emotional state and behaviour. A common tendency is to appraise situations in all-or-nothing ways ('dichotomous reasoning'), for example, either "we're a happy family" or "we're a sad family". Another frequent maladaptive appraisal is to sift out only the components consistent with one's depressive perspective ('selective abstraction'), for example "OK, I've lots of friends, but she doesn't want to know me—my social life is a disaster". Bringing such automatic negative ways of thinking to the clients' attention can go a long way to helping them realize the impact their thought processes are having on their emotions and behaviour.

Behavioural phenotypes in context

There is a balance to be struck between the sharing of specific information on an individual's underlying genetic condition and associated behavioural phenotype on the one hand, and the reality that much intervention and support will be common to most individuals who have a developmental disability on the other (O'Brien 2001a). Families and professionals often have mistaken views regarding the nature of behavioural phenotypes. For example they frequently expect all people with a particular genetic disorder to show certain behavioural traits, or believe that such attributes are immutable and therefore unworthy of therapeutic intervention. Families are also often confused by the multiple labels that become attached to their relative and need help to appreciate that these labels are not mutually exclusive, but reflect different aspects of the person's developmental difficulties.

A particular behaviour in an individual who has learning disability attributable to a genetic anomaly may be explainable in terms of one or more of the following:
• the nature of the genetic abnormality (behavioural phenotype)
• a more general predisposition to having certain neurodevelopmental disorders (often autistic spectrum or attentional) as a consequence of having a genetic anomaly
• the behaviour may be appropriate and understandable in terms of the individual's developmental abilities
• the behaviour can be understood on the basis of the increased vulnerability of people with learning disability to emotional and behavioural disturbance
• the behaviour may be understandable in terms of recent (or not so recent) life events and experiences.

Families have a right to know what developmental and behavioural challenges are more likely given their relative's genetic condition. A 'wait and see' approach should no longer be accepted or tolerated. Equally it should no longer be acceptable to argue that wanting to know the cause of problems reflects individual psychopathology or a selfish lack of empathy towards the client's predicament. Nor should it be acceptable to take the view that having a diagnostic label leads to therapeutic inertia—in fact it is quite the opposite! Families also need to be counselled that such behaviours are not inevitable, and that anticipating such difficulties and preparing for them can go a long way toward minimizing their impact. Conversely, families should be reassured that the appearance of an associated behavioural tendency is not an indicator of their failure in preventative efforts. It needs to be acknowledged that certain behaviours do seem to be associated with particular genetic abnormalities, and that these clusters of associations are not random (O'Brien 1992).

'Diagnosis'
Explanation of what is meant by a diagnosis or diagnostic label is time well spent. Such a label may be:
• aetiological, *e.g.* fragile X syndrome, Down syndrome, fetal alcohol syndrome, congenital rubella
• phenomenological, *e.g.* autism, hyperactivity, self-injury, "challenging behaviour"
• descriptive of degree of intellectual impairment, *e.g.* moderate learning difficulty
• reflective of social factors, *e.g.* inadequate housing or education, abuse or neglect
• reflective of adverse interactions, *e.g.* attachment disorder, family dysfunction, marital disharmony.

Clearly there are many combinations and permutations of the above classes of variables. The greater the number, the greater the complexity of diagnosis and intervention becomes. Research supports the notion that families want to know the truth about causation sooner rather than later, and that they expect honesty and frankness from professionals (Carmichael *et al.* 1999). Nobody wants to learn of bad news—but it is a whole lot better than no news at all. Who breaks the news of a behavioural phenotype-linked condition will vary tremendously. Ideally the physician who ordered the genetic investigation or the clinical geneticist responsible for the test should undertake this. But such individuals have very varying knowledge levels, and are often reliant on rapidly outdated textbooks for their information. The same applies to educational specialists, even those working in the field of special needs (Wilson and Mazzacco 1993, York *et al.*, 1999). Thus families often receive inadequate or indeed inappropriate information on their relative's condition and its implications. The problem here is that in the early stages of recognition of a syndrome it is often the most severely affected individuals who are identified, thereby providing a distorted picture of the prevalence and nature of the associated clinical spectrum (O'Brien 1996a). This emphasizes the need for further large-scale studies on populations ascertained with the minimum of bias. For example, parents have been shocked by the descriptions of nail pulling ('onychotillomania') and object insertion into orifices ('polyembolokoilomania') said to be associated with Smith–Magenis syndrome (Colley *et al.* 1990). More recent research shows that while self-injury does seem to be over-represented in individuals with this condition, the type—or topography—of the said self-injury varies substantially, and is often not severe (Udwin *et al.* 2001). On the other hand, catastrophic sleep disturbance, marked inattentiveness and even autistic features are often witnessed, yet their presence may not raise clinical suspicions of the underlying genetic condition (Vostanis *et al.* 1994). Social and familial causative factors are more frequently considered as postulated causative agents, even to the extent of triggering suspicions of child abuse and neglect rather than biological aetiology (McNaught and Turk 1994). Furthermore, other subtle but important developmental difficulties, such as autistic features, may be overlooked (O'Brien 1996b). This is particularly the case where the already-acknowledged presence of another diagnosis, for example Down syndrome, acts to diagnostically overshadow the possibility of coexisting multiple diagnoses (Rasmussen *et al.* 2001). The presence of dual diagnoses (*e.g.* learning disability plus psychiatric disorder) has been long acknowledged. However, triple diagnoses are also common (*e.g.* learning disability plus autism plus psychiatric disorder) (Barlow and Turk 2001), and these will have a major bearing on upbringing and educational input.

Perhaps above all, it is important to attend carefully to descriptions of problems and behaviour provided by individuals and their carers. This is the basis of sound clinical practice. It is also crucially important in clarifying the nature of an individual's clinical problems—in other words, to be clear just which elements of a possible behavioural phenotype are being discussed, in this individual, at this time and in the setting concerned. Behaviours described may suggest commonly found clinical syndromes, for example hyperactivity or autism (Graham *et al.* 1999). There may be behavioural features that are suggestive of an underlying behavioural phenotype but not diagnostic, for example hand flapping in fragile X syndrome (Turk and Graham 1997) or cocktail party chatter in Williams syndrome (Gosch and Pankau 1997). Other behaviours may be more characteristic of, or specific to, one or other genetic condition—for example, gaze aversion in fragile X syndrome (Cohen *et al.* 1989), presenile Alzheimer dementia in Down syndrome (Holland *et al.* 2000) and spasmodic upper body squeeze in Smith–Magenis syndrome (Finucane *et al.* 1994) have all been described well. In addition, apparently inexplicable improvement in behaviour, demeanour and social functioning in response to a high cholesterol diet in Smith–Lemli–Opitz syndrome has recently been demonstrated (Tierney *et al.* 2001).

Listening and listing by the clinician is not just warmly welcomed by parents and carers; it is expected and indeed is critical in understanding the complex biopsychosocial interaction between neurodevelopmental predisposition and psychosocial moulding of behaviour, cognition and emotions through experience. One of the reasons for the formation of the various syndrome support societies that exist was in response to families feeling that they were *not* being listened to and believed by clinicians. Many important behavioural phenotypes have been clarified and elaborated by the initiatives of families themselves who have organized into societies, and we continue to learn ever more from families and their support societies about the behavioural phenotype syndromes displayed by their members. There is thankfully no sign of this activity abating. Listening out for new problems and new insights is as important as ever. Thus there are many reasons why a diagnosis is important (for further reflections, see Turk and Sales 1996).

In interviews and discussions with parents and carers of individuals who may be affected by behavioural phenotypes, it is important to explain that we need to know exactly which behaviours are occurring. Often, this might seem strange to parents. It may be that, in previous contexts, they merely have had to say that there has been a behaviour problem, without having to give precise details about it. Also, where a child has a difficult or florid behaviour problem—such as self-injury, or aggression or other disruptive behaviours, or a pattern of pronounced social isolation—then it may be that parents will not so readily volunteer all features of other important behaviours. Conversely, many families experience prolonged frustration at the apparent insistence of some clinical services to avoid undertaking a comprehensive detailed assessment of presenting difficulties and developmental history, preferring instead to launch rapidly into systemic discussion of family functioning. There is also an alarming tendency for some professionals to insist on downplaying some of the more negative and challenging behaviours on the basis that only positive attributes should be focused upon. Consequently, it is necessary to enter into a kind of contract with parents and carers, in which we ask them to give us details of a range of important behaviours, and in return we give our attention to the behaviours that they regard as important. Only by this means can clinicians and families cooperate and work collaboratively towards a consensus regarding diagnosis, assessment, intervention and monitoring of treatment effects. This process can be facilitated greatly by the use of structured measurement schedules, as reviewed in Chapter 6.

The need for an individualized approach
To focus on the presence of a possible phenotype and its implications is to respect clients'

individuality. It also acknowledges the need for clear and thorough appraisal and understanding of their problems. When dealing with impairments, disabilities, health problems and behaviours that present in major genetic syndromes, it has long been recognized that there is a danger of adopting too 'clinical' an approach, at the expense of neglecting the individual. In contemporary practice in developmental paediatrics, developmental psychology and psychiatry, and related educational, social and therapeutic endeavours, this is much less common than previously. Clinics and teams are now organized along much more client- and family-friendly lines. However, when discussing development and behaviour with a client's carers, it is timely to remind ourselves to involve the client as much as possible. Always assume understanding of what is being discussed by all who are present—at the very least it is a courtesy to each person at the meeting.

The need for an individualized approach extends beyond assessment to support and intervention. The highly individualistic response of many people with learning disability to a range of psychotropic medication is well documented (Matson *et al.* 2000). However, behavioural and other psychological programmes often flounder because of a lack of appreciation of the need to individualize the programme in order to maximize its personal and clinical relevance to the client and their close ones.

CASE EXAMPLES
An adolescent with autistic spectrum disorder worsened progressively in terms of challenging behaviour including stubbornness, rudeness, aggression and social withdrawal, in response to a 'programme' that involved restriction of social opportunities as a consequence of such undesired tendencies. This was based on the erroneous assumption by staff that the individual being attention-seeking always drove such behaviours. In reality the client was of course solitude seeking, in line with his autistic tendencies. Reversal of the programme so that solitude could be obtained through compliance and appropriate behaviour led to rapid and enduring improvements. Another individual yearned to be back home with her pet dog. She worked towards this by earning 'dog biscuit' shaped tokens which were collected in the form of pasting them on to a drawing of a dog food bowl on a chart—the final target caption being a picture of her home (with adjacent kennel) with the legend "Home at last!"

The importance of the family
It is critical to involve the entire family, nuclear and if possible extended, in the analysis of behavioural phenotypes. This is important for genetic as well as developmental and psychological reasons. The presence of other relevant individuals such as social worker, nurse or special teacher is also desirable—although not always easy to arrange. This illustrates why such work is often far removed from a traditional medical model of patient with one carer (usually mother) facing one clinician across a desk. In dealing with difficult behaviours, it is crucial that key carers—for example, parents, school staff, respite hostel workers—share the same insight and understanding of the behaviours, and adopt consistent, predictable and agreed-upon approaches in order to optimize development and behaviour. Often this is not a problem—many of the families who attend clinics are already motivated and ensure that they attend and comply with what has been agreed—but it is not always

Associated physical difficulties

The disabilities that present in this area of clinical practice are often multiple. Having one disability predisposes to having others. Hence when counselling families and carers of individuals affected by behavioural phenotypes, it is important not to overlook sensory impairments. These usually manifest as hearing and visual problems. They can also relate to taste, smell and touch. Screening for hearing and visual disturbances should be routine in clinical practice with children who have developmental disabilities. However, there are always those who 'slip through the net'. In addition, there is always the risk of 'diagnostic overshadowing'—that is, the tendency to attribute all difficulties to one diagnosis (*e.g.* learning disability) once it has been made. As a result common and treatable problems such as deafness and visual refractory errors are still often missed. It is frequently parents who first suggest this. Indeed, they may query diagnoses such as autism, suggesting that it is in fact hearing impairment that has caused the social and language delays. The two are of course far from being mutually exclusive. Often such an attribution reflects the parental search after meaning—to have a child with a sensory impairment may be perceived as easier to accept and understand than having a child who has autism. Such parental suggestions should always be taken seriously. Testing should always be undertaken, with specialist referral as necessary. Issues should then be worked through within the context of breaking of bad news and the associated 'grief reaction'.

Epilepsy is another common accompaniment of genetic conditions associated with behavioural phenotypes. It should always be enquired after, including specific queries regarding possible 'funny turns', inexplicable behaviours or sudden and bizarre changes in mood or demeanour. There is a raised rate of unusual forms of epilepsy in people with genetically determined learning disability. These include complex partial seizures arising from temporal lobe foci, as well as generalized absence (petit mal) epilepsy which may continue without seizure interruption (status). Sophisticated EEG techniques may be needed to clarify the complexities and to produce clear indicators as to appropriate medication.

Sources of information

Families glean much information from general support groups and agencies (*e.g.* Contact-a-family) and specific syndrome associations. They also make increasing use of internet websites. Some of these latter offer information on seemingly endless lists of conditions and possible interventions, often with quite sensationalist claims for potential cure. Increasingly, parents arrive at clinics with novel and detailed accounts of their child's condition and new treatment possibilities. Usually this is a positive development. Many such websites are developed and run by syndrome support societies and are knowledgeable and reputable. Specialist clinics and information services run many others which may or may not be government sponsored. These too are subject to peer review and provide appropriate and up to date information. Unfortunately, some other websites are less reputable and reliable. At worst, some are in effect marketing vehicles for dubious and even potentially dangerous therapeutic approaches that are unproven and rely more on sensationalist claims, pseudo-logical argument and the draw of expense rather than science. Yet others convey misleading information for other reasons, which are not always clear. The clinician's role here is to support and counsel the family in reaching rational decisions as to where and how to invest their precious mental and physical energies and financial resources to give the greatest likelihood of positive returns. To dismiss any such 'information' out of hand is futile and runs the risk of alienating the family. While time-consuming, it is important to give all such suggestions careful consideration and to explain carefully their potential significance and relevance—or lack thereof. It is equally important to guide parents toward more informative and reliable organizations and websites.

The need for collaboration

One of the hallmarks of good clinical practice and counselling in the behavioural phenotypes field is strong and enduring collaboration between the multidisciplinary professional network and the family. Joint working or settings in which a number of specialists work together are the preferred choice. Service fragmentation leads inevitably to patchy evaluation and formulation with delays in clarification of the individual's problems, their nature, origins and implications. At best such service delivery takes the form of a 'one stop shop' service. This is of overwhelming benefit where individuals have multiple complex needs covering the entire biopsychosocial spectrum. It also allows cross-fertilization of ideas and perspectives with enormous advantages for all concerned.

Part of the collaborative process is the early clarification of what evaluations have already been undertaken and what the results were. Frequently there is a need to revisit tests such as genetic analysis where technology may have progressed substantially over a short time. It is vital that trained and specialist counselling accompanies such efforts. Most, but not all, families will want to know as much detail as possible about their genetic inheritance and its implications. For some, for example where arranged marriages are the rule, such knowledge may be of greater detriment than assistance. There is an urgent need for clinicians to update themselves about the various genetic and chromosomal conditions and their consequences as well as their cultural implications. For example, there is increasing evidence that even fragile X premutations can cause clinically significant developmental, emotional and behavioural problems (Aziz *et al.* 1998). Also, sex chromosome anomalies such as Turner syndrome (El Abd *et al.* 1995) and XYY syndrome (Ratcliffe *et al.* 1991) may be responsible for substantially more developmental difficulties than are usually appreciated.

Terminology is another area bedevilled with problems, which produces challenges when communicating with clients and their families or with other professionals nationally or indeed internationally. In England and Scotland the current equivalent for the standard international term 'mental retardation' is *'learning disability'*, while in Wales, the term *'mental handicap'* is still used. These three terms are synonymous, when used in this way in these countries. However, in most nations—notably in North America—the term 'learning disability' refers to specific developmental delays such as dyslexia, dysgraphia or dyscalculia (numeracy problems). Another term gaining increasing use is *'intellectual disability'*, which refers to individuals who have an IQ under 70 from early in life. As such, it is close to the concept of learning disability/mental retardation, with one exception. Whereas learning disability/mental retardation refers to an IQ of under 70, accompanied by some social in-capacity, intellectual disability does not include from early in life the element of social

161

incapacity. Given that social incapacity is context-determined, this term has some advantages. It also probably comes closest to a useful and meaningful description of the problems experienced by such individuals. *'Developmental disability/delay'* includes all the above, and other developmental problems. It is often adopted in paediatric practice, but has the disadvantage of the inherent implicit suggestion that such difficulties will ultimately be 'grown out of'. It is not surprising then that in clinical practice many parents and fellow professionals become puzzled by our mutually confused terminology (O'Brien 2001b).

Multiple diagnoses

So far we have acknowledged the frequent coexistence of learning disability with other problems such as autistic spectrum disorders and attentional deficits. We have also touched on the fact that further simultaneous diagnoses are frequent and clinically important. High rates of depression and other mood problems are common in individuals with conditions associated with behavioural phenotypes. Parents and carers are often alert to this possibility. They recognize the pattern of social withdrawal, disinterest in accustomed activities, reduction in concentration, sleep and appetite disturbance, tearfulness, and pronounced lack of enjoyment in a host of activities. However, the presence of such a common and treatable psychiatric illness is often mistaken for 'challenging behaviour', an 'attitude problem', or even dementia. Early referral to suitably trained and experienced professionals is essential to clarify the diagnosis and to instigate beneficial medical and psychological therapies.

When dealing with depression (or indeed any other psychological problem) in an individual affected by a behavioural phenotype, it is important to identify what predisposing factors are present, and particularly whether there are any specific precipitants to the episode. Also, what perpetuating factors are maintaining the disturbance? Personal loss or other major changes figure highly here (Hollins and Esterhuyzen 1997), as do substantial transitions such as change of school or accommodation. Identifying the reasons and triggers for emotional disturbance is one thing, treating it effectively is another. Mild depression will often respond to acknowledgement, understanding, psychological support, counselling and attention to living circumstances. Sometimes antidepressant medication will be needed. Medication, when given, should always be in addition to continuing psychological, educational and social interventions and support. It complements rather than replaces these. Medication should always be a means to an end rather than an end in itself. Its use should be monitored carefully with frequent reviews and readiness to stop once its benefits have been consolidated (Turk 1999). Other common behavioural reasons for requesting a combination of psychological and behavioural approaches include severe sleep disturbance. This can be a specific part of a behavioural phenotype as in Smith–Magenis syndrome (Hodapp *et al.* 1998). It is also a frequent accompaniment of development in many individuals who have learning disability. Such problems are common, and the effects on other family members are substantial (Quine 1991). Attention to routine and basic behavioural advice is often effective. Frequently, however, the use of medication is indicated. Sedating antihistamines such as trimeprazine are popular but have a high rate of paradoxical excitation in this population. There is increasing interest in the use of melatonin to induce sleep (Turk and Gringrass 2001). A recent report suggests that the melatonin antagonist acebutolol may also be beneficial in restoring a more normal sleep–wake cycle when taken each morning (De Leersnyder *et al.* 2001). The frequency and impact of severe sleep disturbances in individuals with genetically determined learning disabilities is still grossly underrated. They deserve far more explanation, evaluation, treatment and reassurance when dealing with parents and carers.

In all such diagnostic and therapeutic endeavours there is therefore a need for complete clinical openness. Families often describe how others have not fully appreciated or have underestimated their problems, or simply that agencies have not been interested in their situation. More often than not the agencies concerned have simply not been familiar with such issues as the severity and impact of the presenting difficulties. Consequently, families not uncommonly describe in negative tones their previous experiences with professionals and harbour suspicions as to clinicians' motives and intents. It goes without saying that it is necessary to hear people out and to gain some insight into their situation.

Likewise it is important to recognize one's own 'personal baggage'. For example, a clinician who has detailed knowledge of a given syndrome will carefully explore and assess the various clinical and behavioural problems presented. But it is all too easy to adopt short-cut approaches, particularly where a syndrome is familiar to one. In this respect, the clinician's personal experience can be as much a disadvantage as an advantage. It is critical to remember that certain patterns of behaviour are *characteristic* of a syndrome, but rarely, if ever *diagnostic* or *universal*. For the most part, experienced clinicians will not fall into this trap, at least, not too often. We need to constantly remind ourselves about this, to be open and aware of the range and severity of behaviours that present within individual syndromes, and to maintain humility in our quest for effective and empathic clinical services.

Commonly associated developmental disabilities

Two classes of developmental disabilities recur throughout the behavioural phenotype literature and clinical practice, namely the attention deficit disorders and the autistic spectrum disorders. One of the biggest challenges clinically lies in discussing pervasive developmental disorders such as autism and Asperger syndrome with families. Social disinterest and lack of warmth and affection are some of the most devastating aspects for caring parents. Tact and diplomacy are needed in sharing the neurodevelopmental basis of these disorders and explaining the lack of miracle cures despite the numerous outrageous claims alluded to earlier in this chapter. Common myths such as the proposed link between autism and MMR vaccine should also be dispelled if possible with the aid of compassionate yet logical reasoning. As clinicians we have a duty to explain and thereby enhance understanding of the nature of the condition in question. We need to be able to explain which treatment strategies are likely to be helpful. We must also be ready to refute illogical and often dangerous approaches that may have been proposed. In order to undertake these tasks it is necessary to ensure one holds comprehensive and up-to-date knowledge regarding these disorders.

In explaining autistic spectrum disorders and attention deficit disorders it is useful to focus on two main issues.

1. Even when the general level of developmental delay is taken into account, there are still specific and more striking delays in the areas in question, *i.e.* social and language

functioning in autistic spectrum disorders, and attention skills and freedom from distractibility and impulsivity in the attention deficit disorders.

2. The nature of functioning in these delayed areas is still of a very different *qualitative* type from that which would be expected from straightforward 'developmental delay'. Thus, as in the diagnostic classification descriptions, it is the qualitative as well as quantitative aspects of the delays which characterize the disorder and which can allow for their confident diagnosis even in individuals with moderate to profound learning disability.

Genetic counselling and genetic risk

One of the main reasons for diagnosing the underlying genetic cause of an individual's learning disability concerns the implications for the individual and other family members of further family members with the disorder. Careful, knowledgeable and psychologically adept genetic counselling pre- as well as post-testing are really essential to ensure that families truly understand why they are being tested and what the implications of a positive—or indeed a negative—result might be for them. Genetic counselling in this context is complex. The issue most familiar in the context of dealing with people with genetic disabilities and their families is the risk of future offspring with the same condition. However, when dealing directly with affected individuals and their parents and carers, a different range of risks is frequently discussed. These include the likelihood of attaining or not attaining a degree of independence in adult life through general maturation, or conversely, the risk of remaining or becoming dependent according to the developmental trajectory and/or risks of progression of the condition in question. Other risks include the risk of major physical health problems (and indeed mortality), and the prospect of emerging emotional and behavioural challenges as well as psychiatric problems including degenerative conditions such as dementia.

These issues are never far from the forefront of parents' minds from early on in the consultation process. Increasingly, it is possible to give relatively accurate predictions of risk for further conceptions. For example, even in the absence of an identifiable underlying genetic cause for autistic spectrum disorder in a family member, the risk of this disorder in further offspring rockets from 0.5% to 4% (Bailey *et al.* 1996). Similarly, as many as one-third of first-degree relatives of individuals with attention deficit hyperactivity disorder will have the condition themselves (Biederman *et al.* 1986). What is more appropriate in a behavioural context is to acknowledge that there are concerns and raised likelihoods, and to place them in the context of the individual's condition. That, in turn, indicates the need and opportunities for intervention and preventative work. In this way, discussion of risk is feasible, appropriately turning the issue into one of attainments, prevention of possible secondary handicaps and potential positive outcomes.

Sexual counselling and sexual risk

Counselling over sexuality, relationships and related issues is another area that often dare not speak its name when it comes to family/clinician interactions. However, it must rank amongst the most important of developmental challenges, and as a cause of anxiety and ambivalence amongst family members and clinicians alike. We know from contact with family support societies that parents of children and young people who attend clinics almost invariably hold these thoughts, yet often rely on clinicians to raise them. Many parents and carers have great concerns regarding sexuality, often quite justifiably. These may range from the overwhelmingly practical issue of how to manage periods for a woman with severe learning disability/mental retardation, to concerns regarding exploitation and the potential to develop adequate parenting skills. As with other individuals with delayed intellectual development, there is the real risk of sexual exploitation, and other risks such as those of poorly learned or inappropriate sexual expression. There is a need to acknowledge that these concerns are normal, justifiable and real. Detailed discussion of these matters is always time well spent. Be prepared to think the unthinkable by way of being alert to possible sexual abuse. Such abuse is more common in people with learning disability than in the general population (Turk and Brown 1992, 1993). However, identification rates remain low, and successful perpetrator convictions even lower, despite clear evidence of long-term adverse emotional and behavioural effects on survivors. It is therefore unsurprising that some parents may feel that only close supervision can protect their children from adverse incidents. Even so, attendant risks should be studied carefully and appropriate safeguards instituted, with due regard for both the safety and the right of autonomy and sexual expression of the growing young person with disability.

Honesty and openness

As clinicians we are taught to be knowledgeable and instructive to our clients. But humility is equally important. Families are quick to grasp when clinicians are out of their depth and find this unhelpful. One family, having waited many months to see the 'specialist', were appalled by his opening gambit, "I'm so glad to meet you, I know nothing about your child's condition and am really looking forward to learning more about it from you"! Another parent of a child with fragile X syndrome was bemused by the casualty nursing staffs' insistence on cushioning the child with numerous pillows. It transpired that staff had misunderstood the diagnosis as meaning that the child was physically fragile, presumably attributing a condition such as osteogenesis imperfecta to her. By the natures of our jobs we will intermittently experience unfamiliar problems. Individuals will present with behaviours atypical of their syndrome's phenotype. Families are often well aware of this. This signals an opportunity for investigation of causes other than the main genetic one. Such behaviours may have roots in other eminently treatable problems, be they physical, psychological or social.

Psychometry and professional advocacy

In this area of work, the clinician may be called upon to support (and even fight) for clients' rights to receive appropriate services from other statutory, private and voluntary agencies. Intelligence testing is enjoying a revival in popularity in this connection, in keeping with its importance as one marker of development and intellectual ability. Interestingly, reluctance to employ intelligence testing (which was so widespread) never gained great support with parent groups. Families are generally keen for comprehensive structured assessments to be undertaken as a means to reaching a thorough appraisal of the individual's unique profile of personality attributes, intellectual abilities and other strengths and needs. Discussion of intelligence test results should be done collaboratively with an appropriately trained and experienced psychologist, giving as full and complete an appraisal as possible. This should include details of cognitive profile and any verbal/performance discrepancy as well as full scale IQ. If it is felt that the results are an underestimate of the individual's intellectual level then this should be specified with recommendations for retesting at the appropriate time. Subtle evidence of executive function or attentional deficits, social/symbolic impairments or language difficulties should prompt referral for further more specialized evaluations. Lack of thorough, appropriate multidisciplinary evaluation is one of the most common causes of misunderstanding regarding the individual's abilities, comprehension, language skills and intentions—and of a resultant failure to attain appropriate services.

Conclusion

Clinicians active in this area of clinical practice must be prepared to combine their professional attributes of multidisciplinary knowledge, skill and collaborative working with approaches to clients and their families in which warmth, genuineness, empathy and unconditional positive regard figure highly. On the one hand, there is of course a need for objective clarity regarding the disorders in question, their aetiologies and implications. At the same time, when counselling these individuals and their families, we as clinicians need to be aware of the stigma attached to the clinical labels we use. In fact, it is helpful to go further than this, and to look for opportunities to bolster, or even 'rehumanize' what are commonly dehumanized and devalued individuals and their families. This is best done in the context of a close partnership with the family, sharing closely their experiences and predicaments, and celebrating the maximization of the individual quality of life and social integration. This in turn entails maintaining close links with like-minded professionals and family support groups.

The style of clinical work described in this chapter is deliberately a fairly comprehensive one, in which long-term contact and partnership with families on the part of the informed clinician aims to maximize the individual's development, mental functioning, social adjustment and quality of life. This is only possible through the mutual application of zeal and stamina on the part of the clinician and family. We do not underestimate the time and effort that these processes entail. Nor can we understate the beneficial effects that can be attained, and the satisfaction to be gained by this way of working.

REFERENCES

Aziz M, Turk J, Callias M, Taylor C, Stathopulu E, Patton M, Oostra B, Willemsen R (1998) 'Development and behaviour of boys who have a fragile X premutation or intermediate allele.' Paper presented at the 6th International Fragile X Syndrome Conference, Asheville, NC, USA, 26–29 July 1998.
Bailey A, Phillips W, Rutter M (1996) 'Autism: towards an integration of clinical, genetic, neuropsychological, and neurobiological perspectives.' *Journal of Child Psychology and Psychiatry*, 37, 89–126.
Barlow F, Turk J (2001) 'Adolescents with learning disability and psychiatric illness – two case reports.' *Clinical Child Psychology and Psychiatry*, 6, 125–135.
Biederman J, Munir K, Knee D, Habelow W, Armentano M, Autor S, Hoge SK, Waternaux C (1986) 'A family study of patients with attention deficit disorder and normal controls.' *Journal of Psychiatric Research*, 20, 263–274.

Carmichael B, Pembrey M, Turner G, Barnicoat A.(1999) 'Diagnosis of fragile-X syndrome: the experiences of parents.' *Journal of Intellectual Disability Research*, **43**, 47–53.

Carr J (1980) *Helping Your Handicapped Child.* London: Penguin.

Cohen IL, Vietze PM, Sudhalter V, Jenkins EC, Brown WT (1989) 'Parent–child dyadic gaze patterns in fragile X males and in non-fragile X males with autistic disorder.' *Journal of Child Psychology and Psychiatry*, **30**, 845–856.

Colley AF, Leversha MA, Voullaire LE, Rogers JG (1990) 'Five cases demonstrating the distinctive behavioural features of chromosome deletion 17 (p11.2 p11.2) (Smith–Magenis syndrome).' *Journal of Paediatrics and Child Health*, **26**, 17–21.

Contact-a-Family (2002) *The CaF Directory of Specific Conditions and Rare Disorders 2002.* London: Contact-a-Family.

De Leersnyder H, De Blois M-C, Vekemans M, Sidi D, Villain E, Kindermans C, Munnich A (2001) 'β₁-adrenergic antagonists improve sleep and behavioural disturbances in a circadian disorder, Smith–Magenis syndrome.' *Journal of Medical Genetics*, **38**, 586–590.

Douglas J, Richman N (1984) *My Child Won't Sleep.* London: Penguin.

El Abd S, Turk J, Hill P (1995) 'Psychological characteristics of Turner syndrome.' *Journal of Child Psychology and Psychiatry*, **36**, 1109–1125.

Finucane BM, Konar D, Givler BH, Kurtz MB, Scott LI (1994) 'The spasmodic upper-body squeeze: a characteristic behavior in Smith–Magenis syndrome.' *Developmental Medicine and Child Neurology*, **36**, 70–83.

Gibb C (1992) 'The most common cause of learning difficulties: a profile of fragile-X syndrome and its implications for education.' *Educational Research*, **34**, 221–228.

Gosch A, Pankau R (1997) 'Personality characteristics and behaviour problems in individuals of different ages with Williams syndrome.' *Developmental Medicine and Child Neurology*, **39**, 527–533.

Graham PJ, Turk J, Verhulst F (1999) *Child Psychiatry: A Developmental Approach, 3rd Edn.* Oxford: Oxford University Press.

Hagerman RJ, Cronister A (1996) *Fragile X Syndrome: Diagnosis, Treatment and Research.* Baltimore: Johns Hopkins University Press.

Hodapp RM, Fidler DJ, Smith ACM (1998) 'Stress and coping in families of children with Smith–Magenis syndrome.' *Journal of Intellectual Disability Research*, **42**, 331–340.

Hoffman JB, Dupaul GJ (2000) 'Psychoeducational interventions for children and adolescents with attention-deficit/hyperactivity disorder.' *Child and Adolescent Psychiatric Clinics of North America*, **9**, 647–661.

Holland AJ, Hon J, Huppert FA, Stevens F (2000) 'Incidence and course of dementia in people with Down's syndrome: findings from a population-based study.' *Journal of Intellectual Disability Research*, **44**, 138–146.

Hollins S, Esterhuyzen A (1997) 'Bereavement and grief in adults with learning disabilities.' *British Journal of Psychiatry*, **170**, 497–501.

Jordan R, Powell S (1995) *Understanding and Teaching Children with Autism.* New York: Wiley.

Kewley G (1999) *Attention Deficit Hyperactivity Disorder: Recognition, Reality and Resolution.* Horsham, Sussex: Key 3 Publishers.

Matson JL, Bamburg JW, Mayville EA, Pinkston J, Bielecki J, Kuhn D, Smalls Y, Logan JR (2000) 'Psychopharmacology and mental retardation: a 10 year review.' *Research in Developmental Disabilities*, **21**, 263–296.

McArdle P, O'Brien G, Macmillan A, Kolvin I (2000) 'The peer relations of disruptive children with reference to hyperactivity and conduct disorder.' *European Child and Adolescent Psychiatry*, **9**, 91–99.

McEvoy J (1992) 'Fragile X syndrome: a brief overview.' *Educational Psychology in Practice*, **8**, 146–149.

McNaught A, Turk J (1994) 'A girl with Smith–Magenis syndrome and autistic spectrum disorder misdiagnosed as parental emotional abuse.' Paper presented at the Annual Meeting of the British Paediatric Neurology Association, Birmingham, England, January 6–7, 1994.

O'Brien G (1992) 'Behavioural phenotypes and their measurement.' *Developmental Medicine and Child Neurology*, **34**, 379–381.

O'Brien G (1996a) 'Behavioural problems in disabled children.' *Journal of the Royal Society of Medicine*, **89**, 57–58.

O'Brien G (1996b) 'Psychiatric management of adult autism.' *Advances in Psychiatric Treatment*, **2**, 173–175.

O'Brien G (2000) 'Behavioural phenotypes: their clinical and historical significance.' *Journal of the Royal Society of Medicine*, **93**, 618–620.

O'Brien G (2001a) 'The adult outcome of childhood learning disability.' *Developmental Medicine and Child Neurology*, **43**, 634–638.

167

O'Brien G (2001b) 'The definition of learning disability: what place does intelligence testing have now?' *Developmental Medicine and Child Neurology*, **43**, 570–573.

Quine L (1991) 'Sleep problems in children with mental handicap.' *Journal of Mental Deficiency Research*, **35**, 269–290.

Rasmussen P, Borjesson O, Wentz ?, Gillberg C (2001) 'Autistic disorders in Down syndrome: background factors and clinical correlates.' *Developmental Medicine and Child Neurology*, **43**, 750–754.

Ratcliffe SG, Butler GE, Jones M (1991) 'Edinburgh study of growth and development of children with sex chromosome abnormalities. IV.' *Birth Defects: Original Articles Series*, **26**, 1–44.

Tierney E, Nwokoro N, Porter FD, Bukelis I, Garrett E, Kelley R (2001) 'Smith–Lemli–Opitz syndrome: changes in ADI-R scores with cholesterol supplementation.' Paper presented at the 9th Annual Scientific Meeting of the Society for the Study of Behavioural Phenotypes, Oxford, 15–16 November 2001.

Turk J (1996a) 'Tertiary prevention of childhood mental health problems.' *In:* Kendrick T, Tylee A, Feeling P (eds) *The Prevention of Mental Illness in Primary Care.* Cambridge: Cambridge University Press, pp 265–280.

Turk J (1996b) 'Working with parents of children who have severe learning disabilities.' *Clinical Child Psychology and Psychiatry*, **1**, 581–596.

Turk J (1998) 'Children with learning difficulties and their parents.' *In:* Graham P (ed) *Cognitive Behaviour Therapy for Children and Families.* Cambridge: Cambridge University Press, pp 110–126.

Turk J (1999) 'Drug therapy.' *In:* Graham PJ, Turk J, Verhulst F (1999) *Child Psychiatry: A Developmental Approach, 3rd Edn.* Oxford: Oxford University Press, pp 442–452.

Turk J, Graham P (1997) 'Fragile X syndrome, autism and autistic features.' *Autism*, **1**, 175–197.

Turk J, Gringrass P (2001) 'Melatonin supplementation for severe sleep disturbance in children and adolescents with genetically determined developmental disabilities.' Paper presented at the 9th Annual Scientific Meeting of the Society for the Study of Behavioural Phenotypes, Oxford, 15–16 November 2001.

Turk, J., Sales, J. (1996) 'Behavioural phenotypes and their relevance to child mental health professionals.' *Child Psychology and Psychiatry Review*, **1**, 4–11.

Turk V, Brown H (1992) 'Sexual abuse and adults with learning disabilities: preliminary communication of survey results.' *Mental Handicap*, **20**, 56–58.

Turk V, Brown H (1993) 'The sexual abuse of adults with learning disabilities: results of a two year incidence survey.' *Mental Handicap Research*, **6**, 193–216.

Udwin O, Webber C, Horne I (2001) 'Abilities and attainment in Smith–Magenis syndrome.' *Developmental Medicine and Child Neurology*, **43**, 823–828.

Vostanis P, Harrington R, Prendergast M, Farndon P (1994) 'Case reports of autism with interstitial deletion of chromosome 17 (p11.2 p11.2) and monosomy of chromosome 5 (5pter→5p15.3).' *Psychiatric Genetics*, **4**, 109–111.

Wilson PG, Mazzocco MMM (1993) 'Awareness and knowledge of fragile X syndrome among special educators.' *Mental Retardation*, **31**, 221–227.

Wing L (1996) *The Autistic Spectrum.* London: Constable.

York A, von Fraunhofer N, Turk J, Sedgwick P (1999) 'Fragile X syndrome, Down's syndrome and autism: awareness and knowledge amongst special educators.' *Journal of Intellectual Disability Research*, **43**, 314–324.

8
BEHAVIOURAL PHENOTYPES OF GENETIC SYNDROMES: SUMMARIES, INCLUDING NOTES ON MANAGEMENT AND THERAPY

Louise Barnard, Joanne Pearson, Lisa Rippon and Gregory O'Brien

This section reviews the behavioural phenotypes of the most common and/or important genetic syndromes of learning disability, and their management. The syndromes are arranged in alphabetical order. For each syndrome, there is a brief description, giving:
- any commonly used eponyms or alternative names
- the incidence of the syndrome; for those syndromes for which the incidence is not clearly established, any available information on occurrence is given, and this is indicated by such entries being bracketed
- the mode and mechanism of genetic expression of the condition
- the typical level, or degree of severity, of learning disability associated with the condition
- a brief summary of the principal features of the syndrome, with emphasis on behavioural features, including any that have been recently clarified
- notes on management of the syndrome
- contact details of relevant websites.

For each condition, the description of the principal features is a summary and update of that in O'Brien and Yule (1995).

The aim of the section is to assist clinicians, educators and other specialist carers in their efforts to facilitate maximal development of individuals with the respective syndromes, through consideration and attention to behavioural phenotypes. The focus of the syndrome summaries is therefore on the behavioural features of the conditions, but not exclusively so. The understanding of behaviour, which is the basis of intervention and management of affected individuals, relies on consideration of all factors that might exert an influence on behaviour. In consideration of behavioural phenotypes, the physical and sensory disabilities and the major health problems of the conditions are determinants of the cognitive, linguistic, motor and social expression of the syndrome. Consequently, notes on management are not confined to behavioural and psychiatric interventions.

To some extent, the notes on management are empirically based, inasmuch as they are a response to the behavioural phenotypes in question. For example, in conditions in which autistic-like behaviours feature prominently as part of the behavioural phenotype, management should, at least to some extent, be informed by this. In most such examples, there is no wide base of evidence from which to draw regarding the management of the autistic features of individual syndromes. Where any such information has been identified, it is cited. Also, regarding behavioural and/or psychiatric interventions, such as the application of specific types of behavioural intervention or the use of drug therapy, in many instances specific syndrome-based information is not the guiding hand. Rather, for the most part, decisions on treatment are informed by the nature of the behaviours in question, and their situation and concomitants, taking into careful account the individual's wider circumstances. Additionally, where there is available important evidence on the use of particular behavioural and/or psychiatric approaches to the management of the behaviour of the syndrome in question, this is cited. Similarly, where there is evidence available on the use of other important interventions, which are likely to promote development, and reduce (or facilitate the management of) behavioural problems in these conditions, these are listed. Examples of such interventions range from drug treatment of epilepsy, to surgical procedures aimed at correcting deformity and promoting development, all of which may facilitate behavioural management.

REFERENCE

O'Brien G, Yule W (eds) (1995) *Behavioural Phenotypes, Clinics in Developmental Medicine No 138.* London: Mac Keith Press.

WEBSITES

The following websites are for general use in the area of behavioural phenotypes.
- Ability
  www.ability.org.uk/index1.html
- Birth Disorder Information Directory
  www.bdid.com/sitemap.htm
- Contact a Family
  www.cafamily.org.uk/
- Family Village: A Global Community of Disability-Related Resources
  www.familyvillage.wisc.edu/index.htmlx
- International Birth Defects Information Systems
  www.ibis-birthdefects.org/
- MENCAP
  www.mencap.org.uk/
- Mountain States Genetic Network: Dictionary of Online Genetic Support Groups
  www.mostgene.org/support/index.html
- NCBI Genes and Disease
  www.ncbi.nlm.nih.gov/disease/index.html
- REACH: The Association for Children with Hand or Arm Deficiency
  www.reach.org.uk/
- Society for the Study of Behavioural Phenotypes
  www.psychiatry.cam.ac.uk/ssbp/news.htm
- STEPS, The National Association for Children with Lower Limb Abnormalities
  www.steps-charity.org.uk/

AICARDI SYNDROME

Incidence	200 cases reported by 1997 (Costa *et al.* 1997)
Aetiology/genetics	X-linked dominant disorder
Learning disability	Severe

Aicardi syndrome is a condition of severe disability, necessitating prompt recognition and attention. It is characterized by agenesis of the corpus callosum, severe visual defects (choroidoretinal lacunae), infantile spasms with associated abnormal electroencephalograph (hypsarythmia), and skeletal abnormalities, particularly of the ribs and spine (Altinbasak *et al.* 1993, O'Brien and Yule 1995). The course of the syndrome is characterized by progressive psychomotor slowing, kyphoscoliosis and visual failure, with, typically—up until now—death by early adulthood.

MANAGEMENT

Girls with Aicardi syndrome are usually identified as young babies. The severe epilepsy and other associated severe disabilities of girls who present with the condition mark these infants as cases meriting urgent specialist attention. Referral to a paediatric neurologist is indicated, both for diagnostic assessment and ongoing management.

Perhaps the most prominent of the core issues in the management of this condition is *vigorous, proactive management of epilepsy*. Early treatment with ACTH is indicated, followed by further active treatment, according to progress and severity. There is very convincing evidence that early introduction of ACTH leads to a better prognosis, as does a vigorous approach to the eradication of interictal hypsarrhythmia. Over the course of the disease, it is important to maintain a high index of awareness of the severe epilepsy of this condition, and to respond accordingly. This is especially because affected individuals can be characterized by marked motor slowing and social apathy, to such an extent that may mask ongoing epilepsy.

Active physiotherapy is very important. This serves a range of crucial functions. Firstly, the motor delay of this condition is severe, such as merits programmed physiotherapeutic intervention. Over time, the thrust of intervention will change, from early life emphasis on the acquisition of whatever basic skills are feasible, through ongoing development and maintenance of motor functioning, to a later stage of management of deteriorating motor activity and musculoskeletal state. Importantly, throughout the course of the condition, the physiotherapist works *in partnership with the parents/carers* of the affected individual, who take on a key role in the implementation of the programmed exercises and interventions. Such partnership working is particularly welcomed. The parents of these girls are only too aware of just how severely disabled their children are, and what the future holds, and this knowledge makes active involvement on their parts even more important.

Aicardi syndrome results in severe learning disability, of such a degree that may be difficult to accurately assess. As with any child so severely learning disabled, the thrust of *educational and developmental intervention* should be to look for any islets of ability on which to focus in order to promote generalized development, and also to identify any playful activities that the child appears to enjoy. As with all children, through play and rehearsal comes maximal development. With the pronounced social apathy of children affected by Aicardi syndrome, it is important not to be always too focused on structured developmental tasks, but to find what seems to be fun.

REFERENCES

Altinbasak S, Baytok V, Yalaz M, Onenli N (1993) 'The Aicardi syndrome – a case-report and review of the literature.' *Turkish Journal of Pediatrics*, **35**, 305–312.
Costa T, Greer W, Rysiecki G, Buncic JR, Ray PN (1997) 'Monozygotic twins discordant for Aicardi syndrome.' *Journal of Medical Genetics*, **34**, 688–691.
O'Brien G, Yule W (eds) (1995) *Behavioural Phenotypes. Clinics in Developmental Medicine No. 138.* London: Mac Keith Press.

WEBSITE

• Aicardi Syndrome Foundation
  www.aicardi.com/index.html

ANGELMAN SYNDROME

Incidence   1:30,000
Aetiology/genetics   Usually sporadic, deletion of maternal 15q11–13 (Steinlin 1998)
Learning disability   Severe to profound

Individuals with Angelman syndrome have a typical facial set comprising a long face with a prominent jaw, a wide mouth with widely spaced teeth and a thin upper lip, flat occiput, midface hypoplasia and deep set eyes. Other characteristic features include ataxia, severe learning disability, lack of speech, inappropriate laughter, overactivity, sleep disturbance, limited attention span, microcephaly and epilepsy with associated abnormal electroencephalo-graphic findings (large amplitude slow wave activity persisting in sleep, very large amplitude slow activity in runs more prominent anteriorly, and spikes or sharp waves mixed with large amplitude components posteriorly that are facilitated on eye closure) (Smith *et al.* 1996 Steinlin 1998). Respiratory tract infections, otitis media and obesity are common complications in adulthood (O'Brien and Yule 1995), although epilepsy becomes less prevalent with age. While life expectancy is thought to be normal (O'Brien and Yule 1995), there are few reports of individuals over 50 years of age in the literature, although survival to age 75 years has been documented.

MANAGEMENT

Angelman syndrome can be one of the most rewarding of conditions to manage. The discredited eponym by which the condition used to be known was 'happy puppet syndrome'. This phrase referred to the characteristic combination of ataxia and inappropriate empty laughter, which presents in such a pronounced form as can easily be, mistakenly, regarded as jocular playacting on the part of the affected individual. It is therefore important to give clear and unambiguous advice regarding the condition to parents and carers who strive to understand the perplexing behaviour of individuals affected by Angelman syndrome. This cannot be done in one or two consultations, or through a leaflet or a website—it takes years of contact, and immense patience. The mainstay of management is therefore long-term contact with affected individuals, education on the nature of the condition, and attention to the accompanying health problems, notably epilepsy and respiratory and ear infections, in addition to a social skills acquisition-based behavioural approach, an ongoing programme of development of speech and language, and assisting parents and carers in management of sleep.

In *educating parents and carers* on the nature of Angelman syndrome, it is the characteristic social behaviour of affected children that requires careful explanation. In keeping with the old name of happy puppet syndrome, individuals do smile, giggle and laugh often. However, the smiling, giggling and laughing are not socially dependent, and are often socially inappropriate. Parents often realize this, and are reassured when it is explained to them that this unusual social pattern is recognized.

Close attention to epilepsy is required in almost all cases of Angelman syndrome. The epilepsy can be severe and intractable, and exacerbations of epilepsy are typically associated with sleep disturbance. Recent attention to the epilepsy of Angelman syndrome has focused on a defect in DNA coding for subunits of the gamma-aminobutyric acid (GABA) type A receptor. Anticonvulsant drugs with GABA-ergic properties may therefore be of use in the condition. This was suggested through a trial of topiramate in five children with Angelman syndrome (Franz *et al.* 2000).

Individuals with Angelman syndrome respond well to a long-term programme of *developmental behavioural management*, which focuses on acquisition of social skills. As young children, their traits of overexcitability, overactivity and limited attention span are to some extent compensated for by their propensity to use nonverbal means of communication, including gestures, signs and picture boards. Such a combination responds well to an approach that focuses on development of basic social skills. As the child grows, the impulsivity, overactivity and poor attention span mature and improve. This allows a shift of focus to feeding, dressing and other personal self-care skills.

An ongoing *programme of development of speech and language* is important in Angelman syndrome. Many children have been reported with no speech development. However, there is evidence that this may be due to an underlying oral motor dyspraxia (Penner *et al.* 1993). This finding, combined with the observation that these children appear to be interested in using nonverbal language, indicates the importance of the involvement of the speech and language therapist, in order to facilitate communication—whether this be verbal or nonverbal—according to the child's capabilities.

Assisting parents and carers in the *management of sleep* in Angelman syndrome is important, and often welcomed. In addition to exacerbating epilepsy, the characteristic pattern of sleep disturbance in Angelman syndrome concerns difficulty in the initiation and the maintenance of sleep. It does seem that children with Angelman syndrome require less sleep than other children. This sleep comprises a series of naps for short intervals, with an overall sleep duration of 5–6 hours per night. This has led to trials of intervention on a behavioural and pharmacological basis. While the prime pharmacological consideration is attention to epilepsy, there is evidence that melatonin treatment is of benefit in Angelman syndrome (Zhdanova *et al.* 1999).

REFERENCES

Franz DN, Glauser TA, Tudor C, Williams S (2000) 'Topiramate therapy of epilepsy associated with Angelman's syndrome.' *Neurology*, **54**, 1185–1188.

O'Brien G, Yule W (eds) (1995) *Behavioural Phenotypes. Clinics in Developmental Medicine No. 138.* London: Mac Keith Press.

Penner KA, Johnston J, Faircloth BH, Irish P, Williams CA (1993) 'Communication, cognition and social interaction in the Angelman syndrome.' *American Journal of Medical Genetics*, **46**, 34–39.

Smith A, Wiles C, Haan E, McGill J, Wallis G, Dixon J, Selby R, Colley A, Marks R, Trent RJ (1996) 'Clinical features in 27 patients with Angelman syndrome resulting from DNA deletion.' *Journal of Medical Genetics*, **33**, 107–112.

Steinlin M (1998) 'Non-progressive congenital ataxias.' *Brain and Development*, **20**, 199–208.

Zhdanova IV, Wurtman RJ, Wagstaff J (1999) 'Effects of a low dose of melatonin on sleep in children with Angelman syndrome.' *Journal of Pediatric Endocrinology and Metabolism*, **12**, 57–67.

WEBSITE

• Angelman Syndrome Foundation
  www.angelman.org/

COCKAYNE SYNDROME

Incidence	1:100,000
Genetics	Autosomal recessive—usually mutation on the long arm of chromosome 10 (McElvanney *et al.* 1996); also chromosome 5
Learning disability	Progressive

In Cockayne syndrome there is a deficiency in the capacity for DNA repair following exposure to ultraviolet radiation. There are two accepted expressions of this phenotype: the more common classical (type I), which is apparent after 1 year of age; and congenital (type II), which is apparent from birth. There may also be a third expression, which has a later onset. Cockayne syndrome is characterized by growth failure, hydrocephalus, typical facies—a prematurely aged appearance being the most striking—photosensitive skin, progressive kyphosis, disordered water–salt metabolism, microcephaly, dwarfism, tremor, and hearing and vision impairments (McElvanney *et al.* 1996). There is progressive loss of both mental and physical abilities, which eventually necessitates full-time care (Gilbert 1999). Life expectancy has been correlated to the presence of cataracts in the first three years of life, with an increased expectancy if early cataracts are absent; however, death usually occurs at around 12 years of age (McElvanney *et al.* 1996).

MANAGEMENT

Cockayne syndrome can sometimes be difficult to diagnose in the perinatal period. In some cases, a child may present with all the characteristic features, resulting in prompt recognition of the syndrome. However, often symptoms and signs of the disorder develop insidiously over the first few years of life, and diagnosis can be delayed because of the unfamiliarity of clinicians with this rare condition. Investigations, which can aid in diagnosis, include CT and MRI, which typically show progressive leukodystrophy, thickening of the calvarium, intracranial calcification particularly in the basal ganglia and cerebellum, patchy demyelination and cerebellar atrophy. The sensitivity to ultraviolet radiation necessitates that exposure to sunlight must therefore be avoided. Parents and carers should be made aware of this and of the importance of taking all of the necessary precautions.

Initial management of this condition should include *education and counselling* for parents and carers. A multidisciplinary approach is advantageous in the management of this multisystem disorder. Particular attention should be paid to sensory deficits. Both vision and hearing require regular monitoring in order to track the progressive deterioration of these sensory functions. Some children require hearing aids, and many benefit from sign language training or other *communication aids* depending on visual abilities. It is vital to feedback findings to primary carers so that they can alter their mode of communication with respect to the level of sensory deterioration (Gilbert 1999). Ophthalmic management is difficult in Cockayne syndrome due to the delay in neurological development. Venous access and respiratory difficulties complicate administration of general anaesthetic. Despite these difficulties, cataract extraction is usually performed at an early age (McElvanney *et al.* 1996).

Flexion contractures of joints and kyphosis can occur in Cockayne syndrome. In order to maintain mobility these should be monitored for, and devices such as ankle and foot orthotics can be introduced to assist walking.

REFERENCES

Gilbert PC (1999) *A–Z of Syndromes and Inherited Disorders.* Cheltenham, Gloucestershire: Stanely Thorne.
McElvanney AM, Wooldridge WJ, Khan AA, Ansons AM (1996) 'Ophthalmic management of Cockayne's syndrome.' *Eye*, **10**, 61–64.

WEBSITES

- NCBI Genes and Disease: Cockayne syndrome
  www.ncbi.nlm.nih.gov/disease/Cockayne.html
- Share and Care Cockayne Syndrome Network
  www.cockayne-syndrome.org/

COFFIN–LOWRY SYNDROME

Incidence	More than 100 cases have been reported (SSBP 1996)
Genetics	X-linked with diminished expression in females: Xp22.1–22.2 (SSBP 1996)
Learning disability	Severe in males, females are often normal (SSBP 1996, Gilbert 1999)

Coffin–Lowry syndrome is a systemic connective tissue disorder. Males are more severely affected than females. It is characterized by unusually coarse facies (which become more pronounced with age), learning disability, epilepsy, small stature, generalized hypotonia, characteristic hands (plump, lax, soft hands with tapered, hyperextensible fingers) and metabolic abnormalities of collagen. Motor coordination is poor and causes clumsiness. Scoliosis and kyphosis can emerge during adolescence (Gilbert 1999). With age, the presentation of the syndrome becomes more marked, although it is not a progressive disorder. Life expectancy can be normal—death is commonly attributable to cardiac and respiratory complications (Gilbert 1999).

MANAGEMENT

The early diagnosis of Coffin–Lowry syndrome is essential in managing the complications associated with this syndrome (Merienne *et al.* 1998). It is more difficult to diagnose the condition in females, in whom expression is milder than in males. Once a child has been given a diagnosis of Coffin–Lowry syndrome, s/he should receive a *full developmental assessment* focusing on the multiple disabilities that present. The outcome of this assessment will inform future interventions and will facilitate decisions regarding school placements.

Routine medical examinations should include an assessment of the spine to check for early signs of curvature, which in some cases is present from birth. Kyphosis and vertebral complications can be managed with *orthopaedic intervention*, which in turn can help prevent respiratory problems. The confounding learning disability in this syndrome warrants consistent developmental assessment throughout childhood in order to provide the appropriate level of support. Speech often does develop, although its quality is often poor. *Speech therapy* can be beneficial in promoting language acquisition and developing existing speech (Gilbert 1999). Sign language is also useful for patients with sensorineural deafness.

Parents/carers should be made aware that in this syndrome maladaptive behaviours, such as head banging, are usually symptomatic of underlying physical discomfort, such as chronic ear infection.

Adaptive behaviours such as potty training and self-dressing can be achieved even in boys with Coffin–Lowry syndrome, although the acquisition of these skills will be markedly delayed. Self-dressing can be hampered by poor fine-motor skills, but these can be overcome by providing clothes with Velcro rather than button, zips and laces. Emotional development would seem to be unimpaired in this syndrome, and affected individuals show the whole range of emotions.

REFERENCES

Gilbert PC (1999) *A–Z of Syndromes and Inherited Disorders.* Cheltenham, Gloucestershire: Stanely Thorne.
Merienne K, Jacquot S, Trivier E, Pannetier S, Rossi A, Scott C, Schinzel A, Castellan C, Kress W, Hanauer A (1998) 'Rapid immunoblot and kinase assay tests for a syndromal form of X linked mental retardation: Coffin–Lowry syndrome.' *Journal of Medical Genetics*, **35**, 890–894.
SSBP (1996) *Proceedings of the 4th International Symposium of the Society for the Study of Behavioural Phenotypes, Marino Institute of Education, Dublin, Ireland, 14–16 November 1996..*

WEBSITE

- Coffin–Lowry Syndrome Foundation
  http://clsfoundation.tripod.com/

COFFIN–SIRIS SYNDROME

Incidence	Very low
Genetics	Autosomal recessive
Learning disability	Mild to severe

The main defining feature of Coffin–Siris syndrome is an absent or underdeveloped terminal phalanx and terminal fingernails. Other features include delayed skeletal development leading to retarded growth, scoliosis, hypotonia, gastro-oesophageal abnormalities, teeth, vision and hearing problems, undescended testes, microcephaly, coarse facies and sparse scalp hair with hypertricosis of the face and body. Neurological signs are dependent on the severity of the cranial malformations. Central nervous system complications are secondary to the cranial malformations.

MANAGEMENT

Children with this condition often present with significant oral aversions early in life, which can result in difficulties with sucking and failure to thrive. It is therefore important that the condition is recognized early to support parents and carers in addressing any early *feeding problems*. Gastro-oesophageal reflux can cause pain and discomfort, and this should be monitored for and treated appropriately.

Physiotherapy and occupational therapy are beneficial in treating the difficulties resulting from the skeletal abnormalities and hypotonia. Although affected individuals generally have good receptive skills, most have difficulties with expressive speech and in some cases may not have any speech at all. The input of a *speech and language therapist* is therefore important in the management of Coffin–Siris syndrome.

REFERENCES

DeBassio WA, Kemper TL, Knoefel JE (1985) 'Coffin–Siris syndrome: neuropathologic findings.' *Archives of Neurology*, **42**, 350–353.
Qazi QH, Heckman LS, Markouizos D, Verma RS (1990) 'The Coffin–Siris syndrome.' *Journal of Medical Genetics*, **27**, 333–336.

WEBSITE

- Coffin–Siris Support Group
  http://members.aol.com/CoffinSiri/

CORNELIA DE LANGE SYNDROME

Incidence	1:40,000–1:100,000 (SSBP 2000)
Genetics	Unclear cause, most cases are sporadic (SSBP 2000)
Learning disability	Moderate to severe

Cornelia de Lange syndrome is characterized by typical facies, limb abnormalities and failure to thrive due to gastro-oesophageal reflux (which can lead to aspiration pneumonia and can be fatal). Characteristic facies are present in over three-quarters of affected individuals and include small, upturned nose, anteverted nostrils, neat well-defined arched eyebrows that meet in the middle and may fan out laterally, long curly eyelashes, thin lips and a crescent-shaped mouth, a long philtrum, high arched palate and micrognathia (O'Brien and Yule 1995). The behavioural phenotype can present autistic-like features, particularly stereotypies. Speech usually does not develop beyond the use of single words. There is a recognized dichotomy between a classical and mild phenotype. Both phenotypes have the typical facial characteristics, but the milder form is associated with less severe learning disabilities and less prominent cardiac and limb abnormalities (Berney *et al.* 1999). The classical phenotype is characterized by small stature, self-injury, undescended testes and eye abnormalities. It has been suggested that the lower the birthweight, the more severe the phenotype and the greater the risk of infection (O'Brien and Yule 1995, Salmon 1978). Increasingly, more infants with Cornelia de Lange syndrome survive into childhood and even adulthood as a result of better medical interventions (O'Brien and Yule 1995).

MANAGEMENT

It is important that *parents/carers receive adequate support* upon receiving this diagnosis for their child. The initial diagnosis is usually made by the clinician on the basis of the pattern of abnormalities. It is particularly difficult for parents to come to terms with a diagnosis for a condition that is so rare, and about which there is so little available information. This is where the role of support groups can complement the role of the multidisciplinary team, as knowledge gleaned through these groups, together with the sharing of experience, can be most empowering for families.

Management of this condition can be separated into medical and behavioural components. Although there is no specific treatment for this condition, *early intervention* will help children to reach their full potential, and prompt diagnosis is therefore essential. Good systems of regular communication, between clinicians, educators, families and carers, are important. Caring for a young person suffering from this condition can be extremely difficult, and much of the behavioural intervention that may be needed will take place in the home environment.

Perhaps the most distressing aspect of this condition for parents and carers is *self-injurious behaviour*. There would appear to be an age-related increase in the prevalence of self-injury and this should be anticipated (Berney *et al.* 1999). If self-injury does occur, it is important to ensure that there is appropriate assessment of the physical damage caused, and there must be ongoing vigilance to monitor for evidence of infection. Early behavioural and educational programmes can be beneficial in reducing this behaviour. A *functional* analysis of self-injury is useful, as it has been attributed to physical discomfort, and in particular delayed dentition (Harris 1998). The management of self-injury covers a number of strategies, including restraint, discussing the issue with the affected individual, and removing them from the situation in which the behaviour has occurred. Pharmacological intervention does not appear to be useful in most cases, although a substantial minority (one-third) would seem to find naltrexone, SSRIs and atypical antipsychotics useful (Berney *et al.* 1999).

Aberrant behaviours such as restlessness, aggression, self-injury, overactivity and irritability are thought to be related to gastrointestinal reflux and its resulting physical discomfort. The treatment of gastrointestinal reflux and reflux vomiting therefore helps to alleviate some of the behavioural manifestations of the syndrome. Behavioural therapies are also particularly useful. For example, idiosyncratic behaviours, such as breath holding, respond well to functional analysis and resulting interventions (Kern *et al.* 1995).

Early identification of *hearing impairments* is essential. The degree of the hearing impairment is prognostic—children with more severely impaired hearing show more severe behavioural and language problems (Sataloff *et al.* 1990). Hearing should be assessed regularly. Ongoing speech therapy is vital to facilitate communication skills. Appropriate early educational intervention is also important. Children with Cornelia de Lange syndrome

178

have well-developed visuospatial memory, perceptual organization and fine motor skills. This knowledge is useful when planning teaching strategies for people with the syndrome.

REFERENCES

Berney TP, Ireland M, Burn J (1999) 'Behavioural phenotype of Cornelia de Lange syndrome.' *Archives of Disease in Childhood*, **81**, 333–336.

Harris JC (1998) *Developmental Neuropsychiatry, Vol. II: Assessment, Diagnosis and Treatment of Developmental Disorders.* Oxford: Oxford University Press.

Kern L, Mauk JE, Marder TJ, Mace FC (1995) 'Functional analysis and intervention for breath holding.' *Journal of Applied Behavior Analysis*, **28**, 339–340.

O'Brien G, Yule W (eds) (1995) *Behavioural Phenotypes, Clinics in Developmental Medicine No. 138.* London: Mac Keith Press.

Salmon MA (1978) *Developmental Defects and Syndromes.* London: HMM Publishers.

Sataloff RT, Spiegel JR, Hawkshaw M, Epstein JM, Jackson L (1990) 'Cornelia de Lange syndrome. Otolaryngologic manifestations.' *Archives of Otolaryngology – Head and Neck Surgery*, **116**, 1044–1046.

SSBP (2000) *Proceedings of the 6th International Symposium of the Society for the Study of Behavioural Phenotypes, Venice International University, San Servolo, Italy, 12–14 October 2000.*

WEBSITE

• CDLS–USA Foundation
  www.cdlsusa.org/

CRI DU CHAT SYNDROME (5p– SYNDROME)

Alternative name	5p– syndrome
Incidence	1:50,000 (Cornish *et al.* 1998) to 1:20,000 (Gilbert 1999)
Genetics	Partial deletion of 5p15.2
Learning disability	Severe, no reports of IQ over 35 (Gilbert 1999)

Cri du chat syndrome derives its name from the distinctive high-pitched cat-like cry that is observed in young infants, although this disappears within the first few months of life. The typical phenotypic presentation of cri du chat syndrome is characterized by short stature, microcephaly and cardiac, gastrointestinal and respiratory complications (Cornish and Pigram 1996). Typical facies include a round face with hypertelorism, epicanthal folds, slanting palpebral fissures, posteriorly rotated, low-set ears with preauricular tags, a broad flat nose and microretrognathia (O'Brien and Yule 1995). Psychomotor retardation and primordial growth deficiency are also common features. As patients develop, common complications include failure to thrive, growth retardation and poor muscular development. The location of the deletion on the implicated chromosome is thought to determine the severity of the phenotypic expression—with milder phenotypic expression and a better prognosis being associated with deletions outside of the critical region. Mortality is high in the first few months of life, although life expectancy is increasing due to medical advances (O'Brien and Yule 1995, SSBP 1999). Mortality is commonly attributable to infection.

MANAGEMENT

The initial phase in managing children born with this syndrome is one of medical assessment. The newborn infant must be assessed for the *cardiac and gastrointestinal complications* of this disorder. The need for corrective heart surgery should be assessed if congenital heart defects are present particularly with a view to assessing the severity of the abnormalities. As the child develops s/he should be monitored on a regular basis by the multidisciplinary team, to detect and address any further medical complications that may arise.

Despite the severe learning disability that is associated with cri du chat syndrome, research has shown that early intervention programmes are beneficial to this group, particularly verbal, visual and auditory stimulation. *Early stimulation* can facilitate communication, albeit at a very basic level (Gilbert 1999). *Speech therapy* is useful in assisting in the development of communication skills. Some children with cri du chat syndrome are able to use a few sentences, while others do not develop speech as such, but can use sign language. Constant stimulation can be exhaustive to other family members, and families should be made aware of opportunities for respite care.

Hypotonia, scoliosis and delays in walking are all characteristic of this disorder. These problems can all be improved through regular sessions with a *physiotherapist*. The downward slant of the eyes that is typical in cri du chat syndrome can cause a divergent squint to develop and may necessitate corrective surgery. Surgery is important not just for cosmetic reasons but also to maximize the visual input the child receives (Gilbert 1999).

Cri du chat syndrome can be detected prenatally with chorionic villus sampling. When it is detected in this manner, intensive *genetic counselling* should be offered to parents to help them understand the implications of having a child with this syndrome and to help to prepare them emotionally. They should be provided with information in a clear and matter-of-fact manner and the truth should not be hidden from them.

REFERENCES

Cornish KM, Munir F, Bramble D (1998) 'Adaptive and maladaptive behaviour in children with cri-du-chat syndrome.' *Journal of Applied Research in Intellectual Disabilities*, **11**, 239–246.
Cornish KM, Pigram J (1996) 'Developmental and behavioural characteristics of cri du chat syndrome.' *Archives of Disease in Childhood*, **75**, 448–450.
Gilbert PC (1999) *A–Z of syndromes and Inherited Disorders*. Cheltenham, Gloucestershire: Stanely Thorne.
O'Brien G, Yule W (eds) (1995) *Behavioural Phenotypes. Clinics in Developmental Medicine No. 138*. London: Mac Keith Press.
SSBP (1999) *Proceedings of the 8th Annual Scientific Meeting of the Society for the Study of Behavioural Phenotypes, Beecheres Management Centre, Birmingham, England, 18–19 November 1999.*

WEBSITE

• Cri-du-Chat Syndrome Support Group
  www.cridchat.u-net.com/

CROUZON SYNDROME

Incidence	1:25,000–1:65,000 (Orvidas *et al.* 1999)
Genetics	Autosomal dominant; some cases are sporadic (Gilbert 1999)
Learning disability	Mild to moderate

In Crouzon syndrome, there is premature fusion of the bones in the skull (craniostenosis). This causes microcephaly, increased intracranial pressure and severe midface deformities.

There is resultant hearing, dental and visual involvement, respiratory difficulties (due to nasal involvement) and feeding difficulties. There are two distinct presentations of Crouzon syndrome, one that is primarily characterized with premature craniostenosis and one that is also associated with fusion of elbow, wrist, finger and ankle joints.

MANAGEMENT

The primary issue of concern for the clinician treating a patient with Crouzon syndrome should be the management of craniostenosis and increased intracranial pressure, which can be life threatening. *Increased intracranial pressure* may manifest as headaches, vomiting and convulsions, and these features can be considered symptoms in their own right. Parents should be made fully aware of the signs and symptoms of increased intracranial pressure. Management should involve a multidisciplinary team, particularly a plastic surgeon, neurosurgeon, ophthalmologist, audiologist, orthodontist, octolaryngologist, dentist, geneticist and psychologist. *Surgery is multistage* and may span several years. In the first year of life, surgery should be performed—even in the absence of signs of craniostenosis—to release intracranial pressure and to allow the brain to grow and expand. There is evidence that corrective surgery improves outcome in terms of general development, even when intracranial pressure is not elevated. Skull reshaping may need repeating a number of times as the child grows. Treatment of maxillary hypoplasia and obstructive airways can be conducted only when the child reaches the age of 9 years. Correction of midface deformities is not only for cosmetic reasons but may also facilitate vision, speech, breathing, sleeping and eating.

Other complications arising from craniofacial abnormalities include sleep apnoea and upper airway obstruction. In severe cases tracheotomy may be required (Sculerati *et al.* 1998). It is important to regularly assess both vision and hearing in order to monitor deterioration of these senses as craniofacial abnormalities can lead to damage of the optic nerve (Gilbert 1999).

Although no typical behavioural abnormalities are associated with this syndrome the psychological and emotional development of these young people should be closely monitored. They are at risk from *low self-esteem and poor self-image* because of their appearance and may have to spend prolonged periods in hospital undergoing surgery.

REFERENCES

Gilbert PC (1999) *A–Z of Syndromes and Inherited Disorders.* Cheltenham, Gloucestershire: Stanely Thorpe.
Orvidas LJ, Fabry LB, Diacova S, McDonald TJ (1999) 'Hearing and otopathology in Crouzon syndrome.' *Laryngoscope*, **109**, 1372–1375.
Sculerati N, Gottlieb MD, Zimbler MS, Chibbaro PD, McCarthy JG (1998) 'Airway management in children with major craniofacial anomalies.' *Laryngoscope*, **108**, 1806–1812.

WEBSITE

- Crouzon Support Network
  www.crouzon.org/

DOWN SYNDROME

Incidence	1:600 (Harris 1998)
Genetics	Trisomy 21
Learning disability	Mild to moderate

Down syndrome is the most common genetic condition that gives rise to learning disability (Harris 1998). It is characterized by typical facies, gastrointestinal and congenital heart abnormalities, hyperflexia and short stature. Typical facies include upward- and outward-slanting eyes, epicanthus and wide nasal bridge. Hypotonia is a persistent feature during childhood but gradually becomes less marked with age. Language and speech deficits occur and are independent of the level of learning disability.

Down syndrome has a raised profile in the public domain. This has helped to reduce the stigma of Down syndrome and facilitate acceptance of the syndrome within society. Affected individuals are often portrayed by the media as having a pleasant and happy disposition. However, they can often be prone to aggression and irritability. This is at odds with the stereotyped disposition and families may feel responsible for the negative behaviour (Harris 1998).

MANAGEMENT

Due to the increased *public awareness* of Down syndrome there are many support groups available for parents and carers. These resources are essential in helping the families of affected individuals prepare for the long-term prospects and outcomes of the syndrome. It is essential not to neglect the siblings of affected individuals. Feelings of resentment and a lack of under-standing on behalf of siblings can have an adverse effect on the coping abilities of the family unit. It is important that siblings are made fully aware of what Down syndrome entails and are given appropriate emotional support (Harris 1998). A *referral to counselling* is recommended, not only for siblings but also for the affected person, as watching siblings and peers progress beyond one's own developmental level can be detrimental to self-esteem. A multidisciplinary approach is required when treating the person with Down syndrome, and intervention should commence as early as possible in order to maximize the developmental abilities of the child (Rogers *et al.* 1996).

Attention deficit disorder and other confounding psychiatric disorders co-occur in Down syndrome, but are responsive to *pharmaceutical intervention*. For example, methyl-phenidate, in the usual dose range, is beneficial. Research has suggested that the family environment in which the person with Down syndrome is raised can have a substantial influence on the type of behavioural difficulties exhibited. A chaotic family environment characterized by conflict is associated with a greater risk of antisocial behaviour. A family environment that harbours dependency has been linked to a greater incidence of emotional and mood problems. It is important that both the family and clinician involved in the care of the individual are not only aware of the propensity towards mood disorders, but are also aware that depression may present atypically in this population and that it responds to the usual treatment modalities (Harris 1998). It is also important to establish that the psychiatric disorder is not caused by a medical complication, such as hypothyroidism.

In individuals with Down syndrome over the age of 35 years, there are changes in brain tissue that are identical to the brain-tissue changes seen in people with *Alzheimer's disease*. Alzheimer's disease occurs in one-third of this population.

Congenital heart abnormalities necessitate regular check-ups. In adolescence, further complications may arise, such as orthopaedic problems, auditory impairments and cataracts. These should be medically managed as soon as they arise. There are a number of different strategies for the *management of hearing difficulties*, including antibiotics, placement of ventilation tubes within the middle ear and hearing aids (Rogers *et al.* 1996). Referrals should be made to an orthothalmologist within the first six months of life. It is important to identify visual complications at an early stage, as infantile glaucoma can lead to further substantial visual difficulties. Annual screening for hypothyroidism is also recommended and should commence at 12 months of age.

Despite failure to thrive being common during infancy, there is a propensity towards *obesity* as the child ages, with one-third of individuals with Down syndrome becoming obese by the age of 3 years. In the context of joint laxity and hypotonia, obesity can be a major health issue in this condition. It is therefore vitally important that diet is monitored and exercise and activity are included in the lifestyle of the affected individual (Rogers *et al.* 1996).

Seizures occur in 5% of affected individuals with Down syndrome, with onset usually within the first year of life. Some develop infantile spasms, which respond well to adreno-corticotrophic hormone treatment (Rogers *et al.* 1996).

REFERENCES

Harris JC (1998) *Developmental Neuropsychiatry, Vol. II: Assessment, Diagnosis and Treatment of Developmental Disorders.* Oxford: Oxford University Press.
Rogers PT, Roizen NJ, Capone GT (1996) 'Down syndrome.' In: Capute AJ, Accardo PJ (eds) *Developmental Disabilities in Infancy and Childhood , Vol. II.* Baltimore: Paul H Brookes.

WEBSITES

- Down's Heart Group
  www.downs-heart.downsnet.org/
- Down's Syndrome Association
  www.dsa-uk.com/
- Down's Syndrome Scotland
  www.sdsa.org.uk/
- National Down Syndrome Society (USA)
  www.ndss.org/

DUCHENNE MUSCULAR DYSTROPHY

Incidence	1:3500 male births (Blake and Kroger 2000) (decreasing due to genetic counselling)
Genetics	X-linked (short arm) recessive disorder, or spontaneous mutations
Learning disability	Mild (20–30%) (Blake and Kroger 2000)

There are a number of different forms of muscular dystrophy, all of which are characterized by progressive atrophy of voluntary muscles and muscular weakness. Duchenne muscular dystrophy (DMD) usually affects only boys, but in very rare cases may also affect girls. DMD occurs when a mutated gene on the X chromosome fails to make the protein dystrophin (a different gene mutation on the same chromosome leads to a deficiency of dystrophin: this causes Becker dystrophy). Early signs of muscle weakness are usually evident by 3 years of age. Most children with DMD learn to walk, but lose this ability between 7 and 12 years. Muscle wasting eventually leads to respiratory muscle weakness and increasing respiratory insufficiency. The third of affected individuals who have concomitant mild learning disability do not show any progressive deterioration of cognitive capabilities. Respiratory or cardiac failure are usually fatal in the late teens to mid-twenties (Blake and Kroger 2000) and survival beyond the second decade is rare.

MANAGEMENT

Diagnosis will involve a full personal and familial medical history and a physical examination. It will also usually involve a muscle biopsy. In managing DMD the most important strategies are *exercise and physiotherapy*. It is important that the body be kept as flexible, upright and supple as possible in order to minimize the effects of this condition. Excessive inactivity/bed rest should be avoided whenever possible. Physiotherapy and other exercise, *e.g.* swimming, are highly beneficial.

Muscle deterioration can cause painful contractures of the knee, hip, feet, elbow, wrist and finger joints. 'Range-of-motion' exercises can be performed to help prevent shortening of the tendons. These will be taught by the physiotherapist, and should be performed at home with the help of parents and carers. Hand and lower-leg braces can be useful in intervening against contractures. Surgery aimed at releasing tendons may be useful for advanced contractures—this is often done while the child is still able to walk to prolong mobility.

Spinal curvatures—scoliosis, kyphosis or lordosis—interfere with sitting, sleeping and breathing. These can be partially prevented through physiotherapy and may require corrective surgery. *Pharmacological agents* can be used to slow down the effects of this condition. Catabolic steroids can slow down the loss of muscle function and even increase strength. However, these agents can have serious side-effects that may paradoxically worsen the effects of the disease, and as such their use should be strictly monitored. Adverse reactions may include obesity, which in itself can impair mobility, and thinning of the bones, which can lead to osteoporosis. *Osteoporosis*, in a person who is already especially likely to fall, can lead to an increased risk of fractures. Calcium supplements may be used alongside catabolic steroids to offset osteoporosis.

Mobility aids, such as walking or standing frames and wheelchairs, are particularly useful. It is important that a child with this condition should stand for a couple of hours each day, even if this is done with the aid of a standing frame, in order to help circulation. These aids actually increase mobility rather than restricting it. As cardiomyopathy progresses, the heart should be closely monitored by a cardiologist.

Learning disability affects two key areas of functioning—attention, and verbal learning and memory. There are few specific dietary requirements, other than a high fluid and low sodium intake. A high fibre content is also advisable to prevent against constipation associated with immobility and weakened abdominal muscles. Eating excess protein cannot replace the absent dystrophin. Effects of cardiomyopathy can be diminished with a low-sodium diet.

This distressing and progressive condition is associated with *depression and anxiety*. Diagnosis of these psychiatric disorders may be masked by the motor slowing and muscular dystrophy. Symptoms should be treated appropriately. Affected children benefit from ongoing *emotional and psychological support*, and appropriate antidepressant medication can, at times, be beneficial. In the management of this syndrome, it is vitally important that affected individuals remain mobile. Facial or nasal mask ventilation is often required during sleep to prevent hypoventilation.

REFERENCE

Blake DJ, Kroger S. (2000) 'The neurobiology of Duchenne muscular dystrophy: Learning lessons from muscle?' *Trends in Neuroscience*, **23**, 92–99.

WEBSITES

- Duchenne Family Support Group
  www.dfsg.org.uk/
- Muscular Dystrophy Association
  www.mdausa.org/
- Muscular Dystrophy Campaign
  www.muscular-dystrophy.org/
- Society for Muscular Dystrophy Information International
  www.nsnet.org/smdi/

FRAGILE X SYNDROME

Incidence   1:1000–1:2600 males (Youings *et al.* 2000); 1:4000 females
Genetics   Distal arm Xq27.3; associated with the *FMR-1* gene
Learning disability Mild to moderate

Fragile X syndrome is one of the most common genetic causes of neurodevelopmental disability. It is caused by a large expansion of a sequence of trinucleotide repeats in the first exon of the *FMR-1* gene (Macpherson *et al.* 1995). The increased number of trinucleotide repeats disturbs the *FMR-1* gene and disrupts protein synthesis. FMR protein is required for neuronal connections. Absence of this protein delays neuronal development but does not destroy it. Research has suggested that people with fragile X syndrome can be divided into two groups, those whose IQ remains stable over time and those with a deterioration in cognitive functions (Fisch *et al.* 1992). There are sex differences associated with fragile X syndrome, with milder phenotypic expression, slower deterioration and less severe learning disability in females (fragile XE) (Turner *et al.* 1997, Accardo and Shapiro 1998, Fisch *et al.* 1999). Phenotypic expression includes autistic-like behaviours, pubertal-onset of macroorchidism, typical facies (macrocephaly, large prominent ears and a long face) and connective tissue disorder, which can contribute to heart defects and infections. Affected individuals are socially anxious, and become disturbed in the face of a variety of stressors and environmental changes. Life expectancy is normal but is dependant on the severity of cardiovascular problems.

MANAGEMENT

The difficulties that are associated with fragile X syndrome can be managed through a multidisciplinary approach (Goldson and Hagerman 1992). Following the initial diagnosis a *medical assessment* should be carried out to determine which of the medical complications of the disorder are present. Ongoing monitoring is also essential to screen for further complications. In infancy, patients present with failure to thrive due to gastro-oesophageal reflux and difficulties with sucking. Gastro-oesophageal reflux responds to dietary intervention and medication (de Vries *et al.* 1998). Due to the increased frequency of otitis media and sinusitis, interventions such as the use of antibiotics and polyethylene tubes are frequently used (de Vries *et al.* 1998).

The input from a *speech therapist* can be beneficial in the early years to help with sucking difficulties. Children with fragile X syndrome have particular problems with the pragmatics of language and their difficulties with attention, and behavioural characteristics can result in communication difficulties. The speech and language therapist is therefore essential in facilitating communication skills.

Individuals with fragile X syndrome can often present with a variety of *challenging behaviours*. In infancy, behavioural management should target the temperamental difficulties often associated with this syndrome, specifically sleep difficulties and temper tantrums. It is important to involve parents in all treatment programmes, especially those dealing with the management of behaviours. Individuals with fragile X syndrome can display aggressive behaviour, which is often impulsive and violent. In order to properly assess the cause of these outbursts a functional analysis of behaviour should be carried out to enable an appropriate management plan to be implemented. Often, aggression can be linked to environmental change, anxiety or mood instability. In adolescents, sexual frustration should always be considered as a precipitating factor to aggression. Sex education and the use of more appropriate outlets for their sexual frustration can be useful in this situation.

Behavioural interventions are not only useful for addressing specific behaviours, but also in helping individuals to cope with the demands placed upon them on a day-to-day basis. For example the use of pictured schedules can be beneficial in helping them to navigate the changes that will occur during the day. The use of visual signals can aid the understanding of accompanying verbal requests. Behavioural strategies used in the management of children with ADHD can also be employed for children who suffer from fragile X syndrome. These include the use of visual cues, avoiding distracting situations, sitting near the teacher in class, and planning a number of short sessions between which the individual can get up and move around. People with fragile X syndrome have good abilities in memory, reading and imitation, and special education should capitalize upon these skills, while also providing remedial support for weaker areas (Harris 1998).

Occupational therapy is often beneficial for this group; as well as improving fine motor skills and coordination, when combined with speech therapy it can enhance expressive language and attention span, especially during adolescence when ADHD is more pronounced (Goldson and Hagerman 1992). *Medication* can be used to treat a number of aspects of the disorder. CNS stimulants can be useful in the management of impaired attention and hyperactivity. Methylphenidate has reportedly been prescribed to two-thirds of children with

186

the syndrome (Goldson and Hagerman 1992). SSRIs can be useful in the treatment of anxiety, obsessive–compulsive disorder and impulsivity, and thus help to prevent aggression (Hagerman *et al.* 1994). If aggression occurs in the context of mood instability, mood stabilizers such as lithium carbonate or carbamazepine can be helpful. Although there are few published studies looking at the benefits of atypical antipsychotics in treating aggression in this group, anecdotal evidence suggests that they are of use. The use of medication should always be carefully monitored and should accompany behavioural interventions rather than replacing them.

It has been suggested that overactivity and impulsivity can be reduced with stimulants, although these behaviours naturally decrease with age without pharmacological intervention. The use of folic acid in the syndrome has previously been reported to be effective in helping behavioural symptomatology; however, it is now thought not to be useful.

REFERENCES

Accardo PJ, Shapiro LR (1998) 'FRAXA and FRAXE: to test or not to test?' Journal of Pediatrics, **132**, 762–764.

de Vries BB, Halley DJ, Oostra BA, Niermeijer MF (1998) 'The fragile X syndrome.' *Journal of Medical Genetics*, **35**, 579–589.

Fisch GS, Shapiro LR, Simensen R, Schwartz CE, Fryns JP, Borghgraef M, Curfs LM, Howard-Peebles PN, Arinami T, Mavrou A (1992) 'Longitudinal changes in IQ among fragile X males: Clinical evidence of more than one mutation?' *American Journal of Medical Genetics*, **43**, 28–34.

Fisch GS, Carpenter N, Holden JJA, Howard-Peebles PN, Maddalena A, Borghgraef M, Steyaert J, Fryns J-P (1999) 'Longitudinal changes in cognitive and adaptive behaviour in fragile X females: A prospective multi-centre analysis.' *American Journal of Medical Genetics*, **83**, 308–312.

Goldson E, Hagerman RJ (1992) 'The fragile X syndrome.' *Developmental Medicine and Child Neurology*, **34**, 826–832.

Hagerman RJ, Wilson P, Staley LW, Lang KA, Fan T, Uhlhorn C, Jewell-Smart S, Hull C, Drisko J, Flom K (1994) 'Evaluation of school children at high risk for fragile X syndrome utilizing buccal cell FMR-1 testing.' *American Journal of Medical Genetics*, **51**, 474–481.

Harris JC (1998) *Developmental Neuropsychiatry, Vol. II: Assessment, Diagnosis and Treatment of Developmental Disorders.* Oxford: Oxford University Press.

Macpherson, JN, Curtis G, Crolla JA, Dennis N, Migeon B, Grewal PK, Hirst MC, Davies KE, Jacobs PA (1995) 'Unusual $(CGG)_n$ expansion and recombination in a family with fragile X and DiGeorge syndrome.' *Journal of Medical Genetics*, **32**, 236–239.

Turner G, Robinson H, Wake S, Laing S, Partington M (1997) 'Case finding for the fragile X syndrome and its consequences.' *British Medical Journal*, **315**, 1223–1226.

Youings SA, Murray A, Dennis N, Ennis S, Lewis C, McKechnie N, Pound M, Sharrock A, Jacobs P (2000) 'FRAXA and FRAXE: the results of a five year survey.' *Journal of Medical Genetics*, **37**, 415–421.

WEBSITES

- Fragile X Society
  www.fragilex.org.uk/
- FRAXA Research Foundation
  www.fraxa.org/

GALACTOSAEMIA (CLASSICAL)

Incidence	1:45,000 (Walter *et al.* 1999)
Genetics	Autosomal recessive
Learning disability	Borderline

Galactosaemia is caused by a metabolic error in which there is a deficiency of the enzyme galactose-1-phosphate uridyl transferase (GALT) (Shield *et al.* 2000), resulting in an intolerance to galactose. Long-term dietary restriction of lactose is necessary—failure to do this results in feeding difficulties, vomiting, jaundice and renal-tubular damage (Berry *et al.* 1995). The syndrome usually presents in the first two weeks of life (Hutchesson *et al.* 1999). Complications that can arise if the syndrome is left untreated include liver disease, coagulopathy, septicaemia and encephalopathy (O'Brien and Yule 1995), and these can be fatal. Despite dietary control, a secondary deterioration, characterized by cognitive impairment, speech difficulties, cerebellar ataxia, intention tremor, apraxia and extrapyramidal dysfunction can develop. Fertility in women is also affected; most commonly this manifests as infertility or reduced fertility and ovarian failure, although some galactosaemic women have had natural pregnancies (Berry *et al.* 1995). Fertility and pubertal development in males remains unaffected (Walter *et al.* 1999). When treated, this syndrome is associated with a normal life expectancy. However, if it is not adequately managed, liver failure or infection may be fatal.

MANAGEMENT

Early diagnosis of this condition is essential. If there is any suspicion that an infant is suffering from galactosaemia, galactose must be excluded from their diet until a definitive diagnosis is made. Individuals affected by galactosaemia have the potential to lead normal and fulfilled lives, providing that this galactose is eliminated from the diet. A galactose-free diet must be adhered to for the duration of the life span. An improvement is seen in acute toxicity syndrome within the first 24 hours of removal of galactose from the diet.

Dietary management, however, does not prevent some of the late-onset complications. These include cognitive deterioration, seizures, intention tremor, cataracts, ovarian failure, ataxia, speech deficits and visual–perceptual difficulties. It is thought that these are due to endogenous production of galactose (Berry *et al.* 1995). There would seem to be no relation between the age at which galactosaemia is diagnosed and the diet is introduced, and the severity of these long-term complications (Hutchesson *et al.* 1999). The extent to which these complications are related to compliance is unknown (Hutchesson *et al.* 1999).

The secondary deterioration associated with galactosaemia necessitates regular medical follow-ups. Annual check-ups should also by made by a dietician to monitor the *nutritional value of the diet*, as such a restrictive diet can lead to deficiencies of key nutrients, particularly calcium. Calcium supplements can be used to prevent bone density from decreasing and to protect against osteoporosis (Walter *et al.* 1999). Regular review by an ophthalmologist is recommended as cataracts develop in childhood in one-third of affected individuals. These can be resolved with dietary intervention, and the support of the ophthalmologist ensures that this diagnosis is made promptly. Cognitive impairment, which is a characteristic of this condition, may not manifest until school age. It is therefore important that the cognitive development of children with galactosaemia is regularly monitored. Speech deficits, particularly of expressive speech, often warrant input from a *speech therapist*.

The patient should be under the care of a paediatric endocrinologist by the age of 10 years (Walter *et al.* 1999). Puberty is induced with *hormone treatment* and it is suggested that this treatment should commence by the time the child is 12 years old. Monitoring of bone-age, blood pressure and physical development should be conducted quarterly for the first two years of treatment and every six months thereafter. Measurements of lutenizing hormone, follicle stimulating hormone and oestradiol in females should also be conducted annually.

Many medications contain lactose, and it is important to establish that this is not a component of a drug before it is prescribed (Walter *et al.* 1999).

It has recently been suggested that other interventions should be considered in parallel with dietary control in order to try to prevent deterioration in adulthood. These include augmentation of residual transferase activity (folic acid, progesterone), interdiction of aldose alternative pathways, replacement of depleted metabolites and gene therapy (Harris 1998).

REFERENCES

Berry GT, Nissim I, Lin Z, Mazur AT, Gibson JB, Segal S (1995) 'Endogenous synthesis of galactose in normal men and patients with hereditary galactosaemia.' *Lancet*, **346**, 1073–1074.

Harris JC (1998) *Developmental Neuropsychiatry, Vol. II: Assessment, Diagnosis and Treatment of Developmental Disorders.* Oxford: Oxford University Press.

Hutchesson AC, Murdoch-Davis C, Green A, Preece MA, Allen J, Holton JB, Rylance G (1999) 'Biochemical monitoring of treatment for galactosaemia: biological variability in metabolite concentrations.' *Journal of Inherited Metabolic Disease*, **22**, 139–148.

O'Brien G, Yule W (eds) (1995) *Behavioural Phenotypes. Clinics in Developmental Medicine No. 138.* London: Mac Keith Press.

Shield JPH, Wadsworth EJK, MacDonald A, Stephenson A, Tyfield L, Holton JB, Marlow N (2000) 'The relationship of genotype to cognitive outcome in galactosaemia.' *Archives of Disease in Childhood*, **83**, 248–250.

Walter JH, Collins JE, Leonard JV (1999) 'Recommendations for the management of galactosaemia. UK Galactosaemia Steering Group.' *Archives of Disease in Childhood*, **80**, 93–96.

WEBSITE

• Galactosaemia Support Group UK
  http://www.edinburgh.gov.uk/HEBS/UK_Health_Advice_Groups/uk_health_advice_groups_GALACTOSAEMIA_SUPPORT_GROUP.html

HYPOMELANOSIS OF ITO

Incidence	Unknown—1:1000 new patients in a paediatric neurology service was reported (SSBP 1995)
Genetics	Usually X-linked (Hatchwell 1996)
Learning disability	45% moderate to severe, 15% borderline (O'Brien and Yule 1995)

Hypomelanosis of Ito is the most frequent neuroectodermal disorder; it is more common in males than females (O'Brien and Yule 1995). This multisystem syndrome is characterized by whorls of hypopigmentation around the trunk and in linear patterns down the arms and legs (known as Blaschko's lines). These may be the only features present, or musculoskeletal, central nervous system, hair, dental and visual abnormalities may also occur (Hatchwell 1996, Correa-Cerro *et al.* 1997, Eussen *et al.* 2000). There may also be asymmetrical growth on either side of the body. In adulthood, skin pigmentation becomes less prominent. There would appear to be no correlation between the level of learning disability and the extent of pigmented skin (O'Brien and Yule 1995).

MANAGEMENT

The majority of interventions in this disorder are focused on the management of the medical complications. Individuals should be monitored for *epilepsy* and treated appropriately. Affected individuals can suffer discomfort and gait problems as a consequence of scoliosis. This can be ameliorated by the use of *physiotherapy*. The cosmetic effects of the disorder can result in emotional distress and low self-esteem requiring psychological intervention.

REFERENCES

Correa-Cerro LS, Rivera H, Vasquez AI (1997) 'Functional Xp disomy and de novo t(X;13)(q10;q10) in a girl with hypomelanosis of Ito.' *Journal of Medical Genetics*, **34**, 161–163.
Eussen BH, Bartalini G., Bakker L, Balestri P, Di Lucca C, Van Hemel JO, Dauwerse H, van Den Ouweland AM, Ris-Stalpers C, Verhoef S, Halley DJ, Fois A (2000) 'An unbalanced submicroscopic translocation t(8;16)(q24.3;p13.3)pat associated with tuberous sclerosis complex, adult polycystic kidney disease, and hypomelanosis of Ito.' *Journal of Medical Genetics*, **37**, 287–291.
Hatchwell E (1996) 'Hypomelanosis of Ito and X; autosome translocations: a unifying hypothesis.' *Journal of Medical Genetics*, **33**, 177–183.
O'Brien G, Yule W (eds) (1995) *Behavioural Phenotypes. Clinics in Developmental Medicine No. 138.* London: Mac Keith Press.
SSBP (1995) *Proceedings of the 6th Annual Meeting of the Society for the Study of Behavioural Phenotypes, Edinburgh Conference Centre, Edinburgh, Scotland, 16–17 November 1995.*

JOUBERT SYNDROME

Incidence   Over 100 cases have been reported (SSBP 1996)
Genetics   Autosomal recessive (van Royen-Kerkhof *et al.* 1998)
Learning disability   Mild to moderate

In Joubert syndrome, the cerebellar vermis, which controls balance and coordination, is absent or underdeveloped. The syndrome is characterized by agenesis of the corpus callosum, congenital ataxia, hypotonia, abnormal eye and tongue movements, unstable gait, distinctive breathing patterns and defects of the visual and renal systems (O'Brien and Yule 1995, Steinlin 1998). There is wide variability in the severity of the motor impairment. One-third to one-half of affected individuals die before the age of 2 years (SSBP 1996).

MANAGEMENT

Individuals who exhibit abnormal breathing patterns, including hypercapnoea and sleep apnoea, require regular monitoring. These abnormalities are more prevalent in infancy. A *multidisciplinary approach* to treating the disorder is essential, and should involve occupational therapy, physiotherapy and speech and language therapy. If verbal expressive abilities are poor, alternative methods of communication, such as sign language, can be taught. It is essential that affected infants are provided with a lot of stimulation.

Feeding, eating and speech production can prove difficult due to poor tone in facial muscles. However, *physiotherapy* to massage the muscles of the face and throat, especially prior to feeding, can be beneficial. Physiotherapy involving manipulation of the facial muscles must be done under supervision of a professional and with care, as many children with Joubert syndrome are very sensitive to touch. Individuals with Joubert syndrome often have atypical alignment of muscles. An individualized programme of physiotherapy can correct the alignment, maintaining developed muscles whilst stretching and lengthening underdeveloped muscles. This leads to improvement of posture, gait and balance. A referral to an *orthopaedic specialist* may be necessitated, as some children with this syndrome require the use of ankle and/or foot braces to aid walking. The school environment can also be adapted to suit the child's physical needs, *e.g.* providing appropriate supporting chairs, thus allowing the child to gain maximal access to educational facilities.

Adaptive behaviour skills, balance and motor coordination are often impaired due to abnormalities of the cerebellar vermis. However, *occupational therapy* can help to develop and facilitate these skills. Development of adaptive behaviour skills is vital for the psychological well-being of the affected individual, as it will increase the sense of autonomy. It can also facilitate the ability of the individual to relate and react to the surrounding environments, as the processing abilities in this syndrome are often delayed.

Parents should be made fully aware of the medical complications involved in Joubert syndrome, particularly renal degeneration. This problem is diagnosed through an ERG (electroretinogram).

REFERENCES

O'Brien G, Yule W (eds) (1995) *Behavioural Phenotypes. Clinics in Developmental Medicine No. 138.* London: Mac Keith Press.
SSBP (1996) *Proceedings of the 4th International Symposium of the Society for the Study of Behavioural Phenotypes, Marino Institute of Education, Dublin, Ireland, 14–16 November 1996.*
Steinlin M (1998) 'Non-progressive congenital ataxias.' *Brain and Development*, **20**, 199–208.
van Royen-Kerkhof A, Poll-The BT, Kleijer WJ, van Diggelen OP, Aerts JM., Hopwood JJ, Beemer FA (1998) 'Coexistence of Gaucher disease type 1 and Joubert syndrome.' *Journal of Medical Genetics*, **35**, 965–966.

WEBSITE

- Joubert Syndrome Foundation
  www.joubertfoundation.com/

KALLMANN SYNDROME

Incidence	1:10,000 males; 1:70,000 females
Genetics	Three possible modes of transmission; X-linked, autosomal dominant and autosomal recessive (SSBP 2000)
Learning disability	Normal to borderline (SSBP 2000)

Kallmann syndrome is caused by a failure of fetal gonadotrophin-releasing hormone neurons to migrate to the thalamus. It is more common in males. Typical presentation includes anosmia as a result of agenesis of the olfactory lobes, and hypogonadism. It is difficult to diagnose in the prepubertal child. The literature identifies three types of expression. Type 1 has an X-linked mode of transmission and is characterized by hearing impairment, cerebellar ataxia, renal agenesis and paraplegia. Type 2 is autosomal dominant and is generally associated with congenital heart disease. Type 3 is autosomal recessive and presents with chonal atresia and cleft lip and palate (SSBP 2000). Phenotypic expression is milder in females (Schinzel *et al.* 1995) and is associated with hyposmia, amenorrhoea and lack of breast development (SSBP 2000). Life expectancy is normal (SSBP 2000).

MANAGEMENT

This can be a particularly distressing condition for affected individuals as puberty may have been absent for several years before a referral is made to an *endocrinologist* and the disorder is diagnosed. This syndrome is associated with a total lack of puberty, however, puberty can be artificially induced and the post-pubertal state maintained with synthetic hormones. This syndrome has significant psychological implications, as the failure of the body to develop primary and secondary sexual characteristics can cause low self-esteem, poor self-image and depression, and in many cases can lead to bullying. Affected individuals look extremely young for their age, and low self-esteem can be worsened—often inadvertently—by the actions of others, for example, by offering them children's travel rates. *Specialist counselling* may be particularly appropriate for these symptoms and other issues surrounding sexual and social development (Gilbert 1999).

Hormone replacement therapy is given for two reasons. It is given primarily to induce and maintain puberty, and secondarily to aid fertility. Testosterone treatment is available in a number of forms. Commonly, it is injected once every few weeks; however, this method does not simulate the natural diurnal rhythm of testosterone, and as the effects of the hormone wear off, individuals become fatigued. Skin patches or oral tablets would seem to prevent this.

Males and females with Kallmann syndrome are at an increased risk of insufficient bone calcification, and therefore *osteoporosis*. This increases the propensity to fracture. For this reason, hormone replacement therapy should commence before any signs of decalcified bones manifest. Vigorous, weight-bearing exercise can help to build muscle tissue around weakened bones. This, in combination with calcium supplements, helps to protect against osteoporosis.

Orchidopexy may be necessary to correct undescended testes. When this procedure is performed on patients younger than 6 years of age, chances of fertility are improved. *Fertility treatment* for women affected by this syndrome is particularly effective, with greater than 90% of sufferers becoming pregnant within 6 months of commencing GnRH pulsatile therapy.

There is no cure for anosmia. Bimanual synkinesis is common in non-sporadic cases. This can, for instance, make sports or playing musical instruments difficult, and understanding is needed for this symptom. Gynaecomastia is no more common in this syndrome than in the normal male population.

REFERENCES

Gilbert PC (1999) *A–Z of Syndromes and Inherited Disorders.* Cheltenham, Gloucestershire: Stanely Thorne.
Schinzel A, Lorda-Sanchez I, Binkert F, Carter NP, Bebb CE, Ferguson-Smith MA, Eiholzer U, Zachmann M, Robinson WP (1995) 'Kallmann syndrome in a boy with a t(1;10) translocation detected by reverse chromosome painting.' *Journal of Medical Genetics*, **32**, 957–961.

SSBP (2000) *Proceedings of the 6th International Symposium of the Society for the Study of Behavioural Phenotypes, Venice International University, San Servolo, Italy, 12–14 October 2000.*

WEBSITE

• HYPOHH (Helping You To Be Positive about Hypogonadotrophic Hypogonadism)
  www.hypohh.net/

LESCH–NYHAN SYNDROME

Incidence   1:380,000 (Harris *et al.* 1998)
Genetics   X-linked recessive (McGreevy and Arthur 1987)
Learning disability Mild to moderate (SSBP 2000)

Lesch–Nyhan syndrome is caused by an inborn error of purine nucleotide metabolism, which in turn causes an almost complete deficiency in the enzyme hypoxanthine-guanine phosphoribosyl transferase (HPRT). The more severe the HPRT enzyme deficiency, the greater is the propensity towards more profound learning disability and self-injury (Saito and Takashima 2000). Deficiency of HPRT leads to a build-up of uric acid that can manifest as severe aggression, self-mutilation and gout. The primary behavioural manifestation of this syndrome is severe self-injury. Other typical characteristics include severe motor disability, dystonia, growth retardation, visual impairments, feeding difficulties, involuntary movements, hyponia, seizures and uricaemia (O'Brien and Yule 1995, Harris *et al.* 1998). Infants appear normal at birth and the features of the syndrome do not become prominent until 8–12 months of age. The age of onset predicts the severity of self-mutilation (O'Brien and Yule 1995). Self-injury usually becomes prevalent at 3.5 years of age and typically declines after 10 years of age. Early mortality is due to renal failure, infection and respiration difficulties (O'Brien and Yule 1995); unexpected and sudden death is frequently noted (Saito and Takashima 2000).

MANAGEMENT

Ongoing medical assessment is necessary in this condition to monitor for known medical complications such as renal failure. Allopurinol can be useful to treat increased levels of uric acid and is preventative in the treatment of renal failure and gout, but does not reduce aberrant behaviours (Ernst *et al.* 1996). Renal stones often occur and can be successfully treated with lithotripsy.

The most distressing aspect of this syndrome for most parents and carers is the behavioural manifestations. *Self-injurious behaviour* is a primary feature of the syndrome, directed particularly to the fingers and mouth. There are a number of approaches to reducing self-inflicted injuries, particularly pharmacology, behavioural therapy and restraint. A combination of all these approaches should be used. The most widely used *pharmacological interventions* are naltrexone and benzodiazapines (diazepam) (Saito and Takashima 2000), although SSRIs have also been found to be beneficial in treating self-injury. Prosthetic restraints, such as finger guards and elbow restraints, and physical restraints, prevent the occurrence of self-injury while they are in use, but can be regarded as restrictive (McGreevy and Arthur

1987). In this condition, the self-injury is highly distressing to affected individuals, who are aware of their behaviours but have little control over them. They will actively seek to be restrained to prevent injury and pain, and a state of great anxiety and distress is evoked when restraint is not provided. Behavioural intervention has been used with limited success. It reduces the rate of self-injury, but there is no response generalization to other areas of the body (McGreevy and Arthur 1987). *Behavioural techniques*, such as systematic desensitization, differential reinforcement of other behaviours and extinction, should focus on developing coping mechanisms and should particularly address the distress that manifests when there is no restraint. Overall, families show a preference for positive behavioural techniques, such as redirection. Although an extreme method of intervention, dental extraction is still very commonly used in this syndrome for the prevention of self-injury. In one sample, 60% of affected individuals had had tooth extraction for this reason (Harris 1998).

Stressful events are antecedents of self-injurious behaviour, and can thus be interceded with active engagement in pleasurable activities and social interaction. Most children with this syndrome are aware of the compulsive element of their self-injurious behaviour and adopt *self-regulating coping strategies* to prevent the behaviour occurring and thus reduce anxiety. An example of this type of self-regulation is sitting on their hands. There is an increased rate of anxiety in children with Lesch–Nyhan syndrome, often as a result of awareness of their aggressive and compulsive behaviour (O'Brien and Yule 1995). Aggressive behaviour is often directed towards parents and carers and can be managed with the use of behavioural techniques. The classroom environment can be particularly stressful for individuals suffering from this disorder, thus it is often necessary to devise individual educational programmes.

REFERENCES

Ernst M, Zametkin AJ, Matochik JA, Pascualvaca D, Jons PH, Hardy K, Hankerson JG, Doudet DJ, Cohen RM (1996) 'Presynaptic dopaminergic deficits in Lesch–Nyhan disease.' *New England Journal of Medicine*, **334**, 1568–1572.
Harris JC (1998) *Developmental Neuropsychiatry, Vol. II: Assessment, Diagnosis and Treatment of Developmental Disorders.* Oxford: Oxford University Press.
Harris JC, Lee RR, Jinnah HA, Wong DF, Yaster M, Bryan RN (1998) 'Craniocerebral magnetic resonance imaging measurement and findings in Lesch–Nyhan syndrome.' *Archives of Neurology*, **55**, 547–553.
McGreevy P, Arthur M (1987) 'Effective behavioral treatment of self-biting by a child with Lesch–Nyhan syndrome.' *Developmental Medicine and Child Neurology*, **29**, 536–540.
O'Brien G, Yule W (eds) (1995) *Behavioural Phenotypes, Clinics in Developmental Medicine No. 138.* London: Mac Keith Press.
Saito Y, Takashima S (2000) 'Neurotransmitter changes in the pathophysiology of Lesch–Nyhan syndrome.' *Brain and Development*, **22**, S122–S131.
SSBP (2000) *Proceedings of the 6th International Symposium of the Society for the Study of Behavioural Phenotypes, Venice International University, San Servolo, Italy, 12–14 October 2000.*

WEBSITES

- International Lesch–Nyhan Disease Registry
  www.matheny.org/about/ab_les_reg.html
- Lesch–Nyhan Disease National Registry (USA)
  http://64.93.22.27/
- Purine Research Society
  www2.dgsys.com/~purine/

LOWE SYNDROME

Alternative name	Oculo-cerebro-renal syndrome
Incidence	1:200,000 (O'Brien and Yule 1995)
Genetics	X-linked recessive disorder (Gilbert 1999)
Learning disability	75% have learning disability, usually moderate to severe

Lowe syndrome is a progressive metabolic disorder. It typically affects only males and is characterized by abnormalities of the kidneys, eyes and brain, in addition to muscular–skeletal and serum enzyme abnormalities, typical facies, juvenile stereotypies and self-injury. Renal abnormalities are progressive. Visual deficits are the result of the eyes not growing proportionately to the rest of the face and can lead to limited sight or blindness (Gilbert 1999). Mortality, due to renal failure, dehydration or pneumonia, is high. Affected males do not survive beyond the fourth decade of life. In many cases death occurs in childhood (O'Brien and Yule 1995, Gilbert 1999).

MANAGEMENT
Regular check-ups are vital to monitor vision. Cataracts, squints and glaucoma are the most common visual deficits reported in Lowe syndrome and warrant appropriate treatment. It is important to maximize the potential of the visual system through the use of magnification and good lighting (Gilbert 1999). The most common renal abnormalities are hypophosphataemia and acidosis, both of which require corrective surgery. Early treatment and diagnosis of renal complications can increase life span and improve quality of life (Gilbert 1999). Phosphate and bicarbonate are used to treat renal tubular dysfunction.

Maladaptive behaviours such as screaming, aggression, self-injury and stereotypies are most prevalent in adolescence and decline after the age of 18 years (O'Brien and Yule 1995). In all instances, it is important to enlist the help and support of a clinical psychologist, as most of these behaviours are the result of a delay in immediate gratification (Gilbert 1999). These behaviours have a pervasive impact upon the family, and are especially restrictive when planning family activities. There is no specific treatment for this condition; any treatment is purely symptomatic.

REFERENCES

Gilbert PC (1999) *A–Z of Syndromes and Inherited Disorders.* Cheltenham, Gloucestershire: Stanely Thorne.
O'Brien G, Yule W (eds) (1995) *Behavioural Phenotypes. Clinics in Developmental Medicine No. 138.* London: Mac Keith Press.

WEBSITE

• Lowe Syndrome Association
  www.lowesyndrome.org/

MUCOPOLYSACCHARIDOSES
The group of syndromes classed as mucopolysaccharidoses are lysosomal storage diseases, resulting from deficiencies of various lysosomal enzymes. These enzymes catalyse glycos-

aminoglycans and their deficiency causes mucopolysaccharides to be stored in the body causing progressive damage. Abnormalities of both the lower and upper respiratory tract are common and can lead to sleep apnoea (Leighton *et al.* 2001). Mortality is often the result of cardiorespiratory failure (Leighton *et al.* 2001).

All of the mucopolysaccharidoses are autosomal recessive in transmission with the exception of Hunter syndrome, which is X-linked. Scheie, Hurler and Hurler–Scheie syndromes are phenotypically similar, and although they are separate conditions, they can be viewed on a dimension of severity—Scheie syndrome representing the mildest and Hurler syndrome the most severe of these three, with Hurler–Scheie syndrome being the intermediate phenotype. These three syndromes are all linked to chromosome 4.

Scheie syndrome (MPS IS, formerly MPS V) has an incidence of 1:500,000 (Keith *et al.* 1990). There is usually no learning disability associated with this syndrome; where there is cognitive impairment, it is generally mild. The syndrome is characterized by late childhood onset and is typified by skeletal and cardiac abnormalities, normal life expectancy and typical facies (enlarged tongue and prominent forehead) (O'Brien and Yule 1995, Keith *et al.* 1990). It has a milder expression than Hurler syndrome, despite having an identical biochemical basis (Bredenkamp *et al.* 1992).

Hurler–Scheie syndrome (MPS IH/S) is typically associated with mild learning disability. It commonly presents between the ages of 3 and 8 years. Progressive visual deficits impair vision by the fourth decade (Keith *et al.* 1990). Affected individuals usually survive into adulthood.

Hurler syndrome (MPS IH) has an incidence of 1:100,000 (Gilbert 1999). The level of learning disability is usually moderate to severe. This syndrome is usually diagnosed within the first year of life. It is characterized by severe skeletal, muscular and cognitive deterioration, and mortality usually occurs in the first decade of life. In addition, these individuals have an enlarged liver and spleen, obstructive hydrocephalus and carpal tunnel syndrome. These features, along with weight loss, give rise to high rates of cardiorespiratory infections and complications (O'Brien and Yule 1995, Haddad *et al.* 1997).

Hunter syndrome (MPS II) occurs in 1:132,000 male births (Timms *et al.* 1997). Learning disability varies widely from mild to severe. By the age of 4 years, boys with Hunter syndrome should have received the diagnosis. Hunter syndrome is characterized by a progressive deterioration of physical and mental abilities. Individuals have a highly distinctive facial appearance, enlarged abdomen, liver and spleen, and progressive stiffening of joints that restricts movement (Peters and Krivit 2000). The facial characteristics include a large nose with flattened bridge and flared nostrils, thick lips and a large protruding tongue (O'Brien and Yule 1995). Progressive aural and visual impairments, including recurrent ear infections, are also common. There are two phenotypic expressions of Hunter syndrome. MPS IIA is characterized by cardiac failure and obstructive airway disease, leading to death by the age of 20 years. The less severe expression of the phenotype (MPS IIB) has a slower progression rate, later age of onset and lower rates of early mortality (O'Brien and Yule 1995); affected individuals usually survive into their fifth or sixth decade (Timms *et al.* 1997).

Maroteaux–Lamy syndrome (MPS VI) has an incidence of less than 1:100,000 (Widemann *et al.* 1992) and has been linked to chromosome 5. There is normally no learning disability associated with this syndrome, but where there is, it is mild. The syndrome consists of neurological complications such as carpal tunnel syndrome, cord compression and hydrocephalus. It is not dissimilar from Hurler syndrome, except that life expectancy is greater (mortality usually occurs before 30 years of age), there is less coarse facial dysmorphism and intelligence is preserved (Bredenkamp *et al.* 1992). The physical appearance of affected individuals is marked: due to joint immobility and skeletal abnormalities, they assume a crouched posture.

Morquio syndrome (MPS IV) has a reported incidence 1:100,000 (Gilbert 1999). It is associated with chromosomes 3 and 16. Intelligence is usually preserved, but in some individuals a mild learning disability can occur. There is a classical (IVA) and variant (IVB) form. The variant form is similar to the classical form, but is milder, has a later onset and is not associated with heart murmurs. The classical phenotype is characterized by progressive skeletal deformities, which can cause compression of the cervical cord, leading to quadriplegia or myelopathy (Bredenkamp *et al.* 1992). Growth would seem to cease by 8 years of age. Management of skeletal abnormalities can prolong life expectancy into the third decade of life (O'Brien and Yule 1995).

Sanfilippo syndrome (MPS III) has an incidence of 1:25,000–1:200,000 (Gilbert 1999). It has been linked to chromosomes 7, 12 and 14. In this syndrome skeletal abnormalities are mild. However, there is severe and progressive CNS involvement. Although development is delayed, developmental abnormalities become more obvious at around 4 years of age, and are associated with aggressive hyperactivity and a loss of acquired skills (O'Brien and Yule 1995). Speech is the most severely affected ability and is eventually lost completely. There is a lack of overt somatic symptoms (Bredenkamp *et al.* 1992). At some stage during childhood, most children require tube feeding due to feeding difficulties associated with swallowing incoordination (O'Brien and Yule 1995).

Sly syndrome (MPS VII) is rare, having been documented in only "around 20 patients worldwide" up to 1994 (PEDBASE 1994). It has been linked to chromosome 7. There is vast variability in the phenotypic expression of Sly syndrome, but typically affected patients are described as having deterioration of the auditory and visual systems, typical facies, recurrent respiratory infections, hepatosplenomegaly and inguinal and umbilical hernias and moderate skeletal abnormalities. Milder cases are associated with increased life expectancy.

MANAGEMENT

Following the diagnosis of a mucopolysaccharide syndrome, ongoing medical review is necessary to monitor for the medical complications that can occur, especially cardiorespiratory failure. *Surgery* is often indicated to treat a number of the characteristic features. However, performing surgery on affected individuals is difficult due to the respiratory and airway obstructions that characterize this group of syndromes. Even the simple procedure of laying the person on an operating table may provoke physical discomfort as a result of thoracic kyphoscoliosis and lumbar gibbus (Sjogren *et al.* 1987). Despite these complications, tracheostomy can help manage airway obstruction (Bredenkamp *et al.* 1992). Surgery may also be required to treat hernias that are a commonly reoccurring problem in both Hurler and Hunter syndromes (Gilbert 1999). Spinal fusion of the vertebrae to correct the abnormality of the upper cervical vertebrae is a common method of corrective surgery used with Morquio syndrome. It is vital that parents/carers are well informed about this abnormality so it can be detected at an early stage (Gilbert 1999).

Physiotherapy can be highly beneficial in the treatment of spinal abnormalities, stiff joints and spinal contractures in Morquio, Hurler and Hunter syndromes respectively. Incorporation of hydrotherapy into regular physiotherapy sessions not only enhances the effectiveness of physiotherapy but also provides a pleasurable activity for the child, and facilitates parental involvement (Gilbert 1999).

The *auditory system* deteriorates due to the gradual accumulation of mucopolysaccharides. It is important that the clinician is aware that any decline or plateau in developmental abilities may be a direct result of hearing loss (Wallace *et al.* 1990). Regular monitoring of hearing is vital and the use of hearing aids is often warranted for individuals affected by any of the mucopolysaccharide syndromes (Gilbert 1999). In a sample, 73% of affected individuals suffered from otitis media (Bredenkamp *et al.* 1992). Nonetheless, persistent and systematic treatment of otitis media in tandem with auditory rehabilitation and the teaching of other modes of communication can enhance existing auditory abilities and facilitate communication (Bredenkamp *et al.* 1992).

Evidence has shown that *bone marrow transplantation* in individuals affected by mucopolysaccharidoses slows down the natural progression of these disorders. It improves facial features, reverses upper airway disease and decreases mucopolysacchariduria, thus prolonging longevity (Vellodi *et al.* 1997). However, whilst correcting the enzyme deficiency in white blood cells, it does not alleviate the condition or correct brain abnormalities. The long-term risks and outcomes associated with bone marrow transplantation across the spectrum of mucopolysaccharidoses requires further evaluation (O'Brien and Yule 1995).

As a result of respiratory and skeletal abnormalities, *sleep problems* such as sleep apnoea are especially prevalent in Hurler and Hunter syndromes and are thought to cause the night-time awakening often observed in children with these syndromes. These can be managed through medical procedures such as nocturnal administration of oxygen and nasal continuous positive airway pressure (O'Brien and Yule 1995). However, medical procedures are less effective at treating sleep difficulties in children with Sanfilippo syndrome, for which behavioural and physical intervention strategies are often required. These children engage in disruptive night-time behaviours such as chewing the bedclothes, crying out and, more rarely, wandering around the family home. These behaviours often necessitate the child being physically restrained during the night, and they have a detrimental effect on the quality of sleep of other family members. Medication to induce sleep is reported to have inconsistent effects (O'Brien and Yule 1995).

Regression between 3 and 4 years of age is a common phenomenon in Sanfilippo syndrome. The period of regression marks an increase in *behavioural difficulties*, particularly overactivity, tantrums and aggression, which are typified by lunging for other people. This is thought to be an adverse reaction to the other person invading the personal space of the affected individual (O'Brien and Yule 1995). These behaviours significantly reduce the opportunity for family activities outside the home. It is vital that the family unit has regular access to respite care. Mouthing behaviour is also typical, particularly biting and chewing objects and clothes. Supplying a teething ring in order to reduce this behaviour is an effective management strategy employed by many parents. In spite of this, in order to prevent individuals with Sanfilippo syndrome causing significant damage to themselves and others, the home environment usually has to undergo substantial changes such as removal of breakable objects, providing soft furnishings and surfaces, and fitting windows with toughened glass (O'Brien and Yule 1995).

Psychiatric disturbances have been observed, particularly in individuals affected with Hurler–Scheie syndrome. There is a raised incidence of dementia in individuals with Sanfilippo syndrome (Gilbert 1999), which leads to further progressive deterioration and social and environmental withdrawal (O'Brien and Yule 1995).

Due to small stature and/or wheelchair use, *adaptation of the home or school environment* to suit individual needs is a necessity, in order to create a physical environment to promote maximum potential for both psychological and social development. Regular dental check-ups are crucial for individuals with Morquio syndrome, as the inherent abnormality in dental enamel leaves them susceptible to tooth decay. Early detection of decay is critical for prevention of physical discomfort (Gilbert 1999).

It is crucial for the multidisciplinary team to build up a *good relationship with families* affected by mucopolysaccharidoses. This group of syndromes results in distressing deterioration of the individual, and family members need considerable levels of support to cope with both the progressive nature of the syndromes and the behaviours that can manifest. Parents should be fully informed about the physical profile of the condition so that any deterioration can be detected at an early stage and interceded. They should also have access to a variety of resources that can provide both practical and emotional support, such as respite care and support groups (Harris 1998). However, research has highlighted that parents are not receiving the appropriate level of contact and support from professional agencies. A survey revealed that although 76% of cases had contact with a paediatrician, less than one-third had input from social workers, psychologists or psychiatrists, and only 4% had received a referral to a physiotherapist (Bax and Colville 1995).

REFERENCES

Bax M, Colville GA (1995) 'Behaviour in mucopolysaccharide disorders.' *Archives of Disease in Childhood*, **73**, 77–81.

Bredenkamp JK, Smith ME, Dudley JP, Williams JC, Crumley RL, Crockett DM (1992) 'Otolaryngologic manifestations of the mucopolysaccharidoses.' *Annals of Otology, Rhinology and Laryngology*, **101**, 472–478.

Gilbert PC (1999) *A–Z of Syndromes and Inherited Disorders*. Cheltenham, Gloucestershire: Stanely Thorne.

Haddad FS, Jones DH, Vellodi A, Kane N, Pitt MC (1997) 'Carpal tunnel syndrome in the mucopolysaccharidoses and mucolipidoses.' *Journal of Bone and Joint Surgery. British Volume*, **79**, 576–582.

Harris JC (1998) *Developmental Neuropsychiatry, Vol. II: Assessment, Diagnosis and Treatment of Developmental Disorders*. Oxford: Oxford University Press.

Keith O, Scully C, Weidmann GM (1990) 'Orofacial features of Scheie (Hurler–Scheie) syndrome (alpha-L-iduronidase deficiency).' *Oral Surgery, Oral Medicine and Oral Pathology*, **70**, 70–74.

Leighton SE, Papsin B, Vellodi A, Dinwiddie R, Lane R (2001) 'Disordered breathing during sleep in patients with mucopolysaccharidoses.' *International Journal of Pediatric Otorhinolaryngology*, **58**, 127–138.

O'Brien G, Yule W (eds) (1995) *Behavioural Phenotypes. Clinics in Developmental Medicine No. 138*. London: Mac Keith Press.

PEDBASE (1994) 'Sly syndrome.' Pediatric Database (PEDBASE), electronic fact sheet (http://www.icondata.com/health/pedbase/files/SLYSYNDR.HTM).

Peters C, Krivit W (2000) 'Hematopoietic cell transplantation for mucopolysaccharidosis IIB (Hunter syndrome).' *Bone Marrow Transplantation*, **25**, 1097–1099.

Sjogren P, Pedersen T, Steinmetz H (1987) 'Mucopolysaccharidoses and anaesthetic risks.' *Acta Anaesthesiologica Scandinavica*, **31**, 214–218.

Timms KM, Bondeson ML, Ansari-Lari MA, Lagerstedt K, Muzney MM, Dugan-Rocha SP, Nelson DL, Pettersson U, Gibbs RA (1997) 'Molecular and phenotypic variation in patients with severe Hunter syndrome.' *Human Molecular Genetics*, **6**, 476–486.

Vellodi A, Young EP, Cooper A, Wraith JE, Winchester B, Meaney C, Ramaswami U, Will A (1997) 'Bone marrow transplantation for mucopolysaccharidosis type I: experience of two British centres.' *Archives of Disease in Childhood*, **76**, 92–99.

Wallace SP, Prutting CA, Gerber SE (1990) 'Degeneration of speech, language, and hearing in a patient with mucopolysaccharidosis VII.' *International Journal of Pediatric Otorhinolaryngology*, **19**, 97–107.

Widemann HR, Kunze J, Dibbern H (1992) *An Atlas of Clinical Syndromes: A Visual Aid to Diagnosis.* Stuttgart, Germany: Mosby Wolfe.

WEBSITE

- National MPS Society
  www.mpssociety.org/

MYOTONIC DYSTROPHY (CONGENITAL)

Alternative name	Steinert's disease
Incidence	1:18,000–1:43,000
Genetics	Non-coding region of chromosome 19 (SSBP 2000). Autosomal dominant, almost always maternal transmission
Learning disability	Mild to moderate in 75% of cases (Thornton 1999)

Myotonic dystrophy is a progressive condition that causes muscle wastage and weakness. Affected individuals who survive the neonatal period will develop myotonia at approximately 10 years of age. In this syndrome, affected muscles contract, but are unable to return to a relaxed state (Thornton 1999). Patients surviving into adulthood present with the same symptoms as patients suffering from the late-onset form of myotonic dystrophy (Tanabe and Nonaka 1987). There is considerable neonatal mortality due to severe respiratory problems.

MANAGEMENT

Physiotherapy should be performed on babies to help breathing and lung function and to help improve muscle tone. It is also useful in managing clubfeet, although surgery may also be required for these. Sadly, many babies die within the first few weeks of life; however, babies who do survive show improvements in muscle tone (de Die-Smulders *et al.* 1997).

One particular risk for children with this condition is anaesthesia. The surgeon and anaesthetist should be fully aware of the patient's medical history.

The lack of facial responsiveness can be particularly distressing for parents. However, it does not mean that the child is unresponsive, only that they have weak facial muscles and therefore are unable to make a full range of facial expressions. *Speech therapy* is often required to aid pronunciation. Babies may have swallowing and feeding difficulties, and parents should be advised to try different types of teat. Nasogastric feeding may also be necessary.

Special shoes, walking aids and calipers may be useful.

REFERENCES

de Die-Smulders CE, Smeets HJ, Loots W, Anten HB, Mirandolle JF, Geraedts JP, Howeler CJ (1997) 'Paternal transmission of congenital myotonic dystrophy.' *Journal of Medical Genetics*, **34**, 930–923.

SSBP (2000) *Proceedings of the 6th International Symposium of the Society for the Study of Behavioural Phenotypes, Venice International University, San Servolo, Italy, 12–14 October 2000.*

Tanabe Y, Nonaka I (1987) 'Congenital myotonic dystrophy: changes in muscle pathology with ageing.' *Journal of the Neurological Sciences*, **77**, 59–68.

Thornton C (1999) 'The myotonic dystrophies.' *Seminars in Neurology*, **19**, 25–33.

WEBSITE

• International Myotonic Dystrophy Organization
  www.myotonicdystrophy.org/

NEUROFIBROMATOSIS TYPE 1

Alternative name	von Recklinghausen neurofibromatosis
Incidence	1:2500–1:3500 (DeClue *et al.* 2000)
Genetics	Autosomal dominant, 17q11.2; 50% of cases are sporadic
Learning disability	Borderline

Neurofibromatosis is characterized by tumours on nerve tissues throughout the body. There are two types, type I and type II. Type II is not associated with a recognized behavioural phenotype and will not be discussed here. Neurofibromatosis type 1 is the most common form; it is characterized by the formation of tumours, café-au-lait spots, neurofibromas and Lesch nodules. Café-au-lait spots are caused by an excess of the skin pigment, melanin. The location and number of café-au-lait spots can act as a valuable diagnostic marker for the syndrome, with six or more café-au-lait spots and freckling under the armpits, being signs of the syndrome (Gilbert 1999). It is also associated with macrocephaly, short stature, endocrinological and thorax disorders (Cnossen *et al.* 1998). Benign tumours primarily affect three areas, the eyes, spine and ears. Affected individuals who present with new difficulties in these areas should be examined for possible tumours. Potentially life-threatening complications develop in one-third of affected individuals, including plexiform neurofibromas, coarctation of the aorta, skeletal abnormalities, renal artery stenosis and hypertension. The risk of malignancy is between 3% and 15% (Karnes 1998). The presentation of cutaneous neurofibromas increases with age, but they are seldom reported before mid-adolescence. The occurrence of café-au-lait spots decreases after middle age (Creange *et al.* 1999).

MANAGEMENT

The management of neurofibromatosis requires the involvement of a multidisciplinary team and should include an opthalmologist, paediatric neurologist, psychologist, physiotherapist, dermatologist, speech and language therapist and a paediatrician. The syndrome can thus be tackled on all levels. *Good communication* should be based on an honest and open approach to the complications faced by these individuals, in order to help the affected person and her/his family cope and emotionally prepare.

This syndrome can have a detrimental impact on psychological well-being, particularly if cutaneous neurofibromas occur on the face and other visible areas of the body. The psychological issues are heightened by mobility problems, sensory impairments and communication difficulties, and can result in depression, low self-esteem and social isolation. The psychological distress that these may cause is particularly prominent in adolescence, and the unpredictability and variability of this syndrome can intensify the degree of distress. *Counselling* is often beneficial to help the affected individual to accept her/his illness and to develop appropriate coping strategies. Counselling may also be beneficial for family members as they often report feelings of guilt (Ruggieri 1999). If individuals with neurofibromatosis wish to conceive, genetic counselling is recommended.

Cutaneous neurofibromas require regular monitoring by a dermatologist in order to detect any new growths or changes in the existing neurofibromas, such as bleeding, increased growth or physical discomfort. The nature of the cutaneous neurofibromas means that surgical removal is not advised unless there is physical discomfort, as surgery can lead to scarring. *Cancer* is a major concern for affected individuals. Malignant tumours are four times more common than in the normal population. The treatment of malignant tumours, however, and the associated prognosis, do not differ from the normal population.

Scoliosis, resulting from spinal pressure caused by tumours, is a frequent complication in this syndrome, and becomes more prevalent in adolescence where there is an acceleration in growth rate. Exercise such as swimming, especially during adolescence, can be beneficial (Gilbert 1999). *Physiotherapy* can also be useful in targeting this particular symptom. Many children cope well with mainstream education; however, *special education* can help some children to achieve their full potential. Where there are speech difficulties, input from a *speech and language therapist* may be necessary.

Regular *monitoring of blood pressure* in individuals with neurofibromatosis is recommended, as hypertension can be an indication of lesions on the adrenal gland and renal artery. Assessment by an *ophthalmologist*, to monitor for optic pathway gliomas and associated abnormalities of vision, should occur regularly in order to promote early detection. It has been recommended that until the age of 10 years, this should occur annually, and thereafter biannually (Ruggieri 1999).

REFERENCES

Cnossen MH, de Goede-Bolder A, van den Broek KM, Waasdorp CM, Oranje AP, Stroink H, Simonsz HJ, van den Ouweland AM, Halley DJ, Niermeijer MF (1998) 'A prospective 10 year follow up study of patients with neurofibromatosis type 1.' *Archives of Disease in Childhood*, **78**, 408–412.

Creange A, Zeller J, Rostaing-Rigattieri S, Brugieres P, Degos JD, Revuz J, Wolkenstein P (1999) 'Neurological complications of neurofibromatosis type 1 in adulthood.' *Brain*, **122**, 473–481.

DeClue JE, Heffelfinger S, Benvenuto G, Ling B, Li S, Rui W, Vass WC, Viskochil D, Ratner N (2000) 'Epidermal growth factor receptor expression in neurofibromatosis type 1-related tumors and NF1 animal models.' *Journal of Clinical Investigation*, **105**, 1233–1241.

Gilbert PC (1999) *A–Z of Syndromes and Inherited Disorders*. Cheltenham, Gloucestershire: Stanely Thorne.

Karnes PS (1998) 'Neurofibromatosis: a common neurocutaneous disorder.' *Mayo Clinic Proceedings*, **73**, 1071–1076.
Ruggieri M (1999) 'The different forms of neurofibromatosis.' *Child's Nervous System*, **15**, 295–308.

WEBSITES

- Neurofibromatosis Association
  www.nfa-uk.org.uk/
- Neurofibromatosis (USA) Inc.
  www.nf-inc.org/

NOONAN SYNDROME

Incidence	1:1000–1:5000 (Birth Defects Foundation 2001)
Genetics	Autosomal dominant, chromosome 12; 50% of cases are sporadic
Learning disability	Normal or mild (Noonan 1994)

Noonan syndrome is a multi-malformation disorder, comprising of characteristic facies and short stature, delayed puberty and undescended testes, skeletal and congenital cardio-respiratory abnormalities (Bader-Meunier *et al.* 1997, Noonan 1999). Approximately 80% of babies born with Noonan syndrome will have a heart defect—usually pulmonary stenosis. Usually heart defects are mild or asymptomatic and only 10% of cases with pulmonary stenosis require surgery. At least three-quarters of people with Noonan syndrome will have the following facial features: hypertelorism with downward-slanting palpebral fissures, arched eyebrows, low-set posteriorly rotated ears with a thick helix, and a deeply grooved philtrum with a pronounced top lip (O'Brien and Yule 1995). The nose has a wide base, bulbous tip and a depressed root. Many cases also have a high arched palate and excess nuchal skin with a low posterior hairline (O'Brien and Yule 1995).

Hypertrophic cardiomyopathy is common but usually remains asymptomatic for many years and may improve with age. Patients with an atrial septal defect often require surgery (Birth Defects Foundation 2001). In addition, there are often abnormalities in the lymphatic, visual and hearing system (Bader-Meunier *et al.* 1997). Early feeding difficulties can result in a failure to thrive (Shah *et al.* 1999). Although hypotonia can result in mild motor delay, this usually improves with time (Noonan 1994). Life expectancy is thought to be normal, unless cardiac complications are serious (O'Brien and Yule 1995).

MANAGEMENT

Some cases of Noonan syndrome may be so mild that they go undiagnosed. However, if a diagnosis has been made, a *medical assessment* should be carried out to establish which of the physical abnormalities associated with this condition are present. Congenital heart defects may require rectification and surgical intervention can help prevent infertility in boys who have undescended testes. *Growth hormone therapy* is sometimes used in children and adolescents. However, as most people with Noonan syndrome are not deficient in growth hormone it is not clear whether this treatment has any effect upon adult height.

A substantial minority of people with Noonan syndrome have a *bleeding disorder*, most commonly factor XI deficiency, von Willebrand disease and thrombocytopenia, and they should therefore be evaluated for these prior to surgery (including teeth extraction) (Birth Defects Foundation 2001). Feeding problems can be severe up until the second year of life. These are due to poor sucking reflexes and persistent vomiting. They can lead to failure to thrive if tube feeding is not initiated. However after 2 years, feeding is less of a problem.

Cognitive impairment is usually not present in people with Noonan syndrome, although approximately 10% of affected individuals will have a learning disability and require special educational support (Birth Defects Foundation 2001).

REFERENCES

Bader-Meunier B, Tchernia G, Mielot F, Fontaine JL, Thomas C, Lyonnet S, Lavergne JM, Dommergues JP (1997) 'Occurrence of myeloproliferative disorder in patients with Noonan syndrome.' *Journal of Pediatrics*, **130**, 885–889.
Noonan JA (1994) 'Noonan syndrome: An update and review for the primary pediatrician.' *Clinical Pediatrics*, **33**, 548–555.
Noonan JA (1999) 'Noonan syndrome revisited.' *Journal of Pediatrics*, **135**, 667–668.
O'Brien G, Yule W (eds) (1995) *Behavioural Phenotypes. Clinics in Developmental Medicine No. 138.* London: Mac Keith Press.
Shah N, Rodriguez M, Louis DS, Lindley K, Milla PJ (1999) 'Feeding difficulties and foregut dysmotility in Noonan's syndrome.' *Archives of Disease in Childhood*, **81**, 28–31.

WEBSITES

• Ability
  www.ability.org/Noonan_Syndrome.html
• Birth Defects Foundation
  www.birthdefects.co.uk/bdf_may01/pages/services/noonan_1.htm
• The Noonan Syndrome Support Group
  www.noonansyndrome.org/home.html

PHENYLKETONURIA

Incidence	1:5000–1:14,000 (varies widely according to geographical region) (O'Brien and Yule 1995)
Genetics	Autosomal recessive
Learning disability	Moderate to severe (if untreated)

Individuals with phenylketonuria (PKU) are unable to metabolize the amino acid phenylalanine due to the absence of the enzyme phenylalanine hydroxylase. Treatment consists of a phenylalanine-low diet. The initiation, quality and duration of blood phenylalanine control are the three main parameters of PKU management (Burgard 2000). Discontinuation/non-initiation of the diet prior to the age of 10 years causes learning disability. It is important that the diet should be implemented within the first few weeks of life, but there is wide disagreement over how long the diet should be maintained, with recommendations ranging from four to 45 years (Maddox 1990, Griffiths 2000). If the diet is started early enough, is strict enough and is maintained, life expectancy can be normal. Delayed or inadequate dietary management can result in agitation, restlessness, intention tremor and tics (Harris 1998).

MANAGEMENT

The most important management issue associated with PKU is immediate initiation of a *phenylalanine-free diet*. Modern postnatal assessment protocols (Guthrie test) mean that this syndrome should be detected at birth. Once the phenylalanine-free diet is implemented, blood-phenylalanine should be regularly monitored up to the age of 8 years (Harris 1998). The diet involves the elimination of concentrated sources of protein, including fish, dairy products and meat. A formula providing a synthetic nutritional replacement is available. However, a very small amount of this amino acid is required for protein synthesis. The diet is highly restrictive and this places a great strain on the child and their family. In this condition, the role of the family is vitally important, as they will be required to monitor the child's eating habits. This can impact on the eating habits of the entire family. In adolescence there may be parent–child conflict due to the adolescent wishing to develop a normal social life, to fit in with peers and to assert her/his independence. The diet impacts on all aspects of an individual's life. For example, special considerations should be made when choosing schools, especially for younger children. *Teachers and support workers* should be made aware of the dietary restrictions, as a deterioration in behaviour would be detrimental to academic attainment.

When the condition is left untreated, phenylalanine and its metabolites accumulate in the body. These can lead to *neuropsychiatric symptomatology*—anxiety, depression and thought disorder. Any damage caused to the brain by poor dietary control cannot be reversed, although its effects can be ameliorated by strict dietary control. Even in individuals who have followed a strict phenylalanine-free diet, cognitive, emotional and behavioural difficulties may still arise. It is thought that in particular, problems may occur in learning and this may be related to reduced dopamine metabolism (Harris 1998).

There has been one reported case of resolution of PKU in a child who received liver transplantation as a consequence of cirrhosis (unrelated to the PKU) (cited in Harris 1998).

There is a huge amount of medical controversy regarding the *age at which the diet should be relaxed/terminated*. Initially clinicians recommended that the diet could be relaxed by the age of 10. However, it is now known that this adversely affects intellectual ability, behaviour and personality. It is now believed that the diet should be maintained at least into early adulthood and possibly even for the life span. Blood phenylalanine levels should remain between 2 and 6 mg/dL. Regular check-ups are vital to monitor blood levels.

Affected women who are no longer following the phenylalanine-free diet and wish to conceive are strongly advised to resume the diet prior to *conception*. This is because high levels of maternal phenylalanine can cause congenital abnormalities and learning disability in the neonate. Mothers with PKU give birth to children unaffected by the condition.

REFERENCES

Burgard P (2000) 'Development of intelligence in early treated phenylketonuria.' *European Journal of Pediatrics*, **159**, S74–S79.
Griffiths P (2000) 'Neuropsychological approaches to treatment policy issues in phenylketonuria.' *European Journal of Pediatrics*, **159**, S82–S86.
Harris JC (1998) *Developmental Neuropsychiatry, Vol. II: Assessment, Diagnosis and Treatment of Developmental Disorders.* Oxford: Oxford University Press.

Maddox MA (1990) 'Is there a link between dementia and phenylketonuria?' *Journal of Gerontological Nursing*, 16, 18–23.

O'Brien G, Yule W (eds) (1995) *Behavioural Phenotypes. Clinics in Developmental Medicine No. 138.* Mac Keith Press, London.

WEBSITES

- National PKU News
  http://205.178.182.34/
- National Society for Phenylketonuria (NSPKU)
  http://web.ukonline.co.uk/nspku/

PRADER–WILLI SYNDROME

Incidence	1:10,000 (SSBP 2000)
Genetics	Abnormality in paternal 15q11–13 is observed in 60–70% of cases; most of the remaining cases have maternal uniparental dysomy (Boer and Clarke 1999)
Learning disability	Borderline to moderate

Prader–Willi syndrome is characterized by marked hypotonia, failure to thrive, delayed sexual development, scoliosis, acromicria, small stature and persistent skin picking (Holland 1998, Clarke *et al.* 1995). A flat face, prominent forehead with bitemporal narrowing, almond-shaped eyes and triangular mouth are common facial features (O'Brien and Yule 1995). There are two phases to the disorder: up to 6 months of age the syndrome is characterized by hypotonia, feeding difficulties and sleepiness. Between 1 and 4 years of age hyperphagia develops as a result of hypothalamic abnormalities, and the hypotonia becomes less prominent.

MANAGEMENT

Dietary management is the most fundamental issue for people with this syndrome. Strict behavioural and dietary controls are necessary, as the resulting obesity and its complications (hypertension, cardiovascular symptoms, respiratory difficulties and diabetes) can be fatal (Chu *et al.* 1994). Life expectancy in this condition is dependent upon weight control. *Pharmacological interventions* aimed at hyperphagia can be a useful adjunct to behavioural intervention in controlling dietary intake. Medication tends to have a temporary effect on hyperphagia; one solution to this might be the frequent alternating of different agents. Behavioural programmes should focus on reinforcement and self-monitoring; however, it is also necessary to restrict access to food. This is where the *role of the family* is vitally important, and all treatment strategies should involve parents/carers, siblings and teachers. The necessity of constant supervision for a relatively able person places considerable strain upon the whole family. Family members may report feelings of inadequacy and guilt if the person they are caring for becomes obese. Increased independence at adolescence tends to be accompanied by an increase in problems, as there is less supervision and therefore more opportunity to access food. Hyperphagia has a profound psychological effect and can, in combination with physical disability, lead to emotional and social isolation.

Administration of *human growth hormone* has been used in this condition and has been found to increase growth and decrease fat (Davies *et al.* 1998).

Psychiatric illness, particularly anxiety, depression and paranoid psychosis, and behavioural problems become more prevalent with age in Prader–Willi syndrome. Compulsive and obsessive behaviours are often psychologically based due to relentless hunger, bullying (about obesity) and sexual immaturity. SSRIs, stimulants, neuroleptics and anticonvulsants have been used to target aggression, skin picking and emotional lability (Harris 1998).

REFERENCES

Boer H, Clarke D (1999) 'Development and behaviour in genetic syndromes: Prader–Willi syndrome.' *Journal of Applied Research in Intellectual Disabilities*, **12**, 296–301.

Chu CE, Cooke A, Stephenson JBP, Tolmie JL, Clarke B, Parry-Jones WL, Connor JM, Donaldson MDC (1994) 'Diagnosis in Prader–Willi syndrome.' *Archives of Disease in Childhood*, **71**, 441–442.

Clarke DJ, Boer H, Webb T (1995) 'Genetic and behavioural aspects of Prader–Willi syndrome: A review with a translation of the original paper.' *Mental Handicap Research*, **8**, 38–53.

Davies PS, Evans S, Broomhead S, Clough H, Day JM, Laidlaw A, Barnes ND (1998) 'Effect of growth hormone on height, weight, and body composition in Prader–Willi syndrome.' *Archives of Disease in Childhood*, **78**, 474–476.

Harris JC (1998) *Developmental Neuropsychiatry, Vol. II: Assessment, Diagnosis and Treatment of Developmental Disorders.* Oxford: Oxford University Press.

Holland AJ (1998) 'Understanding the eating disorder affecting people with Prader–Willi syndrome.' *Journal of Applied Research in Intellectual Disabilities*, **11**, 192–206.

O'Brien G, Yule W (eds) (1995) *Behavioural Phenotypes. Clinics in Developmental Medicine No. 138.* London: Mac Keith Press.

SSBP (2000) *Proceedings of the 6th International Symposium of the Society for the Study of Behavioural Phenotypes, Venice International University, San Servolo, Italy, 12–14 October 2000.*

WEBSITES

- Ontario Prader–Willi Syndrome Association
  http://members.attcanada.ca/~opwsa/
- Prader Willi Syndrome Association (UK)
  www.pwsa-uk.demon.co.uk/
- Prader–Willi Syndrome Association (USA)
  www.pwsausa.org/

RETT SYNDROME

Incidence	1:10,000 females (RSRF website)
Genetics	Distal arm of Xq28 (Sandberg *et al.* 2000); 75% of cases are due to mutation of the *MECP2* gene
Learning disability	Profound

Rett syndrome is classed as a pervasive developmental disorder. It usually affects females, but very rarely occurs in males (Sandberg *et al.* 2000). There is controversy as to whether or not it constitutes a degenerative condition. The regression that characterizes the syndrome has usually ceased by the time a diagnosis has been made, and there is no known deterioration in the neurophysiology, as measured by EEGs or evoked potentials (Harris 1998).

Diagnostic criteria for Rett syndrome are: (i) normal development until 6–18 months of age; (ii) deceleration of head growth; (iii) loss of verbal ability; (iv) replacement of purposeful hand movements with stereotypic movements; (v) inability to walk/abnormal gait; and (vi) ataxic movements of torso and limbs that are heightened with distress. About 15% of cases do not meet all of these criteria and are classified as atypical. Regression affects all areas of functioning, particularly, physical (scoliosis and leg deformities), social, linguistic and adaptive behaviours (Clarke 1996).

The rate of regression varies, and onset may be sudden or may progress over a number of months. Movements become jerky and uncoordinated, expressive and receptive language may be lost, and these may be accompanied by social withdrawal. Regression is followed by a period of stabilization and re-emergence of previously lost skills, particularly nonverbal communication and interpersonal skills. In 50% of cases, children relearn to walk.

Rett syndrome is associated with breathing abnormalities, specifically hyperventilation and breath holding (Kerr and Julu 1999), stereotypic hand movements (hand wringing, clapping) and facial grimacing. Physical disabilities, especially joint contractures, muscle wastage, curvature of the spine and stiffness of the lower limbs, present with increasing age. Two-thirds of patients survive beyond the second decade (Ellaway and Christodoulou 1999). Those who do not, tend to be poorly nourished and have chest deformities and greater learning disability; these patients often die during sleep (O'Brien and Yule 1995, Ellaway and Christodoulou 1999).

MANAGEMENT

Following the diagnosis of Rett syndrome, families will often require a great deal of support. They will have cared for an apparently 'normally developing' child for anywhere from 6 to 18 months and will need time to come to terms with and accept the diagnosis. *Parental education* should focus on the stages of the syndrome and should particularly highlight the period of re-emergence of adaptive skills and the capacity to learn following the period of regression.

Muscular hypotonia leads to difficulties with chewing and swallowing. This can cause aspiration and increases susceptibility to respiratory infection. The *behavioural manifestations* of the syndrome vary according to its stage. During regression, there is often sleep disturbance, emotional withdrawal and crying and screaming episodes. These are particularly difficult for parents/carers as they may feel rejected by their child. It is of some consolation that most children growth out of these behaviours. Following the period of regression, characteristic behaviours revolve around abnormalities in breathing and stereotypic hand movements across the midline. The hand movements can be particularly troublesome to manage, as they interfere with all aspects of functioning, including self-feeding and writing. These behaviours intensify during periods of stress. Characteristic breathing abnormalities include hypo- and hyperventilation, breath holding and swallowing of air. Management of breathing abnormalities usually involves ignoring the behaviour.

Treatment is symptomatic. Medical intervention focuses on the *management of epilepsy*. Seizure control is often difficult to achieve and may require multiple antiepileptics. The presentation of epilepsy is severe in early childhood, but reduces with increasing age and may have ceased by the time the affected individual reaches their twenties (Harris 1998).

Physiotherapy can address the difficulties of muscle tone, abnormal gait, scoliosis and ataxia. In addition, physiotherapy *focusing on hand use* will help to develop adaptive behaviours that require the use of hands, such as self-feeding. This can be complemented by the use of hand and arm splints. Exercise should be encouraged in the home environment at whatever level is achievable. Posture and mobility can be improved through the use of walking, sitting and standing aids.

Stress disorder and associated maladaptive behaviours (breathing and hand wringing) respond well to *relaxation techniques*. In particular, music therapy, hydrotherapy and massage may be used. Music therapy is especially useful during the regression stage. Management of these behaviours involves ignoring them and redirecting the person to other activities. *Self-injury* has been assessed with behavioural analysis and seems to serve two purposes, reinforcement by sensory stimulation and escape from social situations (Harris 1998).

REFERENCES

Clarke A (1996) 'Rett syndrome.' *Journal of Medical Genetics*, **33**, 693–639.
Ellaway C, Christodoulou J (1999) 'Rett syndrome: Clinical update and review of recent genetic advances.' *Journal of Paediatric Child Health*, **35**, 419–426.
Harris JC (1998) *Developmental Neuropsychiatry, Vol. II: Assessment, Diagnosis and Treatment of Developmental Disorders*. Oxford: Oxford University Press.
Kerr AM, Julu PO (1999) 'Recent insights into hyperventilation from the study of Rett syndrome.' *Archives of Disease in Childhood*, **80**, 384–387.
O'Brien G, Yule W (eds) (1995) *Behavioural Phenotypes. Clinics in Developmental Medicine No. 138*. London: Mac Keith Press.
Sandberg AD, Ehlers S, Hagbert B, Gillberg C (2000) 'The Rett syndrome complex.' *Autism*, **4**, 249–267.

WEBSITES

- Contact a Family
  www.cafamily.org.uk/
- Rett Resources
  www.rettsyndrome.net/
- Rett Syndrome Association
  www.rettsyndrome.org.uk/
- Rett Syndrome Research Foundation (RSRF)
  www.rsrf.org/

RUBINSTEIN–TAYBI SYNDROME

Alternative name	Broad thumb–great toe syndrome
Incidence	1:125,000 (Boer *et al.* 1999)
Genetics	Autosomal dominant; microdeletion at 16p13.3 (Boer *et al.* 1999)
Learning disability	Mild to severe

The phenotypic make-up of Rubinstein–Taybi syndrome includes broad thumbs and toes, microcephaly, short stature, obesity and facial dysmorphism. Facial features include a prominent beaked nose with a broad fleshy bridge, nasal septum well below the alae with an associated short columella, slightly malformed ears, hypertelorism and downward-slanting palpebral fissures; these are often accompanied by ptosis or thickened eyelids, heavy or highly arched eyebrows and a highly arched palate with a small oral opening and pouting lower lip (O'Brien and Yule 1995). These characteristic facies change predictably with age. Skeletal abnormalities (particularly of the lower vertebrae) can result in an abnormal gait. The behavioural manifestations of the syndrome include stereotypic and self-stimulatory behaviours (rocking and hand-flapping). Medical complications, such as congenital heart, renal and urinary tract abnormalities, can lead to frequent infections and affect morbidity and mortality (Bilir *et al.* 1990).

Management

Sign language and other nonverbal forms of communication can facilitate interaction, and a 'total communication' approach is useful for language training. Frequent night awakenings and breathing abnormalities are common, as are mood swings, self-injury and aggression. There is intolerance to loud noise and a desire for sameness. Affected females show a propensity for obesity, so dietary management is essential. Children with the syndrome are particularly interested in music and derive great pleasure from this. Affected individuals often like to dismantle electronic objects—this could be channelled into a vocation in adulthood (O'Brien and Yule 1995).

REFERENCES

Bilir BM, Bilir N, Wilson GN (1990) 'Intracranial angioblastic meningioma and an aged appearance in a woman with Rubinstein–Taybi syndrome.' *American Journal of Medical Genetics. Supplement*, **6**, 69–72.
Boer H, Langton J, Clarke D (1999) 'Development and behaviour in genetic syndromes: Rubinstein–Taybi syndrome.' *Journal of Applied Research in Intellectual Disabilities*, **12**, 302–307.
O'Brien G, Yule W (eds) (1995) *Behavioural Phenotypes. Clinics in Developmental Medicine No. 138.* London: Mac Keith Press.

WEBSITE

• RTS Support Group
 www.vfrank1701.freeserve.co.uk/

SEX CHROMOSOME ANEUPLOIDIES

Turner syndrome

Alternative names	Ullrich–Turner syndrome; 45X; X/X; X autosomal
Incidence	1:2000–1:2500 female births (SSBP 2000)
Genetics	Total or partial absence of the second X chromosome
Learning disability	No

Turner syndrome is one of the most common chromosomal abnormalities when all conceived fetuses are considered; however, 99% of these fetuses are miscarried (Harris 1998). Affected women usually do not naturally progress through puberty and therefore remain infertile. The condition is usually diagnosed during the first year of life, but some cases remain undiagnosed until the child begins school. Turner syndrome is associated with an increased incidence of osteoporosis, diabetes mellitus, premature ageing of the hearing organs, obesity, cardiovascular disease, hypertension, thyroid dysfunction and strokes (Hultcrantz *et al.*

1994; Garden *et al.* 1996; Gravholt *et al.* 1998a,b). In general, dysmorphic features are subtle, but one-half of cases have a webbed neck, low posterior hairline and broad chest with widely spaced nipples (O'Brien and Yule 1995). Approximately 50% of deaths in Turner syndrome are due to cardiovascular disease, and death occurs 6–13 years earlier than in the general population (Gravholt *et al.* 1998).

MANAGEMENT

Most women with Turner syndrome have the potential to lead *long, healthy and productive lives*. The complications of primary concern to most individuals with Turner syndrome revolve around short stature, puberty and infertility. Short stature is treated with *growth hormone therapy* during childhood, and oestrogen replacement is usually required—this must not be started too early (before 12 years), or adult height may be compromised. It is important to involve the affected individual in the decision as to when to initiate hormone treatment.

As adults, women with Turner syndrome tend to look very young for their age. This can be particularly distressing as it prejudices strangers to treat them as 'children' and to some extent to disregard their feelings. Before the age of 12 years there are no characteristic difficulties in forming peer relations. However, as adults, because of their young appearance and difficulties understanding and interpreting social cues, these women can become socially isolated. *Psychological problems* also stem from feelings of inadequacy and of not being a 'real woman'. These are exacerbated by the fact that many of these women are infertile. *Counselling* that addresses these issues is very useful in this syndrome.

It is important to identify at an early stage if there is a learning disability, so that education can be tailored to the individual's needs. Those suffering from attentional problems should be provided with a highly structured environment, with limited distractions, in order to maximize educational attainment. If necessary, pharmacological agents may be used. Wherever possible, information should be presented verbally rather than visuospatially, as verbal skills are a relative strength (Harris 1998). All opportunities for social development and formation of peer relationships, both within and outside the school environment, should be encouraged.

In treating the *ovarian dysfunction*, both on a medical and psychological level, the prevalence of confounding psychiatric disorders can be reduced. Hyperactivity is common during childhood, but by adolescence an affected individual is more likely to be hypoactive.

Turner syndrome is associated with hypothyroidism and thyroid-stimulating hormone levels should be assessed at least every two years or otherwise when symptoms indicate. Scoliosis, diabetes and hypertension are also associated with Turner syndrome and should be screened for periodically.

There are no real dietary considerations for Turner syndrome other than adequate daily intake of calcium and vitamin D, which are essential to prevent osteoporosis associated with ovarian failure.

REFERENCES

Garden AS, Diver MJ, Fraser WD (1996) 'Undiagnosed morbidity in adult women with Turner syndrome.'

Clinical Endocrinology, **45**, 589–593.

Gravholt CH, Juul S, Naeraa RW, Hansen J (1998a) 'Morbidity in Turner's syndrome.' *Journal of Clinical Epidemiology*, **51**, 147–158.

Gravholt CH, Naeraa RW, Nyholm B, Gerdes LU, Christiansen E, Schmitz O, Christiansen JS (1998b) 'Glucose metabolism, lipid metabolism, and cardiovascular risk factors in adult Turner's syndrome. The impact of sex hormone replacement.' *Diabetes Care*, **21**, 1062–1070.

Harris JC (1998) *Developmental Neuropsychiatry. Vol. II: Assessment, Diagnosis and Treatment of Developmental Disorders.* Oxford: Oxford University Press.

Hultcrantz M, Sylven L, Borg E (1994) 'Ear and hearing problems in 44 middle-aged women with Turner's syndrome.' *Hearing Research*, **76**, 127–132.

O'Brien G, Yule W (eds) (1995) *Behavioural Phenotypes. Clinics in Developmental Medicine No. 138.* London: Mac Keith Press.

SSBP (2000) *Proceedings of the 6th International Symposium of the Society for the Study of Behavioural Phenotypes, Venice International University, San Servolo, Italy, 12–14 October 2000.*

WEBSITES

- The Turner Centre
  www.aaa.dk/turner/engelsk/download.htm
- Turner Syndrome Project (University College London, Behavioural Science Unit)
  www.ich.ucl.ac.uk/units/bsunew/turner.htm
- Turner Syndrome Society of the United States
  www.turner-syndrome-us.org/
- Turner Syndrome Support Society (UK)
  www.tss.org.uk/

Klinefelter syndrome (47XXY; 48XXYY; 49XXXXY)

The most common type of Klinefelter syndrome is 47XXY, which has an incidence of 1:750 male births (SSBP 1999). In 60–70% of cases the extra X chromosome is maternally derived (O'Brien and Yule 1995). Cognitive status of affected individuals ranges from normal to mild learning disability.

48XXYY syndrome is relatively rare, with only 60 documented cases worldwide (O'Brien and Yule 1995). Affected individuals show mild to moderate learning disability.

49XXXXY occurs in 1:85,000 newborn males (Peet *et al.* 1998). It is caused by a maternal non-disjunction. Older publications place the level of learning disability in the moderate to severe range, but recently patients have been found with IQs in the borderline to low-normal range.

Generally the greater the number of replications, the greater the number of associated disabilities. Most males tend to be minimally affected by this condition and consequently it has been predicted that diagnosis is missed in 64% of cases (Ratcliffe 1999). Most cases that do receive a diagnosis do not get this until adolescence (Hachimi-Idrissi *et al.* 1995). Learning disability is not always present in this disorder—where it is it tends to be mild. Symptoms vary in severity, but generally the disorder is characterized by low birthweight, hypogonadism, sparse body hair and microcephaly, followed by enhanced growth velocity, obesity, transient gynaecomastia, androgen deficiency, impaired spermatogenesis and decreased fertility (Smyth and Bremner 1998). There may also be an increased risk of developing breast carcinoma, autoimmune diseases, osteoporosis and psychiatric disorders (Bender *et al.* 1995, Smyth and Bremner 1998).

MANAGEMENT

Many men are unaware that they have this condition until they seek help for *infertility*, although infertility is not an issue for all people with Klinefelter syndrome (due to mosaicism). Testosterone levels are normal during childhood, but fail to rise to the normal adult levels at puberty. At *puberty*, the body may take on a more female appearance with gynecomastia, fatty deposits on the hips, sparse facial hair and low muscle tone. Approximately 40% of boys diagnosed with Klinefelter syndrome will develop gynaecomastia. There are fewer sperm-producing cells (spermatogonia) in the testes prior to puberty, and after puberty fibrosis and hyalinization of the seminiferous tubules occurs, usually leading to infertility.

Particular problems faced by boys with Klinefelter syndrome manifest at puberty. Their feminine physique and poor muscle tone may lead to *bullying* and ultimately social isolation, particularly if they are required to participate in physical education. It is essential that a child is made aware of the full implications of this condition prior to the onset of puberty, so that they can be more intellectually and emotionally prepared, and therefore more able to cope with the condition and with the reactions of their peers. Teachers should be made aware of the physical and psychological consequences of this condition.

Testosterone treatment and even surgery may be considered if gynaecomastia is severe enough, either physically or psychologically. Testosterone supplementation may be useful in adults to help prevent osteoporosis, to reduce fatigue and to enhance sexual activity.

REFERENCES

Bender BG, Harmon RJ, Linden MG, Robinson A (1995) 'Psychosocial adaptation of 39 adolescents with sex chromosome abnormalities.' *Pediatrics*, **96**, 302–308.
Hachimi-Idrissi S, Desmyttere S, Goossens A, Desprechins B, Otten J (1995) 'Retroperitoneal teratoma as first sign of Klinefelter's syndrome.' *Archives of Disease in Childhood*, **72**, 163–164.
O'Brien G, Yule W (eds) (1995) *Behavioural Phenotypes. Clinics in Developmental Medicine No. 138*. London: Mac Keith Press.
Peet J, Weaver DD, Vance GH (1998) '49,XXXXY: a distinct phenotype. Three new cases and review.' *Journal of Medical Genetics*, **35**, 420–424.
Ratcliffe S (1999) 'Long term outcome in children of sex chromosome abnormalities.' *Archives of Disease in Childhood*, **80**, 192–195.
Smyth CM, Bremner WJ (1998) 'Klinefelter syndrome.' *Archives of Internal Medicine*, **158**, 1309–1314.
SSBP (1999) *Proceedings of the 8th Annual Scientific Meeting of the Society for the Study of Behavioural Phenotypes, Beecheres Management Centre, Birmingham, England, 18–19 November 1999.*

WEBSITES

- Klinefelter's Syndrome Association UK
  www.akac70.care4free.net/index.html
- Klinefelter Organisation (formerly the KSCUK)
  www.klinefelter.org.uk/

47XXX, 48XXXX, 49XXXXX

Alternative names	Triple-X syndrome (47XXX)
	Tetra-X syndrome (48XXXX)
	Penta-X syndrome (49XXXXX)
Incidence	47XXX 1:1000 female births (Ratcliffe 1999)
	48XXXX (40 reported cases up to 1995) (O'Brien and Yule 1995)

Genetics	Non-disjunction of the X chromosome
Learning disability	47XXX normal to borderline
	48XXXX borderline to moderate

The majority of women with extra chromosomes have a 47XXX karyotype (50%); 48XXXX occurs in approximately 5% of women who have extra X chromosomes. One-half of 47XXX women have mosaicism. Women with extra X chromosomes have an increased incidence of mothers with advanced maternal age. As babies, these affected individuals are reported to be quiet and passive. Females with a 47XXX karyotype may have had a low birthweight, developmental delays and slightly delayed pubertal development (by 6 months). Microcephaly, social immaturity, and problems with fine motor coordination and balance are also common (Bender *et al.* 1995, Harmon *et al.* 1998). The expression of this syndrome can be mild, and it is postulated that almost three-quarters of cases are never diagnosed (Ratcliffe 1999). Life expectancy is thought to be normal, and fertility does not appear to be affected.

MANAGEMENT

It has been suggested that girls with diagnosed 47XXX have a high incidence of *psychiatric diagnosis*, the most common being depression. In adolescence these girls are characterized as having a high degree of aberrant behaviours and being *socially immature* with poor psychosocial adaptation; these factors can lead to vulnerability and manipulation from others. As a result these girls are more likely to engage in criminal activities and other aberrant behaviours (Bender *et al.* 1995).

Although it has been suggested that women with 47XXX have difficulties with social adaptation, most function at a normal level and can lead fulfilled and independent lives, albeit at a lower level than their peers (Harmon *et al.* 1998). Many marry and have no difficulties with conception associated with their extra X chromosome(s).

Girls with 48XXXX are tall for their age and, similar to 47XYY, this may cause people to assume that they are more mature than they actually are. Back pain and postural deformities are also common, and therefore exercise, particularly swimming, should be actively encouraged from early childhood to strengthen back muscles. Referral to a *speech and language therapist* may be necessary to develop existing speech and overcome articulation difficulties (O'Brien and Yule 1995), as during childhood, speech is delayed in one-half of cases (Ratcliffe 1999). Children born to women with extra X chromosomes have a normal karotype. Previously, it was thought that menopause has an early onset, but this does not now seem to be the case.

In a small number of cases, these conditions can be diagnosed prenatally. As with any genetic condition diagnosed in this manner, it is vitally important that the prospective parents receive specialist *genetic counselling* in order to prepare them for the condition. When counselling for 47XXX, the positive aspects of normal development should be reinforced, at the same time as preparing parents for the developmental difficulties children with this condition may face. It should also highlight the possible interventions that might be required so that these can be implemented in a timely manner in order to be of maximum benefit.

REFERENCES

Bender BG, Harmon RJ, Linden MG, Robinson A (1995) 'Psychosocial adaptation of 39 adolescents with sex chromosome abnormalities.' *Pediatrics*, **96**, 302–308.

Harmon RJ, Bender BG, Linden MG, Robinson A (1998) 'Transition from adolescence to early adulthood: Adaptation and psychiatric status of women with 47,XXX.' *Journal of the American Academy of Child and Adolescent Psychiatry*, **37**, 286–291.

O'Brien G, Yule W (eds) (1995) *Behavioural Phenotypes. Clinics in Developmental Medicine No. 138.* London: Mac Keith Press.

Ratcliffe S (1999) 'Long term outcome in children of sex chromosome abnormalities.' *Archives of Disease in Childhood*, **80**, 192–195.

WEBSITES

• Triple X Syndrome
  www.voicenet.com/~markr/triple.html
• Triplo-X Syndrome
  www.triplo-x.org/

47XYY

Incidence	1:1000 male births (Gotz *et al.* 1999)
Genetics	Non-disjunction of Y chromosome
Learning disability	Borderline

Males with 47XYY will experience accelerated leg and body growth between the ages of 4 and 9 years. The extra Y chromosome has no effect on fertility or testosterone levels. Life expectancy is thought to be normal. The behavioural manifestations of the syndrome include an exaggeration of emotions. For example, these males tend to be impulsive and overexcitable.

MANAGEMENT

Education can be hampered due to overactivity and excitability. Males with this karyotype tend to be strong and physically active. This energy can be *channelled into physical activities* and sport and thus used positively. The need for high levels of activity, in combination with slight learning disability and increased physical stature, can lead to frustration. Emotional immaturity, excitability, clumsiness, boisterousness and increased physical strength can often get these males into trouble. They are vulnerable and can be easily manipulated.

There is a great deal of controversy as to whether people with this syndrome have an increased rate of antisocial and criminal activity. Early reports claimed this to be the case. These were based upon random screening of psychiatric institutions and penal establishments. In these settings there does seem to be a high incidence of 47XYY, but these estimates are biased, as they do not take into account 47XYY males who are undiagnosed or who are not confined to these institutions.

The fact that many people still hold the view that most individuals with 47XYY have violent and aggressive dispositions is the root of many of the *psychological problems* faced by these individuals. This prejudice can be particularly difficult to deal with. This is also the case when the extra chromosome is not known about; for example, when an individual is taken into police custody, his tall stature can lead to more harsh treatment (Gotz *et al.*

1999). In one sample, 47% of individuals had received psychiatric referrals, for mild criminal activities, defiant behaviour and school-related enuresis (Ratcliffe 1999). Temper tantrums may be the result of *communication difficulties* (Ratcliffe 1999).

The tall stature in itself, and the prejudice it incurs, can have a marked psychological effect on the individual. Psychiatric counselling for the individual and their family is useful.

47XYY males would seem to be more prone to acne and this can lead to low self-esteem; where necessary a referral should be made to a dermatologist.

Diagnosis is particularly helpful for parents/carers of affected children as many people wrongfully judge the hyperactivity and excitability of these individuals as the result of poor parenting (O'Brien and Yule 1995).

REFERENCES

Gotz MJ, Johnstone EC, Ratcliffe SG (1999) 'Criminality and antisocial behaviour in unselected men with sex chromosome abnormalities.' *Psychological Medicine*, **29**, 953–962.
O'Brien G, Yule W (eds) (1995) *Behavioural Phenotypes. Clinics in Developmental Medicine No. 138.* London: Mac Keith Press.
Ratcliffe S (1999) 'Long term outcome in children of sex chromosome abnormalities.' *Archives of Disease in Childhood*, **80**, 192–195.

WEBSITE

- Personal 47XYY site
  www.47xyy.com/

SMITH–LEMLI–OPITZ SYNDROME

Alternative name	RSH syndrome
Incidence	1:20,000–1:40,000 (SSBP 2000)
Genetics	Autosomal recessive
Learning disability	Borderline to severe

Smith–Lemli–Opitz syndrome is a metabolic disorder in which there is abnormal metabolism of cholesterol, due to low levels of 7-dehydrocholesterol-reductase (7DHC-reductase), which leads to increased levels of 7-dehydrocholesterol in the blood and tissues. It is a multiple malformation syndrome. Principal abnormalities include distinctive facial dysmorphism: cleft palate, microcephaly, facial capillary haemangiomata, broad nasal bridge and epicanthal folds, ptosis, strabismus, cataracts, anteverted nares, thick alveolar ridges, a small tongue, microgathia and large low-set ears (O'Brien and Yule 1995). Other features include hypotonia and toe syndactyly. More severely affected males have sexual ambiguity. In addition there is growth deficiency, psychomotor delay, recurrent infections, and congenital abnormalities of most major organs including the rectal and urinary tracts and the external genitalia (males only) (de Die-Smulders and Fryns 1992).

MANAGEMENT

The most pressing medical problems are associated with feeding, growth, development and congenital malformations. *Gastrostomy feeding* is often required—sometimes permanently. It is only in the last decade that people have understood that Smith–Lemli–Opitz syndrome is caused by an inability to make cholesterol. As a consequence, research protocols using *cholesterol supplemented diets*, with or without bile acids (cholic acid, chenodeoxycholic acid and ursodeoxycholic acid), are in their infancy but their findings would seem to be encouraging. Commercial milk formulas contain almost no cholesterol, and even breast milk, which is high in cholesterol, does not contain enough cholesterol for a growing baby's needs. Diet can be supplemented with egg yolks, liver and cream. It is important not to over-feed people with this condition, in an attempt to help them grow faster, as they have small stomachs and a lower potential for final height. Cholesterol-supplemented diets not only counter failure-to-thrive but also seem to reduce behavioural features of this syndrome, such as irritability.

Around 70% of individuals with Smith–Lemli–Opitz syndrome have sleep disturbances, which are not responsive to sedatives (Tierney *et al.* 2001).

Surgery will usually be necessary to correct genital abnormalities and may also be considered for extra fingers and webbed toes.

The presentation of Smith–Lemli–Opitz syndrome varies dramatically. Some patients will have only a few congenital malformations whereas others will have many. The possibility of internal anomalies dictates the need for thorough *examination at birth*, particularly of the heart and kidneys.

Many children will not learn to walk or talk, but they do have good comprehension of language.

REFERENCES

de Die-Smulders C, Fryns JP (1992) 'Smith–Lemli–Opitz syndrome: the changing phenotype with age.' *Genetic Counseling*, **3**, 77–82.
O'Brien G, Yule W (eds) (1995) *Behavioural Phenotypes. Clinics in Developmental Medicine No. 138.* London: Mac Keith Press.
SSBP (2000) *Proceedings of the 6th International Symposium of the Society for the Study of Behavioural Phenotypes, Venice International University, San Servolo, Italy, 12–14 October 2000.*
Tierney E, Nwokoro NA, Porter FD, Freund LS, Ghuman JK, Kelley RI (2001) 'Behavior phenotype in the RSH/Smith–Lemli–Opitz syndrome.' *American Journal of Medical Genetics*, **98**, 191–200.

WEBSITES

- Family Village: Smith–Lemli–Opitz
  www.familyvillage.wisc.edu/lib_smith-lemli-opitz.htm
- Smith–Lemli–Opitz Syndrome: Advocacy & Exchange
  http://members.aol.com/slo97/index.html

SMITH–MAGENIS SYNDROME

Incidence	1:25,000 (Dykens and Smith 1998)
Genetics	Partial/complete deletion of band 17p11.2
Learning disability	Moderate

The typical physical presentation of Smith–Magenis syndrome includes multiple congenital abnormalities, hearing and vision difficulties, scoliosis and sleep disturbance (Allanson *et al.* 1999, Potocki *et al.* 2000). Characteristic facies include brachycephaly, broad face and nasal bridge, flat midface, downward-slanting corners of the mouth with a cupid's bow shape to the upper lip, and anomalies of ear shape/positioning (O'Brien and Yule 1995). The behavioural features of this syndrome are the most difficult to manage; these include self-injury, hyperactivity, aggression and an almost insatiable need for one-to-one adult attention. Medical complications seen in a quarter of these patients include hypothyroidism, immuno-globin deficiency and congenital heart defects (Allanson *et al.* 1999). Life expectancy is usually normal.

MANAGEMENT

Increasingly, the greater understanding of Smith–Magenis syndrome that we now have means that it is being diagnosed at increasingly younger ages. However, the years preceding diagnosis can be particularly difficult for parents. It is vitally important that when the syndrome is suspected, even if facial features are subtle, it should be considered.

Although congenital anomalies are prominent in Smith–Magenis syndrome, it is the behavioural phenotype that is most disturbing. Aggression, to both self and others, is severe. *Self-mutilation* often takes unusual forms, such as onychotillomania (pulling of finger- and toenails), and is probably exacerbated by a high pain threshold. *Sleep disturbance* is common and takes a number of forms including difficulty getting to sleep, frequent awakenings, early rising and reduced REM sleep. Melatonin has been successfully used to treat sleep disturbances (Potocki *et al.* 2000)

Behavioural management can be very demanding. Sufferers have an almost *insatiable need for one-to-one adult attention* and may become aggressive and/or self-injurious when attention is given to their peers. They tend to have attention deficit disorders (with or without hyperactivity) and react negatively to changes in their routine. Given this, however, they are usually polite, eager to please and have engaging personalities—they can be among the most popular students in the class. Negative behaviours seem to stem from the need for constant attention. Although positive attention is preferable, if this is not forthcoming, the child will present challenging behaviours (pinching and tantrums) in an attempt to elicit negative attention. As the giving of positive attention stimulates the drive to get attention and the withholding of attention elicits negative behaviours, behavioural management of Smith–Magenis syndrome needs to be carefully designed. Disruptive behaviour should be ignored, and the affected individual should be redirected. Positive attention should be given in a calm manner and only when it has been earned. By doing this consistently the affected individual will know that it is only given when earned. The challenging behaviours can make children with this condition particularly difficult to teach, as teachers may be afraid to let the child monopolize their attention to the detriment of the rest of the class. Teachers should be fully informed about the nature of the condition.

Tantrums can often be diffused before they develop. One key aspect of doing this is identifying and avoiding the triggers for a particular person—very often, changes in routine may trigger tantrums. When a tantrum is developing, the best approach is to remove the child from the situation and to talk to them calmly in a quiet manner. If they are removed from the room when activity is occurring, they regain composure sooner as they are unwilling to 'miss out' on any activities and/or attention that other people may be receiving. People with Smith–Magenis syndrome have difficulties in processing information sequentially;

therefore, any task that requires a number of steps to complete should be given one step at a time, and the next instruction should not be given until the first step has been completed. Where possible, anything to be learnt should be given in diagrammatic form, as people with this condition are visual learners.

REFERENCES

Allanson JE, Greenberg F, Smith AC (1999) 'The face of Smith–Magenis syndrome: a subjective and objective study.' *Journal of Medical Genetics*, **36**, 394–397.
Dykens EM, Smith AC (1998) 'Distinctiveness and correlates of maladaptive behaviour in children and adolescents with Smith–Magenis syndrome.' *Journal of Intellectual Disability Research*, **42**, 481–489.
O'Brien G, Yule W (eds) (1995) *Behavioural Phenotypes. Clinics in Developmental Medicine No. 138.* London: Mac Keith Press.
Potocki L, Glaze D, Tan DX, Park SS, Kashork CD, Shaffer LG, Reiter RJ, Lupski JR (2000) 'Circadian rhythm abnormalities of melatonin in Smith–Magenis syndrome.' *Journal of Medical Genetics*, **37**, 428–433.

WEBSITES

- Ability
  www.ability.org.uk/Smith_Magenis_Syndrome.html
- Parents & Researchers Interested in Smith–Magenis Syndrome (PRISMS)
  www.smithmagenis.org/
- Smith–Magenis Syndrome Foundation
  www.stepstn.com/cgi-win/nord.exe?proc=Redirect&type=org_sum&id=1101.htm

SOTOS SYNDROME

Alternative name	Cerebral gigantism
Incidence	About 200 cases reported (SSBP 2001)
Genetics	Probably autosomal dominant
Learning disability	Borderline to mild

The defining feature of Sotos syndrome is accelerated growth—this begins prenatally and is particularly prominent for the first five years of life (Agwu *et al.* 1999). Other relevant features for diagnosis include a distinctive facial appearance: round face and round, high forehead, frontal bossing, prominent jaw, anteverted nares, high arched palate, antemongoloid slant of the palpebral fissures, premature eruption of the teeth and sparseness of hair (O'Brien and Yule 1995). Facial features coarsen with age. In adolescence, growth rate declines, and, although tall, most adults with this syndrome are within normal height limits. Investigations into the cause of the accelerated growth have so far been inconclusive. Jaundice, early feeding problems and hypotonia present in infants with this condition, and connective tissue anomalies, infections, abnormal EEGs, advanced bone age, asthma and allergies tend to present with increasing age. There are generally no life-threatening complications with this disorder (O'Brien and Yule 1995).

MANAGEMENT
Someone who looks older than they are, but acts younger is at risk of *low self-esteem*. Strangers tend to have unfairly high expectations of people with Sotos syndrome, due to

their tall stature. This, in combination with any learning disability, emotional immaturity and communicative impairment, can lead to frustration and aggression. Development would seem to be slower than normal, but by the time a person with Sotos syndrome reaches adulthood, her/his height and weight are usually within normal limits. Muscle tone improves during late childhood and is accompanied with improvements in articulation. Receptive language is usually better than expressive language, and parents/carers must be aware of this when communicating with their children. Children usually cope with *mainstream schooling* but may need remedial support. Girls may need extra practical and emotional support as menses begins at a younger age than is typical.

Occupational therapy and physiotherapy may be particularly useful to help improve muscle tone. Social skills training is also beneficial. Hormonal treatments, such as oestrogen, somatostatin or testosterone can be given to ensure that final stature is within acceptable limits.

REFERENCES

Agwu JC, Shaw NJ, Kirk J, Chapman S, Ravine D, Cole TR (1999) 'Growth in Sotos syndrome.' *Archives of Disease in Childhood*, **80**, 339–342.
O'Brien G, Yule W (eds) (1995) *Behavioural Phenotypes. Clinics in Developmental Medicine No. 138.* London: Mac Keith Press.
SSBP (2001) 'Sotos syndrome.' Society for the Study of Behavioural Phenotypes, electronic fact sheet (http://www.psychiatry.cam.ac.uk/ssbp/sotos.htm).

WEBSITES

• Call a Family: Sotos Syndrome
  www.cafamily.org.uk/Direct/s36.html
• Sotos Syndrome Support Association
  www.well.com/user/sssa/

TUBEROUS SCLEROSIS

Alternate names	Tuberous sclerosis complex, epiloia
Incidence	1:7000 (Hunt 1998)
Genetics	Autosomal dominant, either chromosome 9q34.3 or 16p13.3 (SSBP 2000)
Learning disability	Half have learning disability, usually severe to profound (Hunt 1998)

Tuberous sclerosis is a complex, non-degenerative, neurocutaneous, multisystem condition. Its manifestation is diverse: some cases are so mild that affected individuals will never be diagnosed, whereas others will be very severely affected. Its name derives from tuber-like growths in the brain that become hard and sclerotic; however, tumours can affect any part of the body. Early infantile spasms and subsequent epilepsy occur in three-quarters of affected individuals. The typical presentation of tuberous sclerosis includes hamartias, hamartomas, true neoplasms, skin lesions, learning disability, behavioural abnormalities and seizures (Jozwiak *et al.* 1998). In addition, facial angiofibromas are usually observable by 5 years of age (O'Brien and Yule 1995). There is a distinct behavioural component to this phenotype, with half of patients exhibiting autistic-like behaviour and/or hyperactivity (irrespective of their level of learning disability). The location of cerebral and peripheral lesions determines life expectancy, with cerebral and renal lesions being the biggest cause of mortality (Cook *et al.* 1996).

MANAGEMENT

There is as yet no cure for tuberous sclerosis, and treatment involves management of the symptoms. Prognosis varies widely from those who are mildly affected and who lead productive lives to those who are severely affected and require intensive support. Severity is often linked to the presence of seizure disorder (Harris 1998). The *control of epilepsy* is of fundamental importance, although in many cases seizures are intractable. Seizures tend to fluctuate, both in type and frequency through life. In one-third of patients, seizure control seems to deteriorate after early childhood; however, a similar number of patients accomplish better seizure control. A limited number of reports have claimed that there is benefit in cortical resection surgery for intractable epilepsy (Avellino *et al.* 1997). There is generally no deterioration in cognitive ability other than that attributable to the natural progression of age.

Management should focus on both the emotional and physical aspects of this disorder. The diversity and unpredictability of the *behavioural difficulties* and sleep disturbances exhibited by affected individuals can place considerable stress upon the family unit, and it is essential that the family receive ongoing support (Harris 1998). Screaming and aggression are related to attentional deficits; these improve with age. In severely learning disabled patients, challenging behaviours may be a reflection of brain tumours (subependymal giant cell astrocytomas). Brain tumours may also manifest as vomiting, headache, lethargy and unsteadiness on the feet (Hunt 1998). Any change in behaviour should be taken seriously, especially where the patient is unable to communicate clearly. For example, the onset of head banging may be indicative of severe headaches caused by tumours. If behaviour does alter, a referral to a neurologist should be sought.

The *characteristic facial rash* (angiofibromas) can cause considerable distress, but there are a number of pharmacological treatments for this and the advice of a dermatologist should be sought. A surprising number of patients are never referred for renal ultrasound for the identification of cysts and growths (angiomyolipomas) or to dermatologists for facial rashes (Hunt 1998). Clinicians should not be reluctant to offer these referrals to patients, particularly if the reason for non-referral is based solely upon the severity of the learning disability.

Speech and language are often areas for concern, even in patients who do not have learning disabilities and these should be assessed where necessary by a speech and language therapist so that appropriate educational systems can be implemented. *Communication aids*, such as Maketon, can be vital in helping patients to express themselves.

When tuberous sclerosis is diagnosed, all immediate members of the family should be screened to see if they are carriers for the condition, as there is a 50% chance that any carrier will pass the affected gene to their offspring.

REFERENCES

Avellino AM, Berger MS, Rostomily RC, Shaw CM, Ojemann GA (1997) 'Surgical management and seizure outcome in patients with tuberous sclerosis.' *Journal of Neurosurgery*, **87**, 391–396.

Cook JA, Oliver K, Mueller RF, Sampson J (1996) 'A cross sectional study of renal involvement in tuberous sclerosis.' *Journal of Medical Genetics*, **33**, 480–484.

Harris JC (1998) *Developmental Neuropsychiatry. Vol. II: Assessment, Diagnosis and Treatment of Developmental Disorders.* Oxford: Oxford University Press.

Hunt A (1998) 'A comparison of the abilities, health and behaviour of 23 people with tuberous sclerosis.' *Journal of Applied Research in Intellectual Disabilities*, **11**, 227–238.

Jozwiak S, Goodman M, Lamm SH (1998) 'Poor mental development in patients with tuberous sclerosis complex: clinical risk factors.' *Archives of Neurology*, **55**, 379–384.

O'Brien G, Yule W (eds) (1995) *Behavioural Phenotypes. Clinics in Developmental Medicine No. 138.* London: Mac Keith Press.

SSBP (2000) *Proceedings of the 6th International Symposium of the Society for the Study of Behavioural Phenotypes, Venice International University, San Servolo, Italy, 12–14 October 2000.*

WEBSITE

• Tuberous Sclerosis Association
www.tuberous-sclerosis.org/

VELOCARDIOFACIAL SYNDROME

Incidence	Estimated at 1:4000 (Murphy *et al.* 1999)
Genetics	Autosomal dominant; submicroscopic deletion at 22q11.2 (85% of cases) (Farrell *et al.* 1999)
Learning disability	Borderline (Wang *et al.* 2000)

Velocardiofacial syndrome has a wide phenotypic expression. There are 180 associated anomalies, and many or just a few may be present in an affected individual. Despite this, the typical presentation of the syndrome involves distinctive facial dysmorphism, congenital heart disease, hypotonia and immune disorders (Goldmuntz and Emanual 1997, Sykes *et al.* 1997). Submucous cleft palate, velopharyngeal insufficiency or cleft palate can result in hypernasal speech (Sykes *et al.* 1997). Infections are common, particularly of the respiratory tract and ear. This is due to an absent or partial absence of the thymus gland. There is a high incidence of schizophrenia in adulthood (Murphy *et al.* 1999). Life expectancy is determined by the severity of heart abnormalities.

MANAGEMENT

Behaviour tends to be extreme—either withdrawn and shy or highly disinhibited and impulsive (Wang *et al.* 2000). The physical appearance, in combination with learning disability, can lead to *low self-esteem and social isolation.* These are real issues and become particularly problematic at puberty, a time when bullying can worsen. It is important that the adolescent receives appropriate emotional support to deal with these issues. In addition to problems with low self-esteem, many affected individuals develop mental health problems after puberty, particularly bipolar affective disorder.

Any person with velocardiofacial syndrome that has an unexplained fit should have their calcium levels assessed. This is because aberrant functioning of the parathyroid gland can lead to hypocalcaemia, which in turn can cause *hypocalcaemic fits*—these are similar to febrile convulsions. It is usually recommended that individuals with velocardiofacial syndrome have regular assessments of calcium levels. It is important to genetically screen for velocardiofacial syndrome in patients presenting with hypocalceamia, as sometimes the other phenotypic features of this syndrome may be mild and the diagnosis may be overlooked (Sykes *et al.* 1997).

Most children present with problems of the palate. These may require *corrective surgery*. However, this is not usually performed before 4 years of age, as it is important for the child to receive speech therapy prior to surgery. If this is the case, any abnormalities of carotid arteries should be identified as they may cause complications. Speech therapy is useful to help children with this condition to understand the pragmatics of language. Language is characterized by autistic-like features, and affected individuals have a literal bias in their understanding of language. It is important to recognize this when communicating with individuals with this syndrome. Alternative methods of communication can facilitate interaction, *e.g.* sign language. When encouraging communication, attention should paid to helping develop nonverbal communication such as eye contact, gaze following and turn-taking.

The missing thymus gland can effect the administering of *immunizations*, and a 'killed' version of live vaccines for poliomyelitis should be given. Careful consideration should also be given to BCG vaccines—a referral to an immunologist should be considered.

Hearing should be regularly monitored as affected individuals suffer from frequent ear infections, with associated hearing loss. A referral to an *ear, nose and throat specialist* is recommended. Ultrasound scans of the kidneys should be performed regardless of whether the child suffers from frequent bladder infections, as this can reveal diseased kidneys. Leg pain is frequently reported, both when asleep and awake. This can be helped with orthopaedic insoles that raise the feet.

Problems with feeding may revolve around a dislike of certain textures, primarily 'adult' food textures—smooth and soft foods are preferred. *Different food textures* can be gradually introduced to the diet through play. Sometimes the help of a nutritionist/dietician can be useful. Children should be encouraged to drink plenty of fluids to help ease the constipation associated with hypotonia.

Cardiac abnormalities may require surgical intervention. This is a highly disturbing and distressing time for the whole family, particularly as surgery is complicated by an increased risk of infection. Once an infection has taken hold, it may often take an excessive amount of time for the individual to recuperate.

Behavioural symptoms of velocardiofacial syndrome such as inattention, poor socialization and concentration difficulties are common and may resemble attention deficit disorder. It is important that *stimulant medications*, such as ritalin, are not prescribed as these can cause particularly severe adverse reactions in velocardiofacial syndrome.

As with all complex medical and behavioural syndromes, the extra parental attention required by the affected individual may leave siblings feeling neglected. This may cause resentment. It is important that the full facts of the syndrome are given in an easily accessible manner to siblings and that questions are answered *openly and honestly*. Siblings may be concerned about whether they can 'catch' the syndrome and at a later age may worry about whether they are carriers. Genetic counselling can address these issues.

REFERENCES

Farrell MJ, Stadt H, Wallis KT, Scambler P, Hixon RL, Wolfe R, Leatherbury L, Kirby ML (1999) 'HIRA, a DiGeorge syndrome candidate gene, is required for cardiac outflow tract septation.' *Circulation Research*, **84**, 127–135.

Goldmuntz E, Emanual BS (1997) 'Genetic disorders of cardiac morphogenesis: The DiGeorge and velocardiofacial syndromes.' *Circulation Research*, **80**, 437–443.

Murphy KC, Jones LA, Owen MJ (1999) 'High rates of schizophrenia in adults with velo-cardio-facial syndrome.' *Archives of General Psychiatry*, **56**, 940–945.

Sykes KS, Bachrach LK, Siegel-Bartelt J, Ipp M, Kooh SW, Cytrynbaum C (1997) 'Velocardiofacial syndrome presenting as hypocalcemia in early adolescence.' *Archives of Pediatrics and Adolescent Medicine*, **151**, 745–747.

Wang PP, Woodin MF, Kreps-Falk R, Moss EM (2000) 'Research on behavioral phenotypes: velocardiofacial syndrome (deletion 22q11.2).' *Developmental Medicine and Child Neurology*, **42**, 422–427.

WEBSITES

- The 22q11 Group
  www.vcfs.net/
- National Institute on Deafness and Other Communication Disorders (NIDCD)
  www.nidcd.nih.gov/textonly/health/pubs_vsl/velocario.htm
- Velo-Cardio-Facial Syndrome Educational Foundation
  www.vcfsef.org/

WILLIAMS SYNDROME

Alternative name	Williams–Beuren syndrome, idiopathic infantile hypercalcaemia
Incidence	1:25,000 (Howlin *et al.* 1998)
Genetics	Usually sporadic; microdeletion on chromosome 7
Learning disability	Moderate

Williams syndrome is a developmental disorder involving vascular, connective tissue and the central nervous system (O'Brien and Yule 1995). Abnormalities can often be detected at birth, particularly low birthweight, cardiac murmurs and feeding problems. Characteristic facial features include a distinctive 'elfin-like' face with prominent cheeks, a wide and long philtrum, a retroussé nose with a flat nasal bridge, heavy orbital ridges, medial eyebrow flair and stellate iris pattern, and dental abnormalities including microdontia, missing teeth and enamel hypoplasia (O'Brien and Yule 1995). A subgroup of infants also have hypercalcaemia. Hernias occur in approximately one third of cases. Skeletal abnormalities, such as joint contractures/laxity can effect gait. The hypotonia seen in infants is often replaced by hypertonia in older children (O'Brien and Yule 1995). Some affected individuals have progressive multisystem involvement of the gastrointestinal, renal and urinary tract systems.

MANAGEMENT

A subgroup of people suffering from Williams syndrome have *idiopathic hypercalcaemia* in infancy. This can be treated successfully with a low-calcium and vitamin D restricted diet, which will also help to stabilize the severe feeding and gastrointestinal problems. Hypercalcaemia spontaneously resolves before 24 months of age. There would seem to be no relationship between the presence/absence of hypercalcaemia and developmental outcome

(O'Brien and Yule 1995). Constipation is a major problem for children and can sometimes lead to rectal prolapse, but it does not seem to be a prominent problem for adults.

Menstruation difficulties, including premenstrual tension and painful periods affect almost all females and can be quite debilitating.

Progressive multisystem anomalies (cardiovascular, gastrointestinal, urinary tract) present in a small number of cases. However, it would seem that the severity of physical complications may have been exaggerated in the literature; for example, in the study by Howlin *et al.* (1998) although 84% of their sample were reported to have cardiac abnormalities, these generally did not require medical intervention.

The *cognitive profile* of Williams syndrome is unusual: affected individuals have highly superior verbal abilities relative to visuospatial abilities (although language may initially be slow to develop). Such superior language abilities may be confusing to parents/carers as command of language is usually far greater than understanding of it. This, in addition to their excessive sociability and engaging personalities, may result in an overestimation of their general cognitive abilities (O'Brien and Yule 1995).

Dilts (1990) proposed that the six most characteristic problems for adults with Williams syndrome are: multiple motor disabilities, cognitive dysfunction, impaired mathematical functioning, unusual language profile, sensory integration dysfunction and hyperactivity.

Although irritable as infants, as they develop through childhood people with Williams syndrome demonstrate *indiscriminate friendliness and talkativeness*. However, despite this, a large survey found that the majority of people with Williams syndrome were isolated. It is important to be aware of this, as attempts to prevent overfamiliar behaviour must take into account the potential for isolation (Davies *et al.* 1998). It should be recognized that people with Williams syndrome are vulnerable, and as such, ongoing support is necessary to protect them from *abuse and manipulation*. Children with Williams syndrome generally have poor peer relations and tend to prefer to spend their time with adults. Depression becomes worse in adulthood and should be suspected if there is any change in behaviour.

Ongoing medical involvement should include periodic monitoring of blood pressure and renal function (Metcalfe 1999).

REFERENCES

Davies M, Udwin O, Howlin P (1998) 'Adults with Williams syndrome. Preliminary study of social, emotional and behavioural difficulties.' *British Journal of Psychiatry*, **172**, 273–276.

Dilts CV, Morris CA, Leonard CO (1990) 'Hypothesis for the development of the behavioural phenotype in Williams syndrome.' *American Journal of Medical Genetics*, **6**, 126–131.

Howlin P, Davies M, Udwin O (1998) 'Syndrome specific characteristics in Williams syndrome: To what extent do early behavioural patterns persist into adult life?' *Journal of Applied Research in Intellectual Disabilities*, **11**, 207–226.

Metcalfe K (1999) 'Williams syndrome: an update on clinical and molecular aspects.' *Archives of Disease in Childhood*, **81**, 198–200.

O'Brien G, Yule W (eds) (1995) *Behavioural Phenotypes. Clinics in Developmental Medicine No. 138.* London: Mac Keith Press.

WEBSITE

- Williams Syndrome Foundation (UK)
  www.williams-syndrome.org.uk/

WOLF–HIRSCHHORN SYNDROME

Incidence	1:50,000 (Lesperance *et al.* 1998)
Genetics	Partial deletion 4p16.3 between D4S43 and D4S142 (Hanley-Lopez *et al.* 1998)
Learning disability	Severe to profound

Wolf–Hirschhorn syndrome is twice as common in females as in males. It is associated with a number of congenital physical and neuromuscular abnormalities. At birth, craniofacial dysmorphism includes severe microcephaly, hypertelorism, highly arched eyebrows, epicanthal folds, a beaked nose with a broad base, a carp-shaped mouth with downturned corners, micrognathia, a prominent glabella and a short philtrum with a cleft lip and palate, large and simple low-set ears and scalp defects (O'Brien and Yule 1995). Babies often have poor muscle tone and are small due to intrauterine growth retardation. Other characteristics of the syndrome include short stature, renal defects, heart and respiratory tract abnormalities and hypotonia (Battaglia *et al.* 1999). These abnormalities increase susceptibility to respiratory infections, and life expectancy is dependent on the number and severity of these malformations. While approximately one-third of infants die before 2 years of age (SSBP 2000) as a result of cardiac failure or bronchopneumonia, there are also reported cases of adults surviving into their third decade.

MANAGEMENT

Cardiac failure and bronchopneumonia are commonly associated with Wolf–Hirschhorn syndrome and, along with *epilepsy*, are the most important symptoms to monitor and treat (O'Brien and Yule 1995). As a high percentage of people with this condition have immuno-deficiencies, monthly immunoglobulin infusions and/or continuous antibiotic therapy can be useful in preventing respiratory and viral infections (Hanley-Lopez *et al.* 1998). Although initially difficult to treat, epilepsy can be well controlled with anticonvulsant medication. Seizures tend to cease by the time the child reaches adolescence (Battaglia *et al.* 1999). Gastrostomy is often required to induce weight gain and protect the airway (Battaglia *et al.* 1999).

This syndrome is associated with *severe to profound learning disability*, and as a result there is a lifelong dependency upon carers. As with any such condition, the child should be presented with stimulating and fun activities. Contrary to many reports, some patients do learn to walk, self-feed, achieve sphincter control and even help to dress themselves. Disorders of affect, such as failure of joint attention, that accompany this syndrome can be particularly distressing for parents/carers—for example, babies often fail to engage in eye contact, even when breastfeeding. Affected individuals also have high levels of anxiety and withdrawal, although these features do resolve somewhat with age.

Battaglia *et al.* (1999) suggest the following standard examinations in infancy: detailed heart examination, ophthalmology, audiology, developmental testing, renal ultrasound and swallowing study, plus EEG if seizures are suspected.

It has been suggested that *hearing loss/impairment* is commonly associated with Wolf–Hirschhorn syndrome, but that this is often overlooked due to early mortality and learning disability (Lesperance *et al.* 1998). Appropriate management of children with this condition should include vision and hearing assessment, including brainstem auditory evoked responses, as soon as the syndrome is identified and then at regular intervals, as hearing loss may be secondary to otitis media. This will allow the implementation of appropriate speech and language techniques for children with hearing impairment.

It may be possible to perform *surgery* to correct physical abnormalities such as club feet and kyphoscoliosis; however, the decision to do this must be taken in light of the fact that the child may still never walk (Battaglia *et al.* 1999).

REFERENCES

Battaglia A, Carey JC, Cederholm P, Viskochil DH, Brothman AR, Galasso C (1999) 'Natural history of Wolf–Hirschhorn syndrome: Experience with 15 cases.' *Pediatrics*, **103**, 830–836.
Hanley-Lopez J, Estabrooks LL, Stiehm R (1998) 'Antibody deficiency in Wolf–Hirschhorn syndrome.' *Journal of Pediatrics*, **133**, 141–143.
Lesperance MM, Grundfast KM, Rosenbaum KN (1998) 'Otologic manifestations of Wolf–Hirschhorn syndrome.' *Archives of Otolaryngology – Head and Neck Surgery*, **124**, 193–196.
O'Brien G, Yule W (eds) (1995) *Behavioural Phenotypes. Clinics in Developmental Medicine No. 138.* London: Mac Keith Press.
SSBP (2000) *Proceedings of the 6th International Symposium of the Society for the Study of Behavioural Phenotypes, Venice International University, San Servolo, Italy, 12–14 October 2000.*

WEBSITE

• Wolf Hirschhorn Support Group UK
  www.whs.webk.co.uk/

INDEX